UNIVERSITY OF BRISTOL
Food Refrigeration and
Process Engineering Research Centre
F R P E R C Churchill Building
Langford, Bristol. BS18 7DY
Tel: + 44 (0)117 928 9239   Fax: + 44 (0)117 928 9314

Minimally Processed Refrigerated Fruits & Vegetables

Minimally Processed Refrigerated Fruits & Vegetables

Edited by

Robert C. Wiley

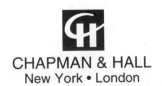

CHAPMAN & HALL
New York • London

First published in 1994 by
Chapman & Hall
One Penn Plaza
New York, NY 10119

Published in Great Britain by
Chapman & Hall
2-6 Boundary Row
London SE1 8HN

Library of Congress Cataloging in Publication Data

Minimally processed refrigerated fruits and vegetables / edited by
   Robert C. Wiley.
      p. cm.
   Includes bibliographical references and index.
   ISBN 0-412-05571-6
   1. Food—Storage. 2. Vegetables—Storage. 3. Cold storage.
   I. Wiley, Robert C., 1924–   .
   TP440.M56 1994   93-40071
   664'.85—dc20   CIP

British Library Cataloguing in Publication Data

Please send your order for this or any other Chapman & Hall book to **Chapman & Hall, 29 West 35th Street, New York, NY 10001, Attn: Customer Service Department.** You may also call our Order Department at 1-212-244-3336 or fax your pur-chase order to 1-800-248-4724.

For a complete listing of Chapman & Hall titles, send your request to **Chapman & Hall, Dept. BC, One Penn Plaza, New York, NY 10119.**

Contents

Preface

The objective of this book is to introduce, organize, and document the scientific, technical and practical aspects involved with the manufacture, storage, distribution and marketing of minimally processed refrigerated (MPR) fruits and vegetables. The overall function of these foods is to provide a convenient, like-fresh product for food service and retail consumers. A high level of quality accompanied by superior safety are essential requisites of MPR fruits and vegetables. Since refrigeration or chilling is essential to the quality and safety of these food products, "refrigeration" is included in the title of this book, i.e. MP*Refrigerated* fruits and vegetables.

This swiftly emerging area of processing requires organization and unification of thinking concerning fruit and vegetable food products which are not considered commercially sterile from a classical standpoint. Fruits and vegetables require very special attention because of the multitude of enzymic and respiratory factors as well as microbiological concerns which impact on the safety of low acid and acidified vegetables and on the economic viability of high acid fruit products of all kinds.

The name of this field, minimally processed (MP) fruits and vegetables, deserves attention in that there is little agreement among processors, produce dealers and merchants and research workers regarding the proper term for these products. Many names are used as synonyms for MP fruits and vegetables, and these include: ready-to-use, pre-cut, lightly processed, fresh-cut, etc; I think it behooves the food industry to settle on a single name and agree on a standard definition of this product. Doing so would benefit research and development efforts, data base searches, nutritional information needs and the like.

The term "refrigerated" as opposed to chilled foods seems to be slightly confusing. These terms are synonymous, but probably one or the other should be selected to avoid confusion. Although the "chilled food" term may be easier to say than "refrigerated food," in the United States (US) at least, "refrigerated" may be more recognizable by consumers.

This volume is designed to serve primarily as a reference book for those interested and involved in the minimally processed refrigerated or chilled fruit and vegetable industry. There has been an attempt to bring together historical information available from many fields developed long before the concept of "minimally processed" foods was considered a viable field of endeavor. I have tried to gather as much knowledge as possible regarding this field but realize there is much more research and development to be completed, and that great opportunities exist in this area of food technology. The lack of information in certain areas has hampered the authors of some of the chapters. If I have been able to summarize the present knowledge of MPR fruits and vegetables and stimulate others to develop this important field in a uniform and concise manner I think we will all feel successful.

I thank all of the contributors to this volume and thank the following individuals for reviewing chapters: Timothy P. Lyddane, Imperial Produce; Dr. John Y. Humber, Kraft General Foods; Dr. Dennis C. Westhoff, University of Maryland; Dr. Harold R. Bolin, USDA-ARS; Dr. Bernard A. Twigg, University of Maryland; Dr. Charles A. McClurg, University of Maryland; and Dr. Charles R. Barmore, W.R. Grace and Co. Thanks also go to Kathleen Hunt, Robert Savoy, Lovant Hicks, David Jones, Ester Lee and all others who read manuscripts, worked with tables and artwork for figures, entered information and data into the computer, and generally made this volume possible.

Finally, I thank Joy Wiley for her help and encouragement during the time that this work was being produced.

Robert C. Wiley, September 22, 1993

Contributors List

Robert E. Brackett
Food Safety and Quality
  Enhancement Laboratory
Georgia Agricultural
Experiment Station
University of Georgia
Griffin, GA 30223-1797

Dennis M. Dignan
Chief, Regulatory Processing
  and Technology Branch
HFS 617
Food and Drug Administration
Washington, DC 20204

Ruth Matthews
U.S. Department of Agriculture
Human Nutrition Information
  Service
Federal Building
Hyattsville, MD 20782

Marie A. McCarthy
U.S. Department of Agriculture
Human Nutrition Information
  Service
Federal Building
Hyattsville, MD 20782

Michael Rooney
Pricipal Research Scientist
CSIRO
Food Research Laboratory
  Division of Food Processing
North Ryde, NSW 2113
AUSTRALIA

Donald V. Schlimme
Department of Nutrition and
  Food Science
University of Maryland
College Park, MD 20742-5611

Theophanes Solomos
Department of Horticulture
University of Maryland
College Park, MD 20742-5611

Patrick Varoquaux
Institut National de la
  Recherche Agronomique
  Center de Recherches
  d'Avignon
Station de Technologie des
Products Vegetaux
Domaine Saint Paul-BP91-84143
Montfavet, FRANCE

Robert C. Wiley
Department of Food Science
  and Technology
1122 Holzapfel Hall
College Park, MD 20742

Faith Yildiz
Department of Food
  Engineering
Middle East Technical
University
Inonu Bulvari-Ankara
TURKEY 0-6531

Minimally Processed Refrigerated Fruits & Vegetables

1

Introduction to Minimally Processed Refrigerated Fruits and Vegetables

Robert C. Wiley

Minimally processed refrigerated (MPR) fruits and vegetables are an important and rapidly developing class of MPR foods. These convenience foods are being produced by unique applications of the basic and food sciences and their supporting technologies and engineering. MPR fruits and vegetables have attracted the interest of many facets of the food industry including such diverse areas as food manufacturers, retail food stores (deli departments), restaurants, carry-out establishments, and commissary units. Much of the developmental work in this field is now being carried out in western Europe, Japan, and the United States in response to strong consumer demand, both individual and institutional, for new types of like-fresh high-quality convenience foods. The purpose of MPR foods is to deliver to the consumer a like-fresh fruit or vegetable product with an extended shelf-life and at the same time ensure food safety and maintain sound nutritional and sensory quality. MPR fruits and vegetables received their original impetus from institutional users but retail applications are gaining favor and are expected to expand rapidly.

Many countries in western Europe are making significant strides toward solving the myriad of problems associated with the manufacturing, distribution, and marketing of MPR fruits and vegetables. This progress appears to be due to strong governmental and food industry support for MPR food applications, a conducive regulatory climate in preparation for the expanding food markets that will be available within the European Community (EC) when the trade and monetary barriers are removed in the near future.

It is clear that investigators in the fields of food science and technology, related disciplines, and engineering have studied and conducted research on the various facets of MPR food for many years, especially in the cold preserved and raw fresh foods areas (Figure 1-1). The early work by (Smock and Neubert 1950) on controlled atmosphere (CA) storage of apples is a good example of the type of research that is now utilized and is being greatly refined with regard to MPR fruits and vegetables. It is now time to look at this field as a concise discipline investigating the continuum of product flow from harvest to consumption (Figures 1-2 and 6-1). As seen in Figure 1-2 the discipline effectively links product production (horticulture production) with manufacturing, packaging, distribution, and consumption. See Morris (1991) and Anon. (1991) for good manufacturing practices (GMP) and Hazard Analysis Critical Control Point (HACCP) Systems for MPR fruits and vegetables and chilled foods in general. A unified approach and thinking of MPR foods as a specific food preservation industry/method as contrasted to canning, freezing, or drying would greatly assist in its development, which is somewhat in its infancy.

As shown in Figure 1-1, the major differences between MPR fruits and vegetables and raw fruits and vegetables are the rather specific processing and preservation steps taken with MPR foods. The MPR fruits and vegetables are usually living respiring tissues (Rolle and Chism 1987) but respiration is greatly increased by cutting, slicing, low temperature heat treatments, and preservatives (Figures 1-3 and 1-4, Anon. 1989a). As seen in Figure 1-3, the intact cell is expected to be much more resistant to oxidative browning and entrance of bacteria as compared to the cut cell. Figure 1-4a shows the intact vegetable product in a package, Figure 1-4b shows the condition of some cut surface cells with the majority of intact interior cells. The latter situation may greatly complicate the modeling of gas exchange

Preservation Category	Not Preserved Raw	Minimally Processed Refrigerated	Cold Preserved	Irradiated	Dehydrated	Heat Preserved
Product Quality	Fresh	Like-Fresh	Slightly Modified*	Slightly Modified*	Slightly to Fully Modified*	Fully Modified*
Process and Preservation Method	Usually Does Not Require Processing or Preservation Methods	Requires Minimal Processing and Preservation Methods	Requires Processing and Cold Preservation Freezing or Refrigeration	Requires Processing and Irradiation Pasteurization/Preservation	Requires Processing and Dehydration	Requires Processing and Heat Preservation
Storage Shelf-Life	May or May Not be Refrigerated	Requires Refrigeration Temperatures	Requires Frozen or Refrigeration Temperatures	Requires Refrigeration or May be Shelf Stable at Ambient Temperatures	Usually Shelf Stable at Ambient Temperatures	Shelf Stable at Ambient Temperatures
Packaging	May or May Not be Packaged	Requires Packaging	Requires Packaging	Requires Packaging	Requires Packaging	Requires Hermetically Sealed Packaging

* Product freshness

Figure 1-1 Spectrum of food preservation systems related to minimally processed refrigerated (MPR) fruits and vegetables.

FRUITS AND VEGETABLES

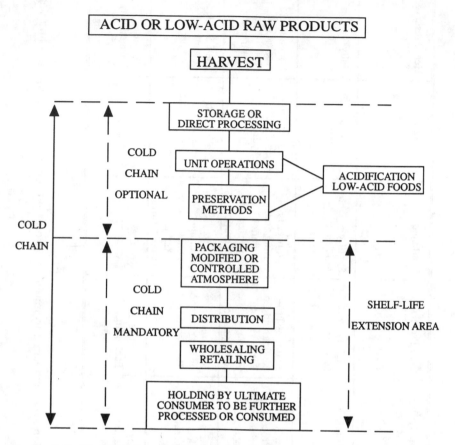

Figure 1-2 General flowsheet for minimally processed refrigerated fruits and vegetables.

in polymeric packages as suggested by Mannapperuma and Singh (1990). Refrigeration and packaging may be optional for raw fresh intact fruits and vegetables but are mandatory for MPR fruits and vegetables.

In this book, the attempt is made to differentiate between intact fresh fruits and vegetables and MPR fruits and vegetables even though the latter are somewhat difficult to define exactly. For example, whole intact apple fruit in CA storage, described by Smock and Neubert (1950), would not be considered an MPR product whereas sliced,

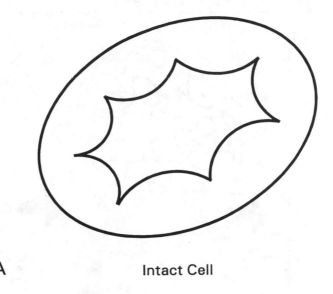

A   Intact Cell

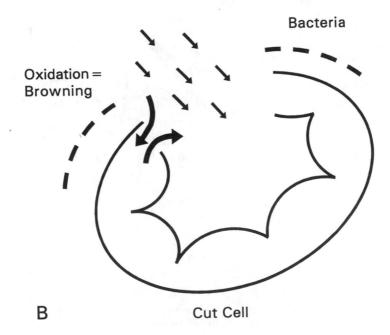

B   Cut Cell

Figure 1-3 Diagrams of intact and processed (cut) fruit or vegetable cell. (From CTIFL, France.)

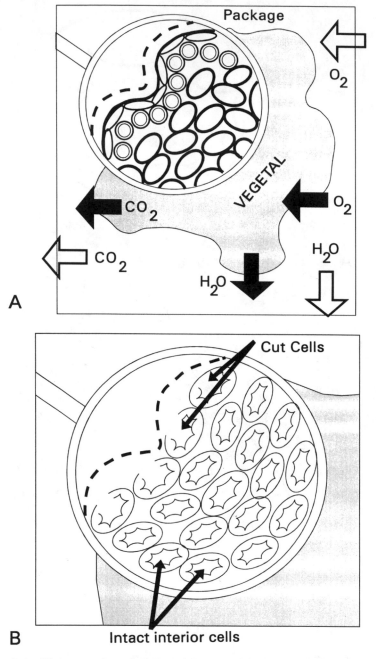

Figure 1-4   Diagram of product in package and product with surface modification such as from peeling or slicing. (From CTIFL, France.)

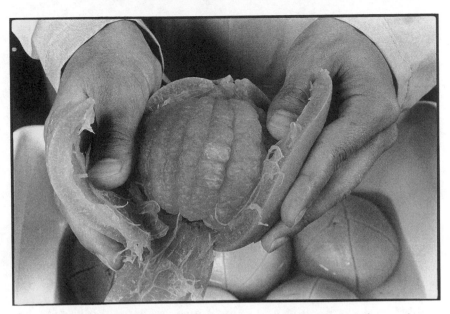

Figure 1-5   Example of vacuum-infusion peeling of grapefruit by pectinase. (From Agricultural Research Service, USDA.)

refrigerated apple slices treated with ascorbic acid and calcium salts, (Ponting Jackson, and Watters 1972) would easily fall into the MPR category. As seen in Figure 1-5, the vacuum-infused peeled grapefruit prepared using pectinase is a good example of minimally processed fruit (Baker and Bruemmer 1987). The fruit can be segmented or handled in a tray pack as a whole fruit. Waldorf salad with diced apples, celery, walnuts, etc. in a dressing and sous vide with a portion of prepared fruits or vegetables would be considered an MPR fruit and vegetable product to carry the concept into prepared foods. See Chapter 2 for an extensive listing of MPR fruits and vegetables.

A more difficult to define, gray area might involve the classification of washed, waxed cucumbers. These products would probably not be considered MPR foods because although they are packaged (waxed), they are also intact. Waxed intact cucumbers could be contrasted with precut or sliced cucumbers which have a relatively short shelf-life and are considered MPR foods. MPR fruits and vegetables should not include fresh intact fruits and vegetables which may undergone normal postharvest handling treatments such as sizing, grading, washing, waxing, CA, or modified atmosphere (MA) storage. (See Figure 1-1.)

Frozen foods make up a portion of products normally classified as cold preserved foods. However, MPR foods are dissimilar to frozen foods in that frozen foods must be transported and stored at $-10°C$ or lower whereas MPR foods require cold-chain refrigerated or slightly higher temperatures depending on the commodity or mixtures of commodities (Anon. 1989b). The overall quality of frozen food is different than the like-fresh quality of MPR food. Many times the consumer can discern differences in texture between frozen and MPR foods. Some manufacturers of sous vide meals, for example, freeze their product, which makes the meal little less than a frozen food in most respects.

MPR foods may be contrasted to irradiated foods although this preservation method may be used as a hurdle to treat MPR foods. In the current regulatory and consumer activist driven climate, irradiation is allowed in the United States to kill insects in wheat flour and to prevent potatoes from sprouting (Kantor 1989). In 1986, the United States Food and Drug Administration (USFDA) (Anon. 1992) approved low-dose irradiation to be used on fresh fruits and vegetables to slow ripening and control insects. Also, the USFDA has recently raised the permissible levels (up to 30 kGy) for killing insects and controlling microorganisms in herbs, spices, seeds, teas, and vegetable seasonings. According to Kantor (1989) 32 countries now use irradiation on about 40 different food products but approval and acceptance has been very slow in the United States. Since irradiation is considered to be a food additive by the USFDA, rather than a preservation method as it is being considered in this book, food treated with irradiation must be labeled "treated with radiation" (Figure 3-11). In MPR foods, irradiation will be considered as a preservation step that may be combined with other preservation methods for manufacture of MPR fruits and vegetables (Figure 1-1). Kader (1986) has published a good review on treatment of fresh intact fruits and vegetables with irradiation.

MPR fruits and vegetables are different from dehydrated fruits and vegetables in terms of texture and water activity (a_w). MPR fruits and vegetables which normally have a_w around 0.97–0.99 are very sensitive to a_w reduction. However, preservatives such as ascorbic acid and citric acid used on dehydrated fruits and vegetables are also used on MPR fruits and vegetables. Dehydrated foods are considered shelf-stable at ambient temperatures and thus do not require the cold-chain delivery system used for MPR foods (Figure 1-2).

An important difference between MPR and thermally processed foods is that MPR foods do not exhibit "commercial sterility" as defined for thermally processed foods. This definition states thermally processed foods are free of microorganisms capable of reproducing under nonrefrigerated conditions and that no viable microorganisms (including spores) of public health significance can reproduce. This "sterility" may be acquired by control of water activity, reducing pH, or application of heat. There is some likelihood that the "commercially sterile" concept may be assigned to those MPR fruits and vegetables that are deemed to be safe. The microbial and enzyme limits for "commercial sterility," or "microbial and enzymatic safety" of MPR fruits and vegetables are yet to be developed, if in fact this term is accepted and is germane to these foods. Thermally processed food cannot be claimed to be like-fresh. Nevertheless, the tremendous amount of research conducted on handling, processing, and preservation of fresh, frozen, irradiated, dehydrated, and thermally processed fruits and vegetables can be applied where appropriate to the relatively new concept of MPR foods.

A major advantage in the development and careful classification of MPR foods is that they provide a basis for separation of the traditional cold preservation field, as described by Potter (1968), into two distinct areas, that is, frozen foods and refrigerated foods. As shown in Figure 1-1 separation of these two areas would greatly simplify the frozen food/refrigerated food classification by placing all frozen foods together and all refrigerated foods in a refrigerated category. No doubt refrigerated as well as other preservation categories should be subclassed into commodity and prepared foods areas. One noticeable difference between MPR fruits and vegetables and many other refrigerated foods is the "living tissue" concept which must be considered in dealing with certain types of MPR fruits and vegetables.

There is the need to update and organize current information developed over many years of research in food science and technology that may apply to MPR foods. In addition, there are demands for research to make MPR foods comparable to the currently more actively used preservation methods for which so many food processing industries are named. The food industry seems interested in making the large family of MPR foods more intensively competitive. It would require several volumes to cover adequately the various food product types that could be interpreted as using the technologies and packaging systems required to produce MPR foods. To narrow the scope of this volume, emphasis will be placed on MPR fruits and vegetables, although in some chapters of the book, particularly in the regulatory and quality control areas, it is difficult to separate MPR fruits and vegetables from other MPR foods. This burgeoning area of food science requires the expertise of horticulturists, plant physiologists and pathologists, biochemists, biotechnologists, microbiologists, food scientists, and food engineers and packaging experts, to name only a few specialties. A truly interdisciplinary effort will be needed to deliver to the markets MPR fruits and vegetables that will have extended high-quality shelf-life beyond 8–10 days, which is usually satisfactory for the retail European market. MPR fruits and vegetables will probably require a minimum shelf-life of 21 days to compete satisfactorily in United States markets (Lioutas 1988). This author is likely referring to name-brand products requiring national distribution, and not to regional operations.

Definitions of MPR Fruits and Vegetables

There have been a number of articles which have defined minimal processing. For example, Rolle and Chism (1987) suggest that minimal processing "includes all unit operations (washing, sorting, peeling, slicing, etc.) that might be used prior to blanching on a conventional processing line." They feel all these products are living tissues. A slightly different approach was taken by Huxsoll and Bolin (1989) in which they felt the "minimally processed product is raw and the cells of the tissues are alive but these characteristics are not required." There was no agreement on the definitions for minimally processed fruits and vegetables at a recent American Chemical Society symposium (Hicks and Sapers 1991). Cantwell (1991) for one, at the symposium, called these products "cut fruits and vegetables which are lightly processed."

It is generally conceded that MPR fruits and vegetables are products that contain live tissues or those that have been only slightly modified from the fresh-condition and are like-fresh in character and quality. These tissues do not exhibit the same physiological responses as normal (raw) untreated intact live plant tissues (Figures 1-3 and 1-4). The cutting, abrasion, or minimal heating of these tissues can cause broadly different responses in various environmental and packaging situations. However, some fruits and vegetables that show little or no physiological activity should also be included in the MPR category. The cold preservation category (Figure 1-1) now encompasses some of these types of foods. MPR fruits probably should include products such as chilled peaches in glass containers in which complete inactivation of cellular metabolism has recently occurred and the product has been quickly transferred to market in the cold chain. Sous vide dishes which may include preheated vegetables or fruit should be included in the MPR food area. In terms of physical state, the tendency has been to include only solids, semisolids, and semiliquids as MPR fruits and vegetables but refrigerated liquids both cloud and clarified juices should be included in this class of foods. The freshly squeezed orange juices and others that are chilled and packaged in plastics, paperboard, or glass are good examples of this type of product. This type of food should probably be included with refrigerated fruit and vegetable products under the like-fresh minimal processing column (Figure 1-1). The USFDA is still considering whether these products should be labelled fresh.

MPR fruits and vegetables (for the purposes of this book) are defined as those prepared by a single or any number of appropriate unit operations such as peeling, slicing, shredding, juicing, etc. given a partial but not end-point preservation treatment including use of minimal heat, a preservative, or radiation. The preservation or hurdle treatment may include pH control, antioxidants, chlorinated water dips, or a combination of these or other treatments (see Chapter 3). It is important to take advantage of the synergies of all preservation treatments. The initial preparation and preservation treatments are usually followed by some kind of controlled/modified atmosphere, vacuum packaging and subjected to reduced temperatures above the freezing point during storage, distribution, marketing, and just prior to preparation for consumption. For safety and greatest retention of sensory and nutritional quality, these products must be distributed and marketed in the cold chain.

Some precut fruits and vegetables (examples are cucumber, eggplant, tomatoes, acid tropicals, and subtropicals) have to be handled at higher temperatures to avoid chilling injury (Appendix, Tables 2 and 3). It should be clear that MPR fruits and vegetables are not intended for ambient shelf-life stability as expected from canned, retorted, or aseptic processed and packaged fruits and vegetables. Nor are they protected from spoilage or quality changes by freezing and being held in frozen storage. There is need for *agreement* by workers in the food field as to the proper description (title) for these foods and definitions thereof. To be successful, MPR foods will have to be high quality, convenient, and safe.

Approach to Studying MPR Fruits and Vegetables

It is becoming increasingly recognized that low temperatures are not the defenses against foodborne illnesses that were previously accepted by the food industry and governmental agencies. The emergence to prominence of non-spore-forming psychrophilic pathogens such as *Listeria monocytogenes* and *Yersinia entercolitica* can cause enormous problems in refrigerated foods (Chapters 7 and 9). Many vegetables, mushrooms, and legume sprouts are considered to be low-acid foods by the USFDA (pH 4.6 and over); thus special measures will have to be taken to make these types of foods free from Type B and Type E *C. botulinum* toxin formation in anaerobic situations brought on by packaging, product density, deaeration, or inert gas injection.

MPR fruits and vegetables have necessarily been studied first on an individual commodity basis and not as mixtures such as precut salads, pizza vegetables, or stir-fry mixtures, sous vide, and the like. A good example of the individual approach is the work on grated carrots in modified atmosphere packaging in France (Carlin et al. 1990). In this research only gaseous packs of thin strips 1.5 mm × 1.5 mm sections of carrots were studied. There is need for studies of convenience foods, that is, complex food mixtures in salads and soup mixtures and the various new products being developed for the market. Also every commodity and its individual cultivars need to be investigated for their applications to MPR foods. It is not clear at this time, for example, whether strawberries for the fresh market or for freezing would be the best suited as a MPR product. Perhaps plant breeders, biotechnologists should be looking for cultivars that are especially suited for minimal processing and refrigerated products. This idea seems to be supported by Rolle and Chism (1987), who have stated that MPR fruits and vegetables are all living respiring tissues in an "energized state." The individualistic concept is also suggested by Labuza and Breene (1989), who feel that is all important to define the end point of high-quality life for each type of fruit and vegetable. Both cultivar and maturity play a very important role in determining these end-point values. It is necessary to collect data on individual commodities, their cultivars, and maturity levels before attempting to work with either simple or complex MPR food mixtures, although this will eventually have to be done by computer modeling. There is no question that complex minimally processed food mixtures are being found in the markets at this time but little information seems to be available about their shelf-life characteristics.

Rolle and Chism (1987) suggested live tissues that have the largest energy reserves such as white potato, topped beetroot, and apple have the longest shelf-life (postharvest) and that the greatest problems are being found with those commodities such as sweet corn, eggplant, raspberries, and strawberries that have the smallest "reserves." Probably more important than the lack or presence of "reserves" is the physical injury received during size reduction operations and the series of preservation steps that will set up a complex series of physiological and microbiological events (Figures 1-3 and 1-4).

It appears that MPR fruits and vegetables of the high-reserve type will have a shorter shelf-life than the intact raw or fresh product, for example, controlled atmosphere stored apples vs. the presliced refrigerated fruit. The former may exhibit a 6- to 8-month or longer satisfactory storage period whereas refrigerated presliced apples may not be usable for more than 2–3 weeks if untreated or up to the average of 10 weeks if treated with 0.5% ascorbic acid and 0.1% Ca (Ponting, Jackson, and Watters 1972). Low-reserve fruits and vegetables are very sensitive to further processing as a means to extend storage and shelf-life and present complex research challenges. There are currently research studies in many parts of the world to address these problems but in most cases the findings are not published or available to the public.

The study of MPR fruits and vegetables will be divided into introductory information, preparatory operations, preservation methods, packaging, biological aspects, and regulatory implications for MPR food products.

References

Anon. 1989a. Caractéristiques techniques des légumes de IVe gamme. In *La Quatrieme Gamme*, pp. 29–30. Paris: Centre Technique Interprofessional des Fruits and Legumes.

Anon. 1989b. Guidelines for the development, production, distribution, and handling of refrigerated foods. Washington, DC: National Food Processors Association. 63 pp.

Anon. 1991. Good Manufacturing Practices for Reddi-Veggies, pp. 1–36. S.A. Salime. Emile Rycheboer and the National Research Institute, Paris.

Anon. 1992. Code of Federal Regulations, Food and Drugs 21 Parts 170–199. Office of the Federal Register National Archieves and Records Administration, Washington, DC.

Baker, R.A. and J.H. Bruemmer. 1989. Quality and stability of enzymatically peeled and sectioned citrus fruit. In *Quality Factors of Fruits and Vegetables*, J.J. Jen (ed.), pp. 140–148, Washington, DC: American Chemical Society.

Carlin, F., C. Nguyen-The, G. Hilbert, and Y. Chambroy. 1990. Modified atmosphere packaging of fresh "Ready-to-use" grated carrots in polymeric films. *J. Food Sci.* **55**:1033–1038.

Cantwell, M. 1991. Physiology of cut fruits and vegetables. Abstract 10. American Chemical Society Annual Meeting, New York, NY.

Hicks, K.B. and G.M. Sapers. 1991. Symposium on minimally processed fruits and vegetables. American Chemical Society Annual Meeting, New York, NY.

Huxsoll, C.C. and H.R. Bolin. 1989. Processing and distribution alternatives for minimally processed fruits and vegetables. *Food Technol.* **43**(3):124–135.

Kader, A.A. 1986. Potential application of ionizing radiation in postharvest handling of fresh fruits and vegetables. *Food Technol.* **40**(6):117–121.

Kantor, MA. 1989. The great food irradiation controversy. *Prof. San. Manag.* **17**(4):29–30.

Labuza, T.P. and W.M. Breene. 1989. Applications of "active" packaging for improvement of shelf-life and nutritional quality of fresh and extended shelf-life food. *J. Food Process. Preserv.* **13**:1–69.

Lioutas, T.S. 1988. Challenges of controlled and modified atmosphere packaging: a food company's perspective. *Food Technol.* **42**(9):78–88.

Mannapperuma, J.D. and R.R. Singh. 1990. Modeling of gas exchange in polymeric packages of fresh fruits and vegetables. Abstract 646. Inst. of Food Technol. Annual Meeting, Dallas, TX.

Morris, C.E. 1991. Designing for chilled foods. *Food Engin.* **63**(5):73–80.

Ponting, J.D., R. Jackson, and G. Watters. 1972. Refrigerated apple slices. Preservative effects of ascorbic acid, calcium and sulfites. *J. Food Sci.* **37**:434–436.

Potter, N.N. 1968. *Food Science*, pp. 177–226. Westport, CT: AVI now Van Nostrand Reinhold.

Rolle, R.S. and G.W. Chism III. 1987. Physiological consequences of minimally processed fruits and vegetables. *J. Food Quality* **10**:157–177.

Smock, R.M. and A.M. Neubert. 1950. *Apple and Apple Products*, pp. 201–207. New York: Interscience.

2

Initial Preparation, Handling, and Distribution of Minimally Processed Refrigerated Fruits and Vegetables

Fatih Yildiz

Introduction

There is a continuous demand for fresh, convenient, high-quality and safely prepared minimally processed refrigerated (MPR) fruits and vegetables throughout the world, but consumption is concentrated in certain areas. On the other hand, most MPR food raw material production is seasonal, usually remote from consumption areas, and concentrated at certain geographical regions where yield and quality can be optimized. In addition, the raw material remains a living entity, and highly perishable, bulky, price, and quantity-variable commodity.

New fruit and vegetable production, storage, processing, packaging, and preparation technologies made year-round availability possible for most products, except perhaps apricots, blueberries, cherries, blackberries, tangerines, carambola, and some others in a global marketing system. An optimum integrated distribution system for MPR foods will minimize energy use, environmental pollution, and cost while maximizing the overall quality and convenience of fruits and vegetables.

Uneven production and processing will be equalized with new transgenic cultivars and improved storage and MPR technologies which will make year-round availability of almost all fruits and vegetables possible in fresh form around the world.

There are over 500,000 species of plants known on which animal and human survival depends. However, if animals and humans ceased to exist on earth, plants would continue not only to survive but also to thrive very well. There are 5,000 genera of plants and 5,000 cultivars (varieties) that might be used to feed the world's people either directly or indirectly. The species is the fundamental unit used to designate groups of plants that can be recognized as distinct kinds. In nature, individuals within one species interbreed, but they do not interbreed with other species because they are separated by some physiological, morphological, or genetic barrier that prevents the interchange of genes between the two species (Hartmann, Kester, and Davies 1990). A cultivar denotes individuals that are distinguished by morphological, physiological, cytological, chemical, or other characteristics significant for the purpose of horticulture and retain their distinguishing features when reproduced. An example of a cultivar is the Jonathan apple. Cultivars also represent different food quality attributes such as color, flavor, texture, and nutritional value. A strain includes those plants of a given cultivar that possess the general varietal characteristics but differ in some minor characteristic or quality. A cultivar with early maturation may be considered a strain within the cultivar. An example of strain is "gray zucchini." As another example, some 70 strawberry cultivars are grown commercially in the United States; only about 10 are truly popular, but these change from year to year as new cultivars are developed by plant breeders (Hartmann et al. 1988). Variations between species, cultivars, and strains can be due either to environmental or to genetic differences. Opportunity exists for a large number of desired transgenic cultivars or strain developments. However, some 200 species of fruits and vegetables are of major importance in world trade.

Raw Product Characteristics and Classification

Raw fruit and vegetable quality and shelf-life depend to a great extent on the preharvest, harvest, and postharvest conditions (Nonnecke 1989). These include:

1. Genetically controlled factors (cultivar, strain)
2. Climatic conditions (light, temperature, percent relative humidity, wind, rain fall, etc.)
3. Soil conditions (type of soil, pH, percent moisture, microflora, mineral composition, etc.)
4. Agricultural practices (use of fertilizers, pesticides, growth regulators, irrigation, and pollination, etc.)
5. Harvesting (mechanical harvest, hand harvest, harvest temperature, etc.)

Currently, most fruits and vegetables are grown in fields, gardens, and greenhouses; however, two very different production (organic and hydroponic) systems are becoming more common.

Before harvest, fruits and vegetables must meet certain minimum maturity requirements. These requirements may vary from one producing area to another and from one product to another but are usually based on (1) color break, (2) minimum juice content, (3) minimum acid content, (4) minimum percentage of total soluble solids, (5) Brix/acid ratio, (6) optimum flavor development, (7) abscission (detachment from parent plant), (8) development of wax on skin, (9) softening (changes in composition of pectic substances), (10) size and shape, and (11) heat units (Pantastico 1975; Wills et al. 1989).

Fruits and vegetables can be classified in different ways for purposes of postharvest storage and processing operations. Classifications of fruits and vegetables according to the use of different plant organs was outlined by Weichmann (1987) as follows:

Root, tuber, and bulb vegetables: Carrot, celeriac, garlic, horseradish, Jerusalem artichoke, onion, parsnip, potato, radish, rutabaga, salsify, scorzonera, sweet potato, table beet, turnip, yam

Leafy vegetables: Brussels sprout, cabbage,
                                     celery, chard, chicory,
                                     Chinese cabbage, collard,
                                     cress, dandelion, endive,
                                     green onion, kale, leek, chive,
                                     lettuce, spinach, parsley

Flower vegetables: Artichoke, broccoli,
                                     cauliflower

Immature fruit vegetables: Bean, cucumber, egg plant,
                                     okra, peas, pepper, squash,
                                     sweet corn

Mature fruit vegetables: Melon, tomato

Seed vegetables: Shelled peas, shelled beans,
                                     corn, lentils

Simple fleshy berry fruits: Banana, grape, date, papaya,
                                     avocado, kiwifruit

Simple fleshy hesperidium fruits: Orange, lemon, lime,
                                     tangerine, grapefruit

Simple drupe (stone) fruits: Peach, plum, cherry, apricot,
                                     almond, olive

Simple pome fruits: Apple, pear, quince

Multiple fleshy berry fruits: Strawberry, blackberry,
                                     raspberry, mulberry, fig,
                                     pineapple, pomegranate

The variation in rates of respiration and transpiration among different commodities is enormous. The various respiration and transpiration properties and temperature sensitivities of horticultural products are compiled in Appendix tables. Table 2-1 lists some climacteric and nonclimacteric fruits according to their respiration patterns (Hardenburg, Watada, and Wang 1986; Kays 1991). All vegetables and fresh herbs can be considered to have a nonclimacteric type of respiratory pattern. Most climacteric, and some nonclimacteric fruits such as pineapple, continue to ripen after separation from the plant. The task in this case is to deliver the fruit to the consumer at an optimal level of quality. Most nonclimacteric and some climacteric products do not ripen after harvest, such as apples, berries, cherries, grapefruit, grapes, lemons, limes, oranges, strawberries,

Table 2-1
Classification of Some Edible Fruits According to their Respiratory Behavior During Ripening

Climacteric Fruits	Nonclimacteric Fruits
Apple	Blackberry
Apricot	Cacao
Avocado	Cashew
Banana	Cherry, sour
Biriba	Cherry, sweet
Bitter melon	Cucumber
Blueberry, highbush	Grape
Blueberry, lowbrush	Grapefruit
Blueberry, rabbiteye	Java plum
Breadfruit	Lemon
Cantaloupe	Litchi
Cherimoya	Mountain apple
Chinese gooseberry	Olive
Corossol sauvage	Orange
Feijoa	Pepper
Fig, common	Pineapple
Guava, "purple strawberry"	Rose apple
Guava, "strawberry"	Satsuma mandarin
Guava, "yellow strawberry"	Star apple
Guava	Strawberry
Honeydew melon	Surinam cherry
Kiwi	Tree tomato
Mammee-apple	
Mango	
Papaw	
Papaya	
Passion fruit	
Peach	
Pear	
Persimmon	
Plum	
Sapote	
Soursop	
Tomato	
Watermelon	

Source: Hardenburg, Watada, and Wang 1986; Kays 1991.

tangerines, and watermelon. In nonclimacteric commodities, quality is optimal at harvest. The task is to minimize quality loss. Quality specifications must be established for the final product by the retailers. The following is a list of changes occurring in fruits and vegetables during harvesting, preparation, and handling:

1. Respiratory, metabolic, and enzymatic activities:
   Heat production
   Climacteric crisis after harvest
   Nonclimacteric metabolism
   Ethylene-induced physiological disorders—russet-spotting
   Reduced O_2- or elevated CO_2-induced physiological disorders, CO_2 injury, blackheart in potatoes
   a. Anaerobic respiration (ethanol–acetaldehyde accumulation causing off-flavors and off-odors)
   b. Lactic acid fermentation at low O_2 concentration in cut products (Juliot, Lindsay, and Ridley 1989).
   Adverse effects of polyphenol oxidases, cellulases, pectolytic enzymes, amylases, peroxidases (discoloration, softening, off-flavors, and off-odors)
2. Transpiration (moisture loss, weight loss)
   Loss of turgidity (firmness)
   Withering and wilting in leafy vegetables
3. Growth phenomena:
   Sprouting
   Root growth (rooting)
   Lignification (toughening)
   Ripening
   Senescence (yellowing, pithiness, feathering opening or floral buds, pink-rib in lettuce)
   Color changes (greening)
   Elongation (asparagus)
   Sloughing (skin loss)
   Wound healing
   Warts
4. Pest and microbial spoilage (nematode, insect, bacteria, yeast, mold, and virus attack and physiological disorders):
   Psyllid yellows
   Insect infestation
   Root knot
   Brown rot
   Stem-end rot

      Gray mold rot
      Rusty brown discoloration
      Downy mildew
      Blossom-end rot
      Blue mold rot

5. Temperature-induced injuries:
      Chill injury (CI)
      Freeze injury
      High-temperature injury
      Solar injury (sunscald, sunburn)

6. Mechanical injuries:
      Wounding
      Latent damage
      Cracking
      Broken tips
      Surface browning
      Cut or bruised products

Temperature is a major, invisible, ever-present factor controlling respiratory, metabolic, and enzymatic activities, transpiration, and the growth of pests and microorganisms. Proper temperature management in the storage of MPR fruit and vegetable tissues can inactivate or retard the physiological defects. A theory developed (Parkin et al. 1989) to explain chill injury was based on low-temperature-induced membrane lipid phase transitions leading to a loss of membrane integrity and physiological dysfunction.

High-temperature and solar injury has been more a concern during the growth and development of plants than in postharvest handling. Hot-water dipping with fungicides is used in certain products to reduce microbial load without injuring the fruit (Harvey 1978; Salunkhe, Bolin, and Reddy 1991).

Mechanical injuries speed up the deterioration of fresh produce by disrupting membranes and increasing enzymatic activity which causes undesirable reactions to occur (Shewfelt 1987). Objectionable quality changes are accelerated by the mechanical rupturing of the cells that occurs during preparation operations such as peeling and cutting, allowing enzymes to intermix with substrates. In addition, cuts and punctures allow for microbial contamination of products as well as moisture loss. Mechanical damage may take place any time a product is handled during harvesting, loading, transportation, sorting, and grading operations. Mechanical stress also stimulates peroxidase activity in cucumbers (Eckert and Ogawa 1988).

Cuts and punctures can be reduced by selecting varieties less susceptible to bruising and by proper shock-absorbing packaging. Harvested fruits and vegetables exhibit considerable resistance to pathogens and decay processes during most of their postharvest life if they are not mechanically damaged.

Most perishable crops increase in susceptibility to infection as they approach senescence, which is a progressive loss of membrane integrity. Treatments that inhibit or delay these processes reduce postharvest decay losses (Eckert and Ogawa 1988).

Susceptibility of fresh fruits and vegetables to freezing injury was summarized by Hardenburg, Watada, and Wang (1986) as follows:

Group 1 Most susceptible	Group 2 Moderately susceptible	Group 3 Least susceptible
Apricots	Apples	Beets
Asparagus	Broccoli, sprouting	Brussels sprouts
Avocados	Cabbage, new	Cabbage, old and
Bananas	Carrots	savoy
Beans, snap	Cauliflower	Dates
Berries (except cran-	Celery	Kale
berries)	Cranberries	Kohlrabi
Cucumbers	Grapefruit	Parsnips
Eggplant	Grapes	Rutabagas
Lemons	Onions (dry)	Salsify
Lettuce	Oranges	Turnips
Limes	Parsley	
Okra	Pears	
Peaches	Peas	
Peppers, sweet	Radishes	
Plums	Spinach	
Potatoes	Squash, winter	
Squash, summer		
Sweet potatoes		
Tomatoes		

It is essential to understand the nature of the harvested fruits and vegetables, and the effects of handling practices, to maintain optimum condition of the product at the market. Due to the diversity of products, it is impossible to suggest a single solution for all fruits and vegetables; rather, the most appropriate practices must be worked out by the individual operator for each commodity and particular situation.

Optimal System Analysis

A systems approach to processing and distribution of MPR fruits and vegetables is essential to optimize storage and handling conditions for individual crops. This offers a challenge and an opportunity for food scientists to develop systems that will attain the lowest overall cost for the system as a whole, while attaining optimum overall quality of fresh horticultural products.

In a systems approach: (1) the steps of unit operations are documented within defined boundaries, (2) the system is analyzed, (3) the system is optimized, and (4) the system coordination and controls are studied. It will be necessary to standardize some components such as container sizes, product size and shapes, labels, etc. for automation of the system.

An analysis of the system must begin with a survey of where the crops are grown and where the products are consumed for specific product and market situations. Each cultivar or closely related cultivars may be considered a system. For minimally processed fruits and vegetables, harvesting, processing, storage, and distribution are accomplished in a fast, highly integrated system to maintain product quality. As a result, postharvest losses have been reduced to a few percentages and manageable transportation distances have been increased up to thousands of kilometers (Meffert 1990). One of the disadvantages of the systems approach is that the understanding of the entire system is emphasized much more than the detailed understanding of each step.

Processing and distribution systems for MPR fruits and vegetables include such issues as processing at the location of production versus at the location of consumption, large versus small processing plants, bulk transportation versus prepackaged shipment other issues include controlled atmosphere (CA)/modified atmosphere (MA)/vacuum/air packaging, storage at the location of production or in the region of consumption of a single commodity versus a multiple fruit and vegetable processing plant.

The alternative processing and distribution systems of minimally processed products affect the kind of initial preparation and distribution that may be used. Once the postharvest handling system has been diagrammed for a specific product, quality attributes are mea-

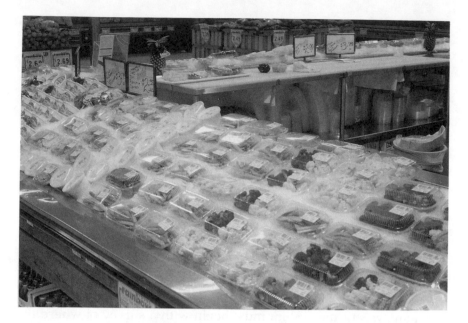

Figure 2-1   A retail display shelf for MPR fruits and vegetables.

sured at each step. Where the greatest quality losses are occurring, they can then be subjected to more intense investigation under controlled conditions. An improved technique can then be evaluated within the context of the entire system and assessed for economic feasibility. In general, quality deterioration occurring in MPR food systems is cumulative (Bogh-Sorensen 1990).

The location of the storage facility will depend greatly on the type of marketing operation and the location of the orchard or field. It is desirable to have wholesale bulk refrigerated storages as close to the production area as possible to dispose of or utilize the waste at nearby areas. On the other hand, retail storage and displays should be in the consumption area (Figure 2-1).

The following type of information should be developed for each product in a systems approach. An example of systems approach to a fresh sliced strawberry processing operation should include at least the following parameters (Rosen and Kader 1989):

1. Cultivar selection: Parjaro are suitable for fresh market

2. Harvest: Hand or mechanical harvesting at full bright red or pink, in swallow tray

3. Precooling:	Rapid forced air or hydro precooling to below 7° C (44.6° F) within 8 min or maximum 2 hrs
4. Field processing:	Dump-wash tank to remove sand, trash eliminator to separate berry from plant, mechanical stemming to remove calyx
5. Transportation:	To packing house with dry ice in shallow baskets or trays around 0° C (32° F)
6. Sorting and grading:	Defectives and color sorting, separation into two sizes (small, large) by a tapered-finger sizing device
7. Processing:	Slicing into quarters, water washing to remove all exudates, dipping into $CaCl_2$ solution, and spin drying
8. Packaging:	Controlled atmosphere (CA) packaging at 12% CO_2, 2% O_2, 95% relative humidity, and 0° C (32° F) packaging into portion, 1-lb, 2-lb, 11-lb (5 kg) size resealable plastic pail packaging for fresh or strawberry shortcake.
9. Storage at warehouse:	95% relative humidity, 0° C (32° F) wholesale warehousing on standard pallets; maximum 7 days
10. Storage and display at retail:	Display cabinets 1 day at 18–20 ° C (64–68 ° F); the first noticeable quality defect is loss of volatiles.

The ideal system will be a completely integrated, computerized, and automated one.

Major Initial Unit Operation of MPR Fruits and Vegetables

The industrial harvesting, handling, processing, preparation, and distribution of fruits and vegetables require a number of steps that are primarily physical in nature, although their effects may contribute to biological, chemical, and physical changes in the products. Many individual processes are required to change or separate horticultural products into various MPR foods. By systematically studying these operations, all processes are unified, simplified, and speeded up. Each operation requires that theory and equipment be considered together. The understanding of the basic physical principles of an operation and the formulation of these principles into a mathematical expression are the first requirements for the application of the unit operation concept. The design and operation of the equipment and the material and energy balance calculations are based on unit operation principles. Major unit operations involved in MPR processing of fruits and vegetables are given in Table 2-2. Packaging and preservation operations are given in other chapters in this book.

Raw Material Handling Operations

Materials handling is movement of MPR foods from the field to the retail display cabinets. It involves the conveying (in all directions) and storage of materials. Hydraulic flow, pneumatic or air flotation methods, conveyors, and forklift trucks are basic to many materials handling systems. An understanding of the characteristics of produce, such as shape, size, density, and hardness, is necessary in designing processes and equipment. Rapid handling, along with precooling and without damage to the product, preserves quality. The product should not be transferred from different containers in the field or in storage that will increase the chance of damage to the product. Palletized unit loads, mobile racking, and lift-trucks reduce the time and labor requirements in handling operations. Therefore, unit loads should be maintained until the final sales point. Unitizing refers to various methods of grouping together shipping containers whereby they can be mechanically handled as a unit load. The most common unitizing method is palletizing; that is, containers are stacked on a pallet. The standard pallet size most commonly used is 1.0 m × 1.2 m and has a thickness of 15 cm. Some of the methods of increasing efficiency in materials handling are (1) to minimize movement, (2) handle in bulk or unit loads, (3) concentrate the products to minimize the quantity of material to be moved, (4) make the operation continuous and mechanized if possible, (5) make units in the proper size. Perishable MPR foods may be damaged by exces-

Table 2-2
Major Unit Operations of MPR Fruit and Vegetable Processing

A. Materials handling operations
  1. Harvesting
  2. Field processing
  3. Transportation
  4. Receiving
B. Preparation operations
  1. Separation and multiphase contacting operations
    a. Separating operations:

Grading	Cleaning
Sorting	Husking
Screening	Heading
Inspection	Topping
Brine separation	Shelling
Culling	Snipping
Dewatering	Silking
Draining	Trimming
Cluster separation	Stemming
Flotation	Skinning
Centrifugation	Peeling
Destoning	Pitting
Dusting	Coring

   b. Mixing operations:

Blending	Mixing with solids
Emulsification	Mixing with liquids

  2. Size reduction operations:

Chopping	Slicing
Cutting	Dicing
Strip-cut	Segmenting
V-cut	Shredding
Flat cut	Pulping
Crinkle cut	Mashing
Halving	Juicing

C. Distribution and utilization operations
  1. Wholesaling: storage and control
    Volume, mass, temperature, time, RH, size measuring, controlling
    CA/MA/air/vacuum storage (O_2, CO_2, N_2, CO, C_2H_4, H_2O controls),
    computer-controlled warehousing
    Wholesale storage
    Retail storage
    Labeling
  2. Physical distribution or movement
  3. Retailing and food service
  4. Communications network

sive temperature fluctuations, severe vibration, or microbial contamination during the handling stage.

Harvesting

Fruit and vegetable harvesting and handling operations are varied and highly dependent on the particular commodity. Lack of uniform ripening can make a one-time-mode harvest difficult but quite manageable. Harvesting at the proper stage of maturity is an extremely exacting operation. Harvest dates may be estimated in advance by crop scheduling systems or the heat unit system. Harvesting at the lowest possible temperature (night or early morning) is advantageous for maintaining fruit quality during handling and storage. Morris (1990) reported that grapes harvested when fruit temperature was high (above 30° C) had a poor color and produced high levels of alcohol and acetic acid, indicating microbial spoilage. The delicate nature of many fruits and vegetables requires careful handling, and many products for the fresh and MPR processed market are hand-harvested. Frequently, mechanical harvesting aids are used. Hydraulic platforms or ladders enable workers to be lifted while harvesting tree fruits. Bulk collection containers or conveyors are used to transfer the harvested products rapidly from fields to the processing unit. Machine harvesting may improve quality over that obtained by hand-harvesting because it is faster and reduces holding time in the fields. In one study, mechanical and hand-harvesting systems bruised 11–40% and 0–18% of apples, respectively (Tennes, Levin, and Wittenberger 1969).

Field Processing

Shelling and threshing of peas, beans, and lentils are done in the field by combines. Beets and carrots are harvested and topped mechanically at the field. Large boom conveyors have been used to carry the harvested pineapple from the pickers to the loading trucks. Potato harvesters dig, lift, clean, and load the product. Field processing includes inspecting for size, defects, maturity, and precooling in the field. Dry sorting in the field removes gross contamination and defective fruit which would otherwise contaminate wash waters. Insects in machine-harvested fruits can be removed by a tank washing technique in which infested fruits pass through water containing a 0.1% nonalkaline anionic wetting agent (Crandall, Shanks, and George 1966). A water spray is then used to remove insects, debris, and wetting agents. Ninety-five percent of the chemical residues such as those arising from the use of pesticides can be removed by this method with no loss of quality (Arthey and Dennis 1991). Precooling may be performed in the field or at the packing house on bulk loads, pallet bin boxes, or shipping containers. Rapid precooling of fruits and vegetables to remove the field heat and the heat of respiration can be achieved by (1) forced air cooling, (2) hydro cooling, (3) hydro air cooling (fine-mist spray combined with forced air cooling), and (4) vacuum cooling.

Significant losses in market life of fresh broccoli were noted (Brennen and Shewfelt 1989) within the 3-h cooling delay after harvest. Some MPR products, such as oranges, strawberries, and honeydew melons, may be hydro-cooled in the field, but green pepper will fill with water if hydro-cooled. However, efficient immediate handling techniques need to be established for chill-sensitive products at the field. Curing or preconditioning, which is holding produce at moderate temperature for a period prior to low-temperature storage, is effective to prevent chill-injury for some fruits such as grapefruit. All harvesting equipment should be maintained in clean condition to prevent deterioration caused by fungi and bacteria. Knives, belts, and other surfaces should be cleaned daily to remove accumulated dirt and soil. Boxes, trays, sacks, and other receptacles for harvested produce should be cleaned daily to reduce microbial load. Metal and plastic receptacles are more easily cleaned than wooden boxes. There are distinct advantages to do as much processing, such as cleaning, trimming, and coring, as possible at the production field as can be done without greatly increasing perishability. This prevents costly disposal problems at metropolitan consumption areas.

Transportation

It is obvious that perishable MPR fruits and vegetables must be quickly and carefully handled during transportation. The choice of shipping in packages or in bulk depends on the product and on market requirements and economics. Bulk transport of some vegetables, such as peas, beans, and sweet corn, presents problems with self-heating due to respiration and cooling may be required before transport. In bulk packaging of leafy and stem vegetables, application of ice-slush lowers the temperature while maintaining high relative humidity in transportation. The containers used in the transport of horticultural products must be so used to avoid any mechanical damage to their contents, both through particle-to-particle or particle-to-container contacts, by load shifting, shock, overhead weight, and vibration. Fleshy berry fruits are placed in shallow boxes to prevent crushing by packing under their own weight. Fast, reliable transportation by air, sea, truck, and rail is an important element in the distribution of minimally processed foods. Mechanically refrigerated CA/MA/ air/vacuum intermodal containers can be transported by truck, rail, ship, or air. Internationally standardized, dry and refrigerated intermodal containers of truck load capacity (20,000–30,000 kg) are now available. Mechanical refrigeration systems consist of a compressor–condenser–evaporator unit that is separated from the load compartment by an insulated bulkhead. The machine section also contains a thermostat for temperature control and an air-temperature indicator.

The air distribution system in a rail car uses a fan to draw air through the evaporator coil and discharge it into a ceiling duct above the load. Air distribution in all refrigerated trailers is normally from front to back. Liquid nitrogen and solid CO_2 have been used for transit refrigeration and modified atmospheres of fresh produce. However, a prepared atmosphere with a specified mixture of N_2, CO_2, O_2, C_2H_2, H_2O, and CO should be tailored to meet the requirements and tolerances of the product treated in air-tight transport vehicles. It is sometimes desirable to initiate the ripening of pears, apples, plums, and tomatoes with a low concentration of ethylene at a controlled temperature during the transit period so that the product is ready for retail sale when it arrives at the market. Regardless of the method of loading, provision should be made for refrigerated, controlled, or modified air to circulate uniformly to all parts of the load. Kays (1991) reported the specific requirements of commodities being transported. The refrigeration requirement is higher during transport than in static storage due to infiltration of air through the container walls, floor, and ceiling. Highly perishable commodities, such as strawberries, apricots, figs, cherries, grapes, lettuce, and mushrooms, may be transported by air in refrigerated cargo containers. Less perishable commodities, such as citrus fruits, potatoes, pears, apples, bananas, tomatoes, and cabbage, may be shipped by sea in refrigerated holds of insulated ships. Fruits and vegetables that require different temperatures, relative humidity (RH) conditions, fumigation, and those that are ethylene producing and non-ethylene-producing, odor absorbing, odor projecting, and possessing different chemical properties should not be loaded into the same container. Grouping of compatible loads is essential in mixed load transportation and storage. Containerization, modulization, unitization, and metrication allow delivery of MPR foods with a minimum of handling and physical injury to the product and a short transit time.

Receiving

At the receiving of MPR product, the cold chain is interrupted; consequently, proper care must be exercised not to lose the quality that has been retained in harvesting and transporting. The efficiency of the receiving operation will be increased by the use of palletized loads. In receiving, produce must be properly segregated to permit adequate grading. Materials should be moved rapidly through the shortest distance possible from the unloading to the storage point to reduce costs. Batch and continuous automatic digital weighing have replaced manual weighing, saving time and labor. Accurate weighing is necessary for proper cost accounting, product formulation, planning, and quality control. Contracts between the supplier and the MPR product processing plant include the required standards. In some cases, contract growing may be necessary as in canning. There is a need to be able to rapidly and nondestructively evaluate the quality of fresh produce at the receiving (Dull 1986) for such safety aspects as pesticide residues, heavy microbial loads, toxic metals, naturally present undesirable compounds, and plant growth regulators.

After products have been received they should be transferred immediately to the proper ($-1°$ C to $+6°$ C, or $+6°$ to $13°$ C or $+13°$ C to $18°$ C) storage areas depending on the chill characteristics of the product.

Preparation Operations

Ready-to-cook, ready-to-eat, and ready-to-use type convenience fruits and vegetables require many preparation operations. Most of these involve physical changes, but chemical reactions also take place. The weight of the prepared cooked final product may be 50–99% of the raw material as shown in Table 2-3 (USDA 1984).

Vegetables in the following food groups are prepared for ready-to-use MPR products (Figures 2-2, 2-3, and 2-4).

F. Yildiz

Table 2-3
Raw or Cooked Yield of Edible Portion (EP) Per Pound of Selected
Fruits and Vegetables as Purchased (AP)

Food Items	Yield (Pounds of EP)
Apples, fresh peeled	0.92
Bananas, with peel	0.65
Beans, green (cooked)	0.88
Broccoli	0.81
Cabbage	0.87
Cantaloupe	0.52
Carrots	0.70
Carrots (cooked)	0.60
Corn on cob (cooked)	0.55
Lettuce, head	0.76
Mushrooms	0.98
Onions	0.88
Peaches	0.76
Pears, pared	0.78
Pineapple	0.54
Plums	0.94
Potato, baked with skin (cooked)	0.81
Potato, mashed (cooked)	0.81
Spinach (cooked)	0.81
Sweet potato, baked with skin (cooked)	0.61
Tomato	0.99
Watermelon	0.57

Source: USDA 1984.

Snack vegetables:	Whole and sliced onion, celery strip, cut carrots, sliced cucumbers, whole lettuce
Stew vegetables:	Cut green beans, sliced onions, diced potatoes, corn, diced tomatoes, asparagus, riba, diced peppers, peas, diced broccoli stalks, diced mushrooms, brussel sprouts, crinkle-sliced eggplants, whole okra

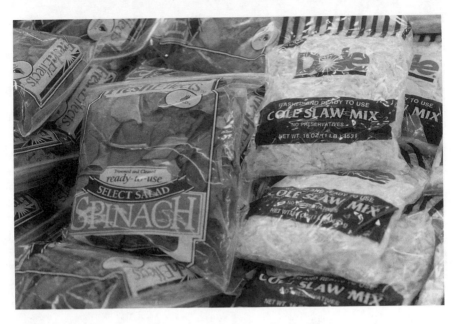

Figure 2-2   Fresh ready-to-cook spinach and coleslaw.

Salad vegetables:	Shredded carrots, shredded cabbage for cole slaw, halved and cored pepper, diced onions, sliced red cabbage, shredded lettuce, whole parsley, sliced tomatoes, endive, chicory
Soup vegetables:	Diced peppers, diced mushrooms, diced onions, strip-cut parsley, crinkle-cut celery, diced garlic, cross-cut leeks
Sandwich vegetables:	Sliced tomatoes, shredded lettuce
Ready-to-cook vegetables:	Sliced potatoes, strip cuts for french fries, stir-fry vegetables
Sauce and gravy vegetables:	Diced peppers, diced mushrooms, diced onions and garlic, strip-cut peppermint, diced tomatoes, etc.

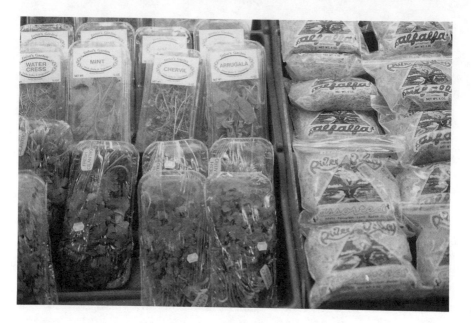

Figure 2-3   Some fresh ready-to-use herbs and sprouts.

Puree and juice vegetables:	Shredded potatoes, mashed potatoes, diced tomatoes, diced carrots, diced celery, diced beets, diced eggplants
Pizza topping vegetables:	Strip-cut peppers, sliced mushrooms, sliced tomatoes

Fruits in the following groups are prepared for MPR products in the end-use form (Figures 2-5 and 2-6)

Fruits cocktail:	Diced peaches, diced pears, whole seedless grapes, diced pineapples, pitted cherries, diced apples
Fruits pies:	Apple slices, peeled peach halves, peeled apricot halves
Fruit salads:	Diced peaches, diced pears, seedless grapes, diced pineapple, pitted cherry halves, sliced bananas in 20° Brix syrup, citrus salads, segmented oranges, segmented mandarins, halved grapefruits, etc.

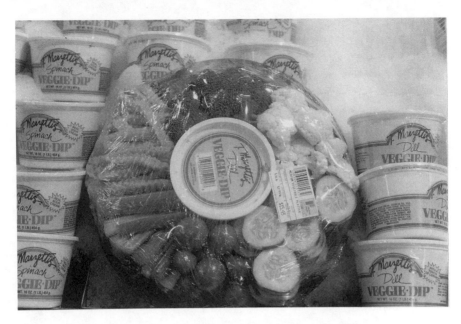

Figure 2-4   Ready-to-eat mixed snack vegetables with dip.

Fruit soups:	Pitted prunes, pitted cherries, sliced peaches, sliced apricots, etc.
Fruit cakes:	Sliced strawberries, peeled bananas, pitted cherries, sliced apricots
Fruit jellos:	Whole strawberries, sliced bananas, pitted cherries, seedless grapes, sliced oranges
Fruit puddings:	Cut strawberries, sliced bananas, pitted cherry halves
Snack fruits:	Sliced melons, pitted plums, peeled oranges
Fruit sauce/puree/juice:	Shredded apples for puree or sauce, prune sauce, whole or cut oranges, lemons, grapefruits for juice

The preparation functions may be simplified by using assembly-line concepts and related equipment to enable mass production. The primary objective of industrial food preparation is to ensure ultimate

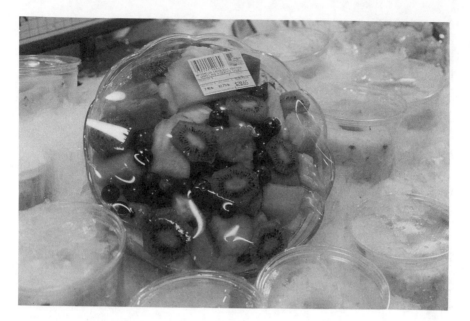

Figure 2-5   Ready-to-eat fruit salad platter on an ice-slush display cabinet in a retail store.

consumer safety (nutritional and health), quality, convenience, and innovation at minimum cost. Preparation of MPR fruits and vegetables for ready-to-use form involves washing, cutting, rinsing, conditioning, packaging, and storage operations as illustrated in Figure 2-7 (Anon. 1988d).

In addition to general methods of doing these operations for some products, specialized equipment is required such as green bean snippers and centrifugal spin driers, special cutters, and aseptic assembly and filling rooms. In the design of a processing line for MPR products, the major economic consideration is the cost of operation and the amount of time the equipment is being utilized. The initial investment cost is usually secondary to the costs of operation. Operating costs on a per-unit of product processed basis take into account the type and use of energy, the labor employed, the amount and type of water used, and the cost of effluent disposal and innovation at minimum cost.

Separation and Multiphase Contacting Operations

In MPR food preparation, solid–solid, solid–liquid, and solid–gas contacting systems are utilized for separation and mixing opera-

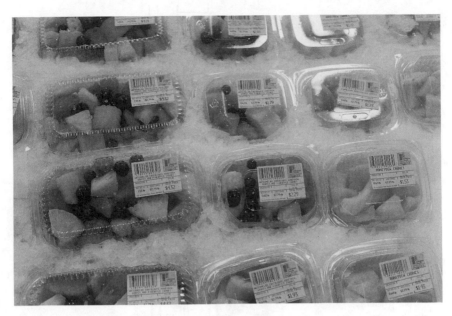

Figure 2-6   Ready-to-eat watermelon, grape, and honeydew mix and honeydew chunks on an ice-slush display cabinet.

tions. Process equipment for such systems is designed to achieve the appropriate transfer operations with a minimum expenditure of energy and capital investment. Screening is the solid–solid separation of a mixture of various sizes of fruits. Blending of ingredients may be the main objective of a solid–solid mixing. Leaching or simple washing is a separation of solid–liquid system which consists of the displacement of dirt by a liquid in which it is soluble. Separation and multiphase contacting operations of this kind are carried out in single or multiple steps or stages. A stage may be defined as a unit of equipment in which two dissimilar phases are brought into contact with each other and then are mechanically separated. Gravity sedimentation operations are also solid–liquid separations. Solid–liquid mixing is involved in fruit juice and puree preparations. Modified and controlled atmosphere storage and packaging involves gas–solid mixing operations. The solid phase is usually in a static condition. The gas phase flows or circulates more or less freely around the solid particles. Gas–solid separation is involved in dust collection, aspiration, dewatering, O_2 scavenging, CO_2 scavenging, and ethylene emitting.

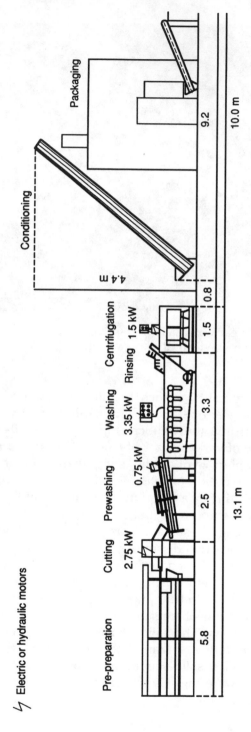

Figure 2-7   Diagram of an MPR salad production line (Anon. 1987.)

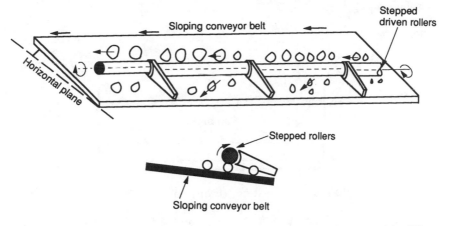

Figure 2-8   The operating principle of a belt and roller sorter: (a) oblique view; (b) section across conveyor belt. (From Brennan et al. 1990.)

Solid materials such as horticultural produce may be separated by virtue of differences in density, shape, size, color, surface characteristics (surface area, electrostatic charge), and solubility. In general, separating includes the following operations: grading, cleaning, washing, screening, sorting, peeling, coring, draining, paring, pitting, stemming, sedimenting, trimming, and centrifuging. The MPR products processing industry uses separators of various kinds. Solid–solid separators include screens, sizers, classifiers, magnetic separators, and cluster separators. Solid–liquid separators are exemplified by the commonly used clarifiers, basket centrifuges, strainers, and percolators. Also, solid–gas separators such as driers, dehumidifiers, aspirators, cyclone separators, air filters, electrical precipitators, dust collectors, and ethylene-removing catalyzers are used.

Sorting, Sizing, and Grading

Figures 2-8 and 2-9 show separation of raw materials into size and weight quality groups. This provides uniformity and standardization of the finished products for buying and selling. The most important grade factors are size, shape, color, firmness, flavor, friability, bruises, cut surfaces, chemical composition, disease, and soundness. Overripe, undersized, and blemished products are separated from those of acceptable quality. Grading and sorting com-

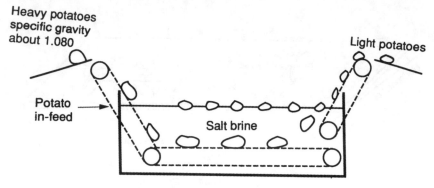

Figure 2-9 Potato handling system. (From Farrel 1976.)

prise the last separation stage before processing. Damage and spoilage therefore are likely to be transmitted to the finished product if the bad products are not removed. The emptying of field containers onto sorting belts and dropping of product units from sorters can cause extensive damage if it is not controlled. Screening is the separation of a mixture of various sizes of produce such as peaches, strawberries, apricots, or oranges into two or more portions by means of a screening surface. Material that remains on a given screening surface is the normal size and that passing through the screening surface is the undersize material. Vibrating bar screens are used for coarse size separation and dewatering at 4-mesh (4.76 mm) and larger screening operations. Smaller than 4-mesh and larger than 48-mesh (0.29 mm or 297 μm) is referred to as fine separation. Ultrafine separation screens are smaller than 48-mesh size (Perry, Green, and Maloney 1989). In the grading and sorting of fruits and vegetables, various devices and types of apparatus are used to facilitate and mechanize grading operations. Screens of various design are used. Flatbeds, drums, rollers, vibrating screens, and belt and roller sorters are a few examples of industrial operations. Light reflectance and transmittance sorting is used for nondestructively sorting and internal examination of foods (Dull 1986). Some grading is carried out manually by trained personnel who are able to assess a number of grading factors simultaneously. Automated grading has the advantages of speed, reliability, and low labor cost. The consumer recognizes, in descending order of preference, fancy, choice, standard, and seconds for most fruits and vegetables. A fancy product is normally one that can be secured only from the most nearly perfectly grown crop in a given season.

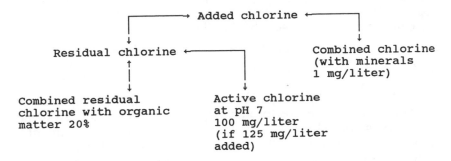

Figure 2-10   Chlorination of wash water for MPR fruits and vegetables. (Anon. 1988d.)

Cleaning, Washing, and Disinfection

Cleaning and washing may be the only preservation treatments in most of the MPR fruits and vegetables. Cleaning refers to the removal of foreign materials. As a unit operation, cleaning is a form of separation concerned with the removal of twigs, stalks, dirt, sand, soil, insects, pesticides, and fertilizer residues from fruits and vegetables, as well as containers and equipment, as the first step in processing. The cleaning process also involves separation of light from heavy materials by gravity, destoning, flotation, picking, screening, dewatering, and others.

In an MPR fruit and vegetable process line, washing is generally done in an isolated chamber with a restricted number of entrances; human contact to product is limited which is in sharp contrast with the previous operations. At this stage the product becomes ready-to-eat and ready for preservation. To this end, the product is washed and freed of the majority of microorganisms by chlorine treatment up to 200 ppm allowed in the United States. The MPR product is immersed in a bath in which bubbling is maintained by a jet of air. This turbulence permits one to eliminate practically all traces of earth and foreign matter without bruising the product. The addition of various forms of chlorine to wash waters helps to prevent microbial contamination. Chlorine is the only technological washing aid permitted (Anon. 1988d); it is eliminated from the product by a final step (Figure 2-10).

Water is one of the key elements in the quality of the MPR products. The source and quality of water must be considered. Three parameters are controlled in washing MPR fruits and vegetables (Anon. 1986):

1. Quantity of water used: 5–10 L/kg of product
2. Temperature of water: 4° C to cool the product
3. Concentration of active chlorine: 100 mg/L

Two forms of chlorine may be used in water treatment. Gaseous chlorine is a 100% active form. It is easy to control and automate but requires special equipment; therefore, additional investment is necessary (National Food Processors Assoc. 1968). Chlorine is only slightly soluble in water. Calcium and sodium hypochlorites are widely used for chlorination of wash waters in MPR fruits and vegetables. The sodium hypochlorites are sold as liquids, whereas the calcium hypochlorites are sold in powder form. Hypochlorites are easily used without special equipment, but the dosage regulation is approximate. The germicidal activity of hypochlorites declines with concentration, especially if the water is alkaline (pH >8.5). It is therefore necessary to regulate the pH level of the water. When added to water, chlorine gas and the hypochlorites readily produce hypochlorous acid which is considered to be the germicidal agent. Germicidal activity is directly proportional to the concentration of unionized HOCl in the solution (Jay 1992).

After washing, centrifugal drying depends on the speed and time of rotation of the centrifuge (Figure 2-11). A few minutes of centrifugal drying is sufficient for most products. Theoretically, antioxidants can be used after washing, but few chemicals are permitted to be used with MPR foods in European Community countries (Anon. 1988d). Ascorbic acid and its salts, and citric acid and its salts at a maximum of 300 ppm (mg/L or mg/kg) are permitted.

Use of sulfites and sulfurous anhydrides are awaiting approval in the EEC (Anon. 1986) and have been granted provisional status limited to potatoes and vegetables destined to be cooked, with a residual dosage of 50 ppm. (See the discussion of sulfite bans on fresh vegetables in Chapter 3.) All processing operations of MPR fruits and vegetables, that is, cutting, washing, and centrifugal drying, can be done in 20 min. The cleaning properties of water can be improved by the use of physical and mechanical aids. MPR fruits and vegetables can be washed by soaking in still or moving water or brines, using water sprays, rotary drums, rotating brushes, or shaker washers. In the design of suitable washing equipment, one should keep in mind the nature of horticultural products, the need for maximum dirt removal with minimum water, avoidance of injury to the product, and rate of output. Some products such as mature onions,

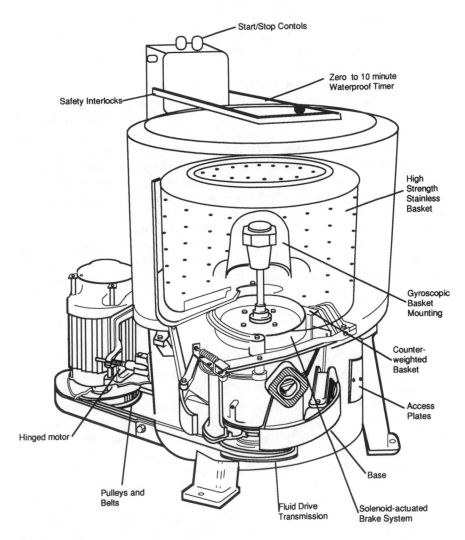

Figure 2-11   A basket loading type stainless steel food processing centrifuge for spin drying of MPR foods. (Source: Bock Centrifugal Systems, Toledo, Ohio.)

mushrooms, potatoes, and sweet potatoes are never washed or are washed after storage since added moisture is undesirable. Dry cleaning methods such as screening, brushing, aspiration, abrasion, and magnetic separation can be applied. The automatic aeroseparator for spinach and leafy vegetables removes foreign matter such as worms, insects, stones, wood pieces, etc. (Femia Industries, S. A., France, Anon. 1990b).

The washing operation has been studied for specific products (Gould 1974), and such steps as the soak period, spray pressure, and use and concentration of detergents added to the soak tank have been optimized. Rotary drum washers are used for cleaning apples, pears, peaches, potatoes, turnips, beets; high-pressure water is sprayed over the product and it never comes in contact with dirty water. In wire-cylinder leafy vegetable washers, medium pressure sprays of fresh water are used for washing spinach, lettuce, parsley, and leeks.

Because free moisture and cellular exudates on the surface of horticultural products tend to stimulate the growth of yeasts, molds, and bacteria, many types of driers (dewaterers, centrifuges, screens, dehumidifiers) have been used to remove water after washing.

Peeling

The removal of the outer layer of a fruit or vegetable is referred to as peeling, paring, skinning, husking, shelling, etc. Peeling may be done (1) by hand, (2) with steam or boiling water, (3) with lye or alkalies (NaOH, KOH), (4) by dry caustic peeling with infrared heat, (5) by flame, (6) by mechanical means, (7) by high pressure steam, (8) by freezing, and (9) with acids (Lopez 1987). Industrial peeling of large volumes of products can be accomplished mechanically, chemically, or in high-pressure steam peelers. Root vegetables such as potatoes, beets, carrots, turnips, and onions may be peeled mechanically or lye peeled. Lye peeling of peaches, pears, apricots, and tomatoes causes less loss of fruit and permits rapid handling but requires a large water supply, NaOH, and a source of heat. Hand peeling is slow, costly, and wasteful of the product. Husking of corn, shelling of peas, and snipping of beans may be done by high-speed machines. Silking is an operation applied exclusively to corn. An apple preparation system has been developed by FMC (Anon. 1988a) that automatically peels, cores, and slices apples in a high-speed continuous operation (Figure 2-12).

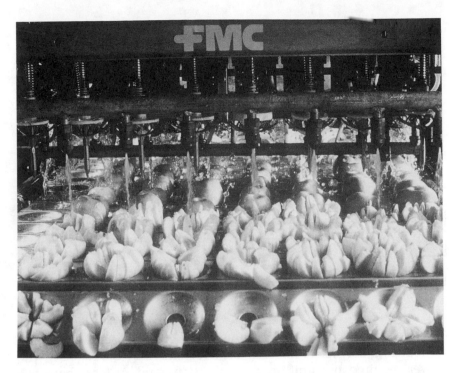

Figure 2-12   Automatic apple washing, peeling, coring, and slicing machine. (Source: FMC, Anon., 1988a.)

Size Reduction Operation

Size reduction describes all means by which fruits and vegetables are cut or broken into smaller and uniform pieces of definite shape and size (Figure 2-13). Size reduction may be an essential step to improve taste, digestibility, ease of handling, and effective heat transfer, but it has accompanying disadvantages.

Cutting

Cutting accelerates respiration, causes mechanical damage, and softens plant tissue. Cut tissues have lower barriers to gas diffusion and they tolerate higher concentrations of CO_2 and lower O_2 levels than intact commodities. Therefore, the products must be taken to a 4° C room immediately after cutting. Four types of force are generally recognized in cutting machines. They are (1) compression, (2)

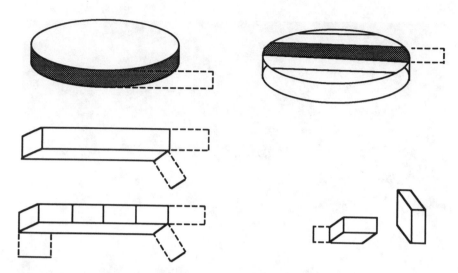

Figure 2-13   Cutting, giving a definite size and shape to the product.

impact, (3) attrition, and (4) cutting. The performance of a machine
for reducing the size of material is characterized by the capacity, the
power required per unit of material, shape and surface characteristics of the product, and the optimum size (Perry, Green, and Maloney 1989).

MPR fruits and vegetables are moved on a belt or centrifugally to
vertical or horizontal cutting blades (Figure 2-14). Size reduction
equipment is divided into grinders for grinding, pulping, mashing,
and juicing. Cutting machines are divided for chopping, slicing, dicing, and shredding of horticultural products. Grinders break large
pieces, then the products pass through a 200-mesh screen that cuts
them into particles 1–50 µm in size. The smallest size attainable by
wet grinding with suitable surfactants is 0.5 µm, but in dry grinding
it is 1 µm (Perry, Green, and Maloney 1989).

Fresh horticultural products are automatically sliced, diced, and
strip cut with high-speed centrifugal machines. A slicing knife, circular knife, spindle, and crosscut knife spindle are used for dicing.
Changing the size of the cubes is done by using the required cutting
spindles and adjusting the slice thickness. Strip cuts of any product
can be made by removing the crosscut knife from the machine. The
length of the strips will depend on the size of the original product
(Figure 2-14, Anon. 1988b).

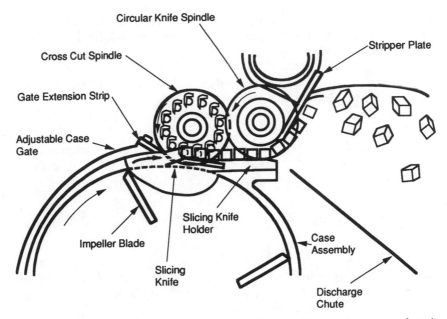

Figure 2-14 Automatic high-speed centrifugal slicing, dicing, and strip cutting machine. (Urschel Laboratories, Inc.; Anon. 1988b.)

The use of power is a major expense in size reduction operations. Cutters give products of definite size and shape (fixed dimensions). The most satisfactory cutting device is a knife of extreme sharpness and as thin as structurally possible. In general, impact and shearing forces applied via a cutting edge are used in the disintegration of fibrous materials. Cutting machines are constructed of 18-8 stainless steel that contacts the product. The slicing knives are made of high-carbon stainless-steel alloys. Most knives are ground to one of three shapes: fully tapered, partially tapered, or hollow-ground. The knives of a cutter must be kept sharp and usually must be sharpened after each 8-h operation. The effects of cutting angle, cutting speed, and core diameter on energy requirement have been studied. It was concluded that the energy and the peak force are not affected by the cutting speed (Kulshreshtha, Pathak, and Sarkar 1988). The energy requirement is minimum for a cutting angle of about 21°. The cutting angle corresponding to the minimum peak force is dependent on the diameter. Cutting and grinding equipment must be thoroughly washed after each operation. It is possible to produce aseptically diced or sliced products by using sterile knives and aseptic conditions. Thorough washing with water alone to remove the free cellular contents that are released by cutting was found to be important in prolonging the shelf-life of cut carrots (Bolin and Huxsoll 1991).

Water knives are a new innovation where the fruits and vegetables are cut by a fine jet of high-pressure water (3,000 kPa). Heiland, Konstance, and Craig (1990) investigated the use of water knives as a high-capacity, high-speed, accurate, and automatically controlled cutting equipment for fruits and vegetables. Cell exudates were washed away by the very stream that produced them. The cost study showed that, at the high capacity, water knives may be economical.

Mixing and Assembling

Combined foods such as salads and ready-to-eat meals all require mixing and assembling before packaging. The object of mixing in fruit and vegetable processing is to ensure that a homogeneous mixture is formed and maintained with as low an energy input as possible at the lowest overall cost. Blending, coating, and dipping operations all require solid–solid mixing. Salad dressings are emulsions that are a mixture of liquids. Stable emulsions are formed by homogenizing. The three basic mechanisms by which solid particles are mixed are diffusive mixing, convective mixing, and shearing. There are several types of solid mixing machines. Tumblers are suitable for gentle blending of solids. Ribbon mixers are effective blenders for thin pastes and for solids that do not flow readily. The power they require is moderate. Agitators are used for slow-speed mixing with a number of paddles and baffles. The mixing efficiency of an industrial mixer is judged by the time required (mixing time) and power load (power consumption) and the properties of the product. If two or more gases are brought together, complete blending is achieved instantly. In gas–solid mixtures, the diffusion of gas molecules and the convective currents will cause slow but certain mixing. The simplest approach to mixing gases with liquid foods is to introduce the gas with a sparger at the bottom of the tank containing the liquid food and to permit it to bubble up through the liquid. Whippers and beaters are used for the mixing of gases with low-viscosity liquids. The colloid mill is a special mixing device for mixing extremely fine suspensions of either solids or liquids in a liquid. Mayonnaise, salad dressing, seasoning blends, fruit cocktail, and fruit and vegetable sauces all require mixing and emulsification.

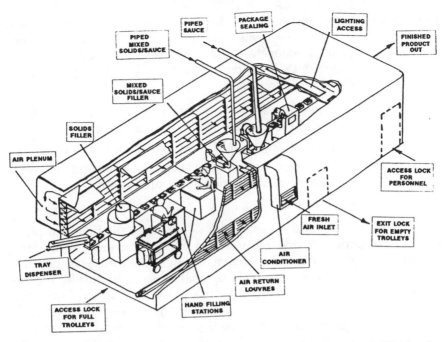

Figure 2-15   An aseptic assembly and packaging room for MPR foods. (Source: Arthey and Dennis 1991.)

The final operation in the processing of MPR foods takes place in the assembly and packaging room. Shredded lettuce, sliced carrots, peeled oranges, or mixtures of fresh vegetable or fruit ingredients are combined to produce a palatable mixture with dressing, mayonnaise, and other ingredients. Cook–chill meals and pizza mixes are prepared, portioned, plated, and filled in consumer packaging containers. The assembly room is the most critical zone in the processing chain and aseptic techniques are employed. A schematic diagram of an assembly and packaging room is given in Figure 2-15. Operators working in the assembly room wear special dress, mouth masks, hair caps, and gloves. Inside the assembly room, a positive air pressure is maintained with filtered air; ambient temperature is controlled at 10–12° C and humidity is 60–70% RH.

Distribution and Utilization of MPR Fruits and Vegetables

Distribution, in general, may be defined as the fast and efficient movement and handling of fruits and vegetables from the farm gate to the point of consumption. This involves collecting 30 million tons of produce from 196,035 farms and distributing into 234,575 food stores and 727,000 foodservice establishments in the United States (Figure 2-16; How 1991). Distribution and utilization of MPR foods include the following operations:

1. Production center operations: raw and processed fruit and vegetable storage and control, central processing operations
2. Physical distribution: intra- and intercity transportation
3. Consumption center operations: food distribution centers, wholesaling, retailing, and foodservice operations
4. Communication network

   MPR food distribution systems seek to maximize the time and place utility or economic value of products by getting and having the products where they are wanted, at the time they are wanted, at a reasonable cost. The exact marketing channels differ with each commodity and change in pattern over the years. Quality and quantity of MPR food losses occur in the field, at the processing plants, in shipment to warehouses, and in the retail stores. Pilferage and tampering losses occur primarily in retail outlets and, to some extent, in truck and rail shipments. It has been reported (Kays 1991) that 3.62% of durable products such as dried fruits, nuts, and potatoes; 5.42% of fruits; and 10.3% of fresh vegetables are lost during transportation. Total distribution systems should reduce food losses and standardize the product in wholesale, retail, and consumer packaging. This would also increase the speed of distribution.

   The selection and establishment of a distribution system is a key decision area as it usually binds the firm long term, involves heavy investment, and can be the deciding factor in determining the success or failure of a marketing strategy. If a product is to sell, it must be made readily available to target segments such as fast-food chains, supermarkets, restaurants, hotels, institutional cafeterias, and caterers. The extensiveness of the distribution system is the foundation of marketing in the industrialized countries. The system must be able to adjust the supply of commodities to market demands quickly and easily as either supply or demand changes. During the 3- to 10-day distribution time, the product is often handled four to six times in loading, warehousing, and unloading at the retail outlet (Anon. 1978).

   Quality maintenance is aided by the following procedures in distribution channels:

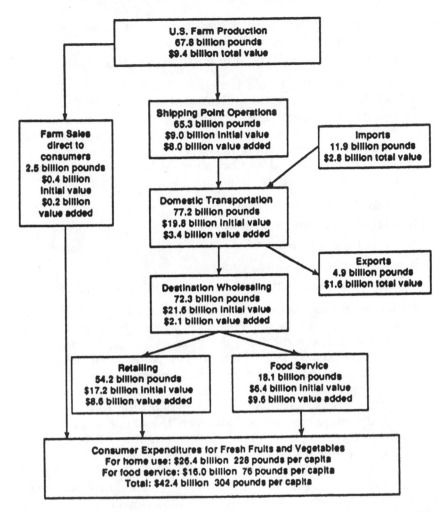

Figure 2-16   United States fresh fruit and vegetable marketing system. (How 1991.)

1.   Minimize handling frequency.

2.   Provide continued control of temperature, % RH, modified atmosphere (MA)/controlled atmosphere (CA) conditions (total environmental control) during storage and transportation.

3.   Always transfer product from truck to refrigerated storage immediately.

4. Always rotate product on a first-in/first-out basis; rotate the complete inventory on a weekly basis.

5. Never stack individual cases more than five cases high.

Proper control of storage and transportation will extend the shelf-life of MPR fruits and vegetables. Extended shelf-life MPR foods can reduce number and magnitude of returned products, extend the distribution range of products, and will reduce the frequency of deliveries to retail from two or three per week to one per week.

Currently, the MPR food section offers at least 300–400 items in retail display cabinets. These items include:

Ready-to-eat fruits and vegetables

Ready-to-cook fruits and vegetables

Ready-to-cook mixed meals

Fresh ready-to-use herbs and sprouts

Fresh ready-to-eat specialty fruits and vegetables (tropical plants)

An alternative processing and distribution system for MPR foods is given in Figure 2-17. A single item or a few items may be more efficiently handled, but the more the produce items the more complex are the problems of distribution. The MPR foods are of low unit value and purchased frequently as convenience foods, which are usually eaten within 2 days of purchase. An intensive distribution system seeks maximum market penetration to increase, attract, or retain more customers. However, the adoption of this system reduces the incentive for a retailer. On the other hand, an exclusive or selective distribution system may be used for some high-priced items to push the product to retail outlets. High-image products, for example, some tropical fruits, vegetables, or fresh herbs, may not be distributed to every retailer who is willing to buy but only to up-scale retailers and restaurants. There may be a conflict of interest between fresh produce distribution channels and MPR foods distribution channels in local, regional, national, or even international markets.

A. Production Center Operations

Functions performed at production centers can be divided into two categories: first, physical operations which include harvesting, cooling, sizing, ripening, cutting, preservation, packaging, storing, and shipping; and second, related service operations which include buy-

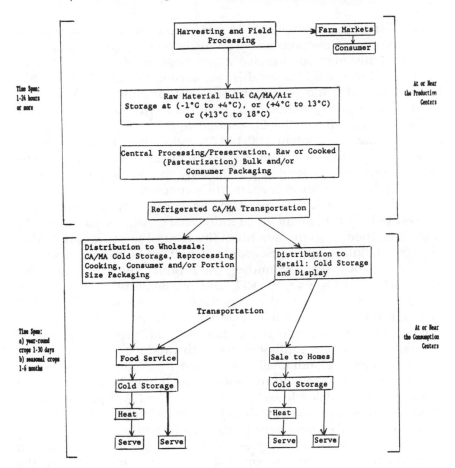

Figure 2-17   An alternative processing and distribution system for MPR fruits and vegetables.

ing, selling, financing, market finding, inspecting, and regulating. Production center operations will vary from product to product and from place to place. In the processing of MPR foods, two important functions may be distinguished: (1) raw material or processed products CA/MA/air/vacuum packaged storage operations (storage and control); and (2) central processing and preservation operations.

Storage and Control Operations

Fresh fruits and vegetables are stored in bulk or in prepackaged forms in conventional refrigerated storage. In addition to refrigeration at certain relative humidity, CA/MA/air/vacuum and low pressure or hypobaric storage methods are used for improving quality and shelf-life. The latter methods involve a combination of lowering the O_2 level from the usual 21% level in air, raising the CO_2 level to 20% in a gas mixture, and controlling the level of ethylene (Wills et al. 1989). Newer storage methods include the low-oxygen (LO) storage method which reduces the O_2 content to 2.0–1.5% by volume and maintains the CO_2 content at 0.1–0.2% below the O_2 value. The ul-tra-low-oxygen (ULO) storage method reduces O_2 content to the bi-ological compatibility level of 1.2–0.8% by volume. The CO_2 content should be held at a lower level than O_2 concentration (Anon. 1989). All of these methods are practiced in completely air-tight ware-houses, in bulk containers, or in individual consumer packages. All storage methods also involve humidity control to prevent dehydra-tion and maintain turgor. Stacking of unit loads must provide for free passage of gases surrounding the product during storage. Op-timum levels of O_2, CO_2, % RH, and temperature must be estab-lished for each precut fruit or vegetable variety. Because CA/MA storage leaves no undesirable residues on the products, its use for minimally processed products will increase. Much research is needed to establish optimum conditions for each product.

The marketing of minimally processed fruits and vegetables re-quires storages for the long and short term and for bulk or packaged products at the wholesale and retail levels. The CA/MA storage can affect all forms of postharvest deterioration of fresh produce directly or indirectly and, consequently, its quality and postharvest shelf-life. The composition of the gases in a closed space may be altered by increasing the concentration of some gases while reducing the concentration of others. This can be accomplished by scrubbing the atmosphere of CO_2 or O_2 by controlled venting and, if only O_2 is lowered, by continuous evacuation of the storage space. Individual gases can be added from pressurized cylinders or insulated tanks or by catalytic burners that consume O_2 and produce CO_2. Mem-brane air separation systems may be employed for lowering the O_2 level or increasing CO_2 level in CA storage. Air filtration is used in storage rooms to prevent microbial contamination.

The CA/MA storage rooms must be constructed similarly to con-ventional refrigerated storages with adequate insulation and vapor barriers and enough cooling surface to ensure high humidities and air circulation. The most reliable method of making a room gas-tight is to line the walls and ceiling with 28-gauge galvanized steel and connect it into the floor. The metal sheets must be fastened tightly to the walls and ceiling and the joints between sheets must be well sealed. A method of testing for gas tightness is to build up a pressure in the room 1 inch of water (gauge) and to observe the rate of pressure drop. If at the end of 1 h 0.10–0.2 inch of water (gauge) remains, the room is tight enough (Anon. 1990b).

In cold-storage rooms with ceiling evaporators, the following clearances should be respected: (1) between rows of pallets in the direction of air flow, 5–10 cm (2–4 inches); (2) wall to evaporator, 40 cm (15.7 inches); (3) under evaporator, 30 cm (11.8 inches); and (4) side walls, 40 cm (15.7 inches). Commodities should never be stacked higher than the lower edge of the evaporator.

Control systems are used to regulate mass, volume, temperature, pressure, time, %RH, $\%O_2$, $\%CO_2$, $\%C_2H_2$ concentrations and other controllable variables to minimize total cost and maintain product quality. The refrigeration system should be designed such that the thermostats work with very small switching differences if possible. Because new storage methods require drastic reduction in the O_2 level, as in the ULO process, while at the same time maintaining CO_2 at certain levels, highly accurate measuring and control systems are needed to ensure efficient control and to prevent damage to the stored products.

Microprocessor-controlled systems have been designed for the refrigeration CA/MA system to monitor the entire cooling installation and regulate cooling, ventilation, defrosting, and compressor utilization, balancing all of these different factors for maximum efficiency, which results in significant energy savings. The levels of C_2H_4, CO_2, and O_2 are measured by special analyzers and displayed digitally. At the same time, the stored data are compared with target set points for CO_2, C_2H_4, and O_2 levels for the relevant storeroom. Any differences between set points and actual levels are recorded and the system sends instructions to the CO_2 adsorption, O_2 reduction, or ethylene removing units to make the necessary corrections. So far, no suitable sensors have been designed for measuring the relative humidity. The data recorded by the microcontrollers are continuously displayed on the terminal monitor. Besides temperature, all analytical data pertaining to the CA/MA refrigeration system, total defrosting time, temperature readings, set point values, adsorbers running times, and O_2 supply times are printed out automatically on the printer. The electronic analyzer should be checked once a week with portable electronic devices as a manual emergency control for a fully automatic system.

The quality of minimally processed food products is dependent on their temperature history, from production through distribution and storage to consumption. Therefore, time–temperature indicator labels are an integral part of the storage and packaging; they monitor changes in food quality arising from poor temperature maintenance during storage and distribution of MPR foods (Labuza and Breene 1989).

Central Processing Operations

The processing and preservation center at the raw material production areas will expand or replace conventional packing house operation in the MPR food system. Certain economic scale of operation is required for the establishment of a central processing plant for single or multiple commodities. A minimum efficient scale plant is the smallest sized plant at which minimum unit cost is achieved (Marion 1986). At the processing center, MPR foods will go through the processing stages of handling, cleaning, and washing and many of the following operations.

Grading and inspection: size, shape, quality grading can be done mechanically or by hand. Pesticide residue and other contaminants are tested.

Cutting, preparation, and mixing

Preservation operations: chemical preservatives, mild heat treatments, pasteurization, pH modification, water activity reduction, ionizing radiation or other minimal treatments.

CA/MA/vacuum packaging

Storage: a few commodities, such as winter apples and potatoes, can be stored for long periods. However, most items must be shipped and sold as soon as possible.

Loading and shipping

Physical Distribution

Physical distribution refers to the portion of the total distribution system concerned with long- or short-distance transportation of MPR products from the producer to the consumer under the cold chain including local delivery. Knowledge of the available transportation systems and the ability to select the most appropriate mode of transportation for each product and destination is essential to minimize cost while optimizing quality and shelf-life. Over 80% of produce is shipped by truck; the remainder travels mostly by rail, water, or air (Imming 1985). Sanitation is a major factor in food transportation. Inadequate cleaning of trucks or rail cars may lead to food spoilage and waste. Freight cars designed specifically for MPR foods need to be used. These are called "reefer containers." The temperature range is adjustable, between $-25°$ C to $+25°$ C ($-15°$ F to $+75°$ F $\pm 1°$ F). This degree of temperature control may be done by the use of platinum sensors and integrated circuits. The microbial risks in CA/MA/ vacuum packaged products are much greater in the absence of proper sanitation and temperature control (Jay 1992).

New multicomponent trailers and containers offer the possibility of combined, cold ($-1°$ C to $+4°$ C), chilled ($+4°$ C to $+13°$ C), and ambient ($+13°$ C to $+18°$ C) transportation. Radio-linked computers installed in all trucks give operators a direct link to the stock control computer telling them which pallets are required for each dispatch (Goad 1989).

When the transport vehicle travels over land, sea, or air at a constant speed, some degree of vibration and sudden compression impact (shock) is always present. Transportation shocks and vibrations are transmitted from the vehicle through the packaging to the product inside, causing injury during long journeys from production areas to markets. Therefore, optimum package design is essential for maximum protection of MPR products in transportation.

Consumption Center Operations

Fresh, minimally processed products arrive at terminal market facilities which include food distribution centers, wholesalers, retailers, and foodservices.

Food Distribution Center Operations

National or international food distribution centers are important for MPR foods to extend the season and to facilitate the distribution. The typical distribution center operations include receiving, storing, order picking, wholesale packaging, and final shipment. The intermodal terminal food distribution centers are large facilities designed to receive unit trains of produce or MPR food containers, truck lots, and shipment by nearby air or water ports. The operation would

require short-time storage and standardized or containerized shipment allowing for easy and efficient intermodal transfer for local
distribution.

Wholesaling

The wholesaling function consists of procurement, ripening of some
products, warehousing, repacking, and reselling smaller amounts to
many different types of customers. Local warehouses stock items
close to the consumers to provide immediate availability. Automat-
ing warehouse operations allows for faster handling of larger volumes of product with less labor. Repacking or some reprocessing
of MPR products in consumer units is done at all marketing levels
including warehouses.

Retailing and Foodservice

Retail stores and foodservice establishments are the final link in the
distribution of MPR foods. A small portion (3–5%) of fresh produce
are directly marketed by farmers to consumers. The principal ways
are through farmers' markets, pick-your-own operations on the farm,
and roadside markets. Retailing is a very specialized operation involving all business activities that are concerned with selling the
MPR products to final consumers for at-home use. In general, MPR
products are priced 10% above conventional produce at the retail
level, but products are 100% useable and there is no waste (Swientek 1991). A retail storewide computer system that uses data derived
from an automated checkout system and controls physical facilities
for heating, lighting, and refrigeration and interfaces electronically
with suppliers will increase efficiency and speed of operation. Standardization of retail packages, cases, and pallets has been advocated
(Kadoya 1990) as a means for improving efficiency in handling products moving through the marketing system by reducing the number
of different sizes and shapes, improving modularity, and making
palletizing more efficient. There is a need for a better design of the
location and layout of the MPR foods section within the retail outlets. Figure 2-18 gives an alternative layout for an MPR food section
in a supermarket.

   Foodservice operations can be divided into commercial or noncommercial eating places. Commercial operations consist of cafeterias, catering, fast-food outlets, restaurants, and other eating places.
Noncommercial foodservices include schools, hospitals, military es-

BACK ROOM PREPARATION AND STORAGE AREA		
Sliding	Mirror	Windows
Cold Section* (-1°C to +3°C)	Chilled Section (+4°C to +12°C)	Dry-Cool Section (+13°C to +18°C)
Fresh fruit/ vegetable juices Precut fruits and vegetables Ready-to-cook meals Green salads	Cut pepper, tomato or cucumbers Fresh herbs	Bananas Tropical fruits Sweet potatoes

*Ice-slush or mechanically cooled cabinet.

Potatoes Onions Cut pumpkin	Oranges Lemons Limes	Apples Pears Melons

Seasonal ambient temperature display area

Figure 2-18   An alternative MPR foods display section layout within the store.

tablishments, and other facilities. Sales of food to eat away from home are increasing (How 1991). The increase in the foodservice market has been attributed to rising income, increase in two-income families, and demographic factors. Fast-food chains are good examples of mass production and service of certain MPR products, especially salad bar technology (Figure 2-19). For example, McDonalds requires that its lettuce suppliers harvest a week earlier than

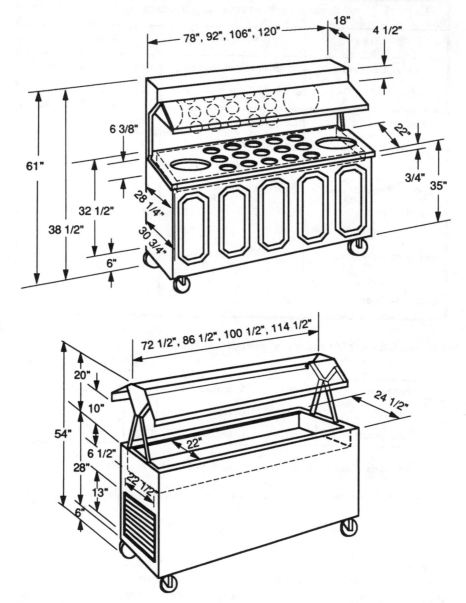

Figure 2-19 Two types of mobile mechanically cooled salad serving equipment: (a) mirrored back salad bar; (b) two-sided salad bar. (Source: Duke Manufacturing Co.; Anon. 1988c.)

normal to prevent the core from becoming too crunchy. A company grows lettuce year-round exclusively for McDonalds. About 175 acres of lettuce is cut each week, leaving about 25% in the field that failed to meet the quality standards. Following harvest the lettuce is promptly cooled and then shipped to McDonalds' 10 central salad processing plants strategically located around the country. Lettuce and other salad vegetables are processed. Processing involves chopping, washing, drying, and packaging in 3 1/2-1b. bags, each holding the equivalent of four heads. The product is then shipped to 1500 stores, some as far as 300 miles from the processing plant. To meet the quality standards the lettuce must be used within 10 days. The lettuce is harvested and delivered to the processor within 5 days. Processing takes about 1 day, so the store must sell the product within 4 days.

Delivery of complete meals to the home is a possible extension of changing lifestyles and MPR technology. The sous-vide concept has been tried with several variations for feeding elderly or handicapped individuals and children in special programs (Schafheifle 1990).

Sous-vide processing involves vacuum packaging of prepared raw or par-cooked meals or meal components, pasteurizing them under controlled time–temperature conditions (closed-pack pasteurization), chilling, then storage under 3° C until reheating and serving.

Communication Network

Communications provide the exchange of information among the distribution channel members. Information as accurate and up to date as possible on supply, demand, and price is essential for anyone directly or indirectly involved in the production, processing, and consumption of MPR foods. The ability to identify what information is important and how to use it will be the key for success of managers.

The National Agricultural Statistics Service (NASS) gathers and disseminates official information on the production, storage stocks, and seasonal average price of major commodities. Government grades and international standards provide impartial general information about the individual product.

MPR food prices fluctuate widely from day to day and between places due to many factors. However, knowledge of differences in price elasticities of demand for a commodity in different markets may be used to raise total returns in those markets.

Information between firms needs to be exchanged for compatibility, transport type, scheduling, unit load requirements, warehousing, product availability, package size and type, delivery dates, and order quantity. Inventories exist as a necessary device to coordinate supply and demand. It is information that adjusts the relationship between orders, inventory, and production output (O'Shaughnessy 1988).

Advertising and promotion provides consumers with information and an incentive to purchase the advertised product. There are three major types of advertising programs directed specifically at buyers of MPR products. First, generic advertising is directed at expanding the market for a commodity or group of commodities grown in a specific area or country-wide, such as Washington State hazelnuts and the national potato program. Second, brand advertising seeks to increase sales and prices for a commodity or commodities sold by a specific company, such as Sunkist oranges. Third, private label advertising is used to expand sales of product under the label or brand of a chain retailer or foodservice wholesaler. Use of a private label does not bind retailers to purchase branded products from any particular seller, and so they can shop around for the best buy. The private label package does not have to support as heavy an advertising budget as branded products and so can be sold at a lower price.

The MPR fruit and vegetable processing company deals with a host of environmental elements that influence physical distribution planning and operations. Technological changes can have a great effect on distribution systems. Changes can be received through an appropriate information channel. The gross national product, population, inflation, economic growth, changing lifestyles, competition, changes in labor rates, and political changes all affect distribution in a variety of ways.

References

Anon. 1978. U.S. Congress, Office of Technology Assessment. Emerging food marketing technologies: a preliminary analysis. Washington, DC: U.S. Government Printing Office.

Anon. 1988a. FMC Food Machinery Cat. No. 209-661-3200. Madera, CA.

Anon. 1988b. Guide to size reduction equipment. Urschel Laboratories, Inc., Valparaiso, IN.

Anon. 1988c. Duke Manufacturing Co. Catalog Nos. 886 and 887. St. Louis, MO.

Anon. 1988d. *Infos.* Centre technique interprofessional des fruits et legumes. Hors Serie, 4e gamme. Paris, France.

Anon. 1989. Technology. *International Fruit World I*, pp. 194–207. Aeschengraben 16, Basel, Switzerland: Agropress.

Anon. 1990a. Technology. *International Fruit World I*, pp. 1–199. Aeschengraben 16, Basel, Switzerland. Agropress.

Anon. 1990b. FEMIA. The vegetable processing machinery engineers. *Food Trade Rev.* 60(5):257. Kent, England: Homesdale Press.

Arthey, D. and C. Dennis. 1991. *Vegetable Processing.* New York: VCH Publishers.

Bogh-Sorensen, L. 1990. The TTT-PPP concept for chilled foods, in processing and quality of foods. In *Chilled Foods: The Revolution in Freshness*, Vol. 3, pp. 3.42–3.52. London: Elsevier-Applied Science.

Bolin, H.R. and C.C. Huxsoll. 1991. Control of minimally processed carrot (*Daucus carota*) surface discoloration caused by abrasion peeling. *J. Food Sci.* 56:416–418.

Brennan, G.J., J.R. Butters, N.D. Cowell, and A.E. Lilly. 1990. *Food Engineering Operations*, 2nd edit. London: Applied Science.

Brennen, P.S. and R.L. Shewfelt. 1989. Effect of cooling delay at harvest on broccoli quality during postharvest storage. *J. Food Quality* 12:13–22.

Burton, W.G. 1982. *Postharvest Physiology of Food Crops.* London and New York: Longman Publishing.

Crandall, P.C., C.H. Shanks, Jr., and J.E. George, Jr. 1966. Mechanically harvesting red raspberries and removal of insects from the harvested product. *Proc. Am. Soc. Horticult. Sci.* 89:295.

Dull, G.G. 1986. Nondestructive evaluation of quality of stored fruits and vegetables. *Food Technol.* 40(5):106–110.

Eckert, W.J. and J.M. Ogawa. 1988. The chemical control of postharvest diseases: deciduous fruits, berries, vegetables and root/tuber crops. *Ann. Rev. Phytopathol.* 26:433–469.

Farrel, A.W. 1976. *Food Engineering Systems*, Vol. 1. *Operations.* Westport, CT: AVI now Van Nostrand Reinhold.

Goad, P. 1989. *The Chill Chain Food Processing*, pp. 41–45. Kent, England: Techpress Publishing.

Gould, W.A. 1974. *Tomato Production, Processing and Quality Evaluation.* Westport, CT: AVI now Van Nostrand Reinhold.

Hardenburg, R.E., A.E. Watada, and C.Y. Wang. 1986. The Commercial Storage of Fruits, Vegetables and Florist and Nursery Stocks. Ag. Handbook No. 66. Washington, DC: U.S. Dept. of Agriculture.

Hartmann, H.T., A.M. Kofranck, V.E. Rubatzky, and W.J. Flocker. 1988. *Plant Science Growth, Development and Utilization of Cultivated Plants*, 2nd edit. Englewood Cliffs, NJ: Prentice-Hall.

Hartmann, T.H., D.E. Kester, and F.T. Davies. 1990. *Plant Propagation Principles and Practices*, 5th edit. Englewood Cliffs, NJ: Prentice Hall.

Harvey, J.M. 1978. Reduction of losses in fresh market foods and vegetables. *Ann. Rev. Phytopathol.* 16:321–341.

Heiland, W.K., R.P. Konstance, and J.C. Craig, Jr. 1990. Robotic high pressure water jet cutting of chunk slices. *J. Food Proc. Engin.* **12**:131–136.

How, B.R. 1991. *Marketing of Fresh Fruits and Vegetables.* New York: Van Nostrand Reinhold.

Imming, B.J. 1985. *Produce Management and Operations.* Ithaca, NY: Cornell University Press.

Jay, M.J. 1992. *Modern Food Microbiology,* 6th edit. New York: Van Nostrand Reinhold.

Juliot, K.N., R.C. Lindsay, and S.C. Ridley. 1989. Directly acidified carrot slices for ingredients in refrigerated vegetable salads. *J. Food Sci.* **54**:90–93.

Kadoya, T. 1990. *Food Packaging.* New York: Academic Press.

Kays, S.J. 1991. *Postharvest Physiology of Perishable Plant Products.* New York: Van Nostrand Reinhold.

Kulshreshtha, M., A.K. Pathak, and B.C. Sarkar. 1988. Energy and peak force requirement in potato slicing. *Indian J. Food Sci. Technol.* **25**:259–262.

Labuza, T.P. and W.M. Breene. 1989. Application of active packaging for improvement of shelf-life and nutritional quality of fresh and extended shelf-life foods. *J. Food Proc. Preserv.* **13**:1–69.

Lopez, A. 1987. *A Complete Course in Canning,* 12th edit., Vol. III. Baltimore: The Canning Trade.

Marion, B.W. 1986. *The Organization and Performance of the U.S. Food System.* Lexington, MA: Lexington Books.

Meffert, H.F.T. 1990. Chilled foods in the market place in processing and quality of foods. In *Chilled Foods: The Revolution in Freshness,* Vol. 3, P. Zeuthen, J.C. Cheftel, C. Ericksson, T.R. Gormley, P. Linko, and K. Paulus (eds.), p. 3.12. London: Elsevier-Applied Science.

Morris, J.R. 1990. Fruit and vegetable harvest mechanization. *Food Technol.* **44**(2):97–100.

National Food Processors Assoc. 1968. *Laboratory Manual for Food Canners and Processors,* Vol. 1. Westport, CT: AVI now Van Nostrand Reinhold.

Nonnecke, I.L. 1989. *Vegetable Production.* New York: Van Nostrand Reinhold.

O'Shaughnessy, J. 1988. *Competitive Marketing: A Strategic Approach,* 2nd edit. Glenview, IL: Scott, Foresman.

Pantastico, B. 1975. *Postharvest Physiology, Handling and Utilization of Tropical and Subtropical Fruits and Vegetables.* Westport CT: AVI now Van Nostrand Reinhold.

Parkin, K.L., A. Marangoni, R.L. Jackman, R.Y. Yada, and D.W. Stanley. 1989. Chilling injury: a review of possible mechanisms. *J. Food Biochem.* **13**:127–153.

Perry, R.H., W.D. Green, and O.J. Maloney. 1989. *Perry's Chemical Engineers Handbook,* 6th edit. New York: McGraw-Hill.

Robinson, J.F. and C.H. Hills. 1959. Preservation of fruit products by sodium sorbate and mild heat. *Food Technol.* **13**:251–254.

Robinson, J.F., K.M. Browne, and W.G. Burton. 1975. Storage characteristics of some vegetables and soft foods. *Ann. Appl. Biol.* **81**:399–420.

Rolle, R.S. and G.W. Chism III. 1987. Physiological consequences of minimally processed fruits and vegetables. *J. Food Quality* **10**:157–177.

Rosen, C.J. and A.A. Kader. 1989. Postharvest physiology and quality maintenance of sliced pear and strawberry fruits. *J. Food Sci.* **54**:656–659.

Ryall, A.L. and W.J. Lipton. 1979. Handling transportation and storage of fruits and vegetables. In *Vegetables and Melons*, 2nd edit., Vol. 1. Westport, CT: AVI now Van Nostrand Reinhold.

Salunkhe, D.K., H.R. Bolin, and N.R. Reddy. 1991. Storage, processing and nutritional quality of fruits and vegetables. In *Fresh Fruits and Vegetables*, 2nd edit., Vol. I, p. 223. Boca Raton, FL: CRC Press.

Schafheifle, M.J. 1990. The sous-vide system for preparing chilled meals. *Br. Food J.* **92**:23–28.

Shewfelt, R.L. 1987. Quality of minimally processed fruits and vegetables. *J. Food Qual.* **10**:143–156.

Swientek, R.J. 1991. Produce power. *Food Processing* **10**:54–58.

Tennes, B.R., J.H. Levin, and R. Wittenberger. 1969. New developments in mechanical harvesting of apples in Michigan. *Proc. New York State Horticult. Soc.* p. 115–120.

USDA. 1984. Food buying guide for child nutrition programs. Program Aid No. 1331. Washington, DC: Food and Nutrition Service.

Weichmann, J. 1987. *Postharvest Physiology of Vegetables*. New York and Basel. Marcel Dekker.

Wills, R.B.H., W.B. McGlasson, D. Graham, T.H. Lee, and E.G. Hall. 1989. *Postharvest: An Introduction to the Physiology and Handling of Fruit and Vegetables*. New York: Van Nostrand Reinhold.

3

Preservation Methods for Minimally Processed Refrigerated Fruits and Vegetables

Robert C. Wiley

Introduction

The preservation of foods, an important manufacturing step that is used to provide food safety, maintain quality, extend shelf-life, and prevent spoilage, has long been called "food processing." In the context of this book "process" is an operation or treatment, and especially in manufacture, a procedure for forward movement such as cutting, slicing, dicing, washing, etc. (Anon., Webster's 1987). To "preserve" is the act or process of preserving, by canning, pickling, or similarly preparing food for future use (Anon., Webster's 1987). Preservation methods then are the "actual" acts of preserving to reduce spoilage. Nicolas Appert in 1810 was probably the first person to explain preservation methods primarily by heating in his treatise "The Art of Preserving Animal and Vegetable Substances." He originally stated (before the completion of his work) that preserving foods could be reduced to two principal methods, "one in which desiccation is employed and the other in which more or less of a characteristic foreign substance is added to prevent fermentation and putrefaction." In his book the latter treatment refers to the use of sugar, vinegar, or salt. His primary method of preservation was "1st. to enclose in the bottle or jar the substances that one wishes to preserve; 2d, to cork these different vessels with the greatest care because success depends chiefly on the closing; 3d, to submit these substances thus enclosed to the action of boiling water in a water-bath for more or less time according to their nature in the manner that I shall indicate for each kind of food; 4th. to remove the bottles from the water-bath at the time prescribed." This method is obviously heat preservation; current synonyms are canning, thermal processing, or heat processing. The inception of minimally processed refrigerated (MPR) foods that in one way or another may undergo all of the preservation methods referred to in Appert's book, and the many more to follow in this text, are examples of the great sophistication that has developed in the field of food science and technology over the last 200 years.

Some workers in the field tend to equate the word preservation before, during, or after packaging with (1) near end-point destruction of all microorganisms and (2) end-point destruction of all enzyme systems. Others use a broader interpretation of the word preservation to describe a procedure in which some but not all species of microorganisms are reduced in count and specific enzyme systems may be partially or fully inactivated in the package or prior to packaging. In this text, MPR preservation is considered in the latter context and is developed with the purpose of providing maximum food safety, like-fresh quality, and substantial increase in shelf-life.

The question arises whether packaging per se is a preservation method. Packaging acts as a vehicle to protect or provide a suitable atmosphere for MPR fruits and vegetables but does not usually constitute the "actual" act of preserving (see Chapters 4 and 5). The actual preservation method, however, may precede packaging or may occur by treating the food material and packaging simultaneously. Other options include treatment immediately after packaging or continuously during the shelf-life period. In the latter case, it is the modified atmosphere developed during packaging that gives a degree of preservation. Refrigeration also is a good example of this kind of situation. Packaging is inherent in the protection of food to prevent spoilage and this idea seems to have been put forth first by Appert (1810).

MPR fruits and vegetables must be held continuously at refrigeration temperatures and guarded from temperature abuse in distribution and retailing. Refrigeration probably should be considered an active act of preservation which is well known to reduce adverse quality and nutritional changes and greatly extend shelf-life of many food product types including dehydrated, canned, and irradiated foods as well as minimally processed fruits and vegetables. Refrigeration itself is not a requirement, however, for dehydrated, canned, and some other types of food products.

Preservation of MPR fruits and vegetables is especially complex in that treatment is required for damaged or killed plant cells as well as those cells that are intact and not wounded or damaged (Figure 1-3). In other words, some cells are respiring at normal rates, some damaged cells may be respiring at very high rates, and other cells are virtually dead or inactive (Rolle and Chism 1987). The volume-to-surface ratio of a whole minimally processed product that has been subjected to size reduction operations, for example, might be used to give an accurate prediction of the kind of preservation methods that would be most effective to extend shelf-life. Human and plant pathogens as well as endogenous enzyme systems found in fruits and vegetables should be susceptible to the "hurdles" or "barriers" concept (Scott 1989).

Preservation methods to extend shelf-life of MPR fruits and vegetables can utilize many of the classic procedures to preserve foods. These well-known methods which may be used to target MPR foods include heat preservation, utilizing mild heat treatments with quick cooling; chemical preservation, including acidulants, antioxidants, chlorine, antimicrobials, and the like; gas and controlled modified atmosphere preservation; refrigeration preservation, preservation by irradiation; oxidation/reduction potential (O/R) preservation; and in some cases, moisture reduction by lowering water activity (a_w), which in MPR fruits and vegetables would seriously reduce turgidity and crispness of the product. Combinations of the above preservation methods in specific or random order, taking advantage of the synergisms of the various preservation hurdles or barriers, may be used. These barriers have to consider intact or damaged enzyme systems in the living tissues, particularly polyphenoloxidases (PPOs), peroxidases (POs), and the various pectinases, polygalacturonases (PGs) and pectinesterases (PE) and respiratory-related enzymes (Table 3-1).

Freezing preservation should not be used for most MPR foods because freezing tends to cause changes in texture and other like-

Table 3-1
Enzymes Related to Food Quality

Enzyme	Catalyzed Reaction	Quality Defect
Flavor		
Lipolytic acyl hydro-lase (lipase, ester-ase, etc.)	Hydrolysis of lipids	Hydrolytic rancidity (soapy flavor)
Lipoxygenase	Oxidation of polyun-saturated fatty acids	Oxidative rancidity ("green" flavor)
Peroxidase/catalase	?	"Off-flavor" (?)
Protease	Hydrolysis of proteins	Bitterness
Color		
Polyphenol oxidase	Oxidation of phenols	Dark color
Texture consistency		
Amylase	Hydrolysis of starch	Softness/loss in viscosity
Pectin methylester-ase	Hydrolysis of pectin to pectic acid and methanol	Softness/loss in viscosity
Polygalacturonase	Hydrolysis of x-1,4 glycosidic linkages in pectic acid	Softness/loss in viscosity
Nutritional value		
Abscorbic acid oxi-dase	Oxidation of L-ascorbic acid	Loss in vitamin C content
Thiaminase	Hydrolysis of thiamine	Loss in vitamin B_1 content

(From Svensson, 1977.)

fresh characteristics. However, from a safety standpoint it is clear that certain MPR foods (entrees) are being frozen to avoid regulatory problems in the United States. Freezing is a preservation method that manufacturers should not use if they wish to market an authentic MPR food. Precut salads, sliced tomatoes, fresh soup mixes, and the like do not lend themselves well to freezing as an alternate preservation method because of the above-mentioned quality constraints. This is not an attempt to downgrade freezing as a preservation method, but is simply intended to emphasize that MPR fruits and vegetables should be considered a specific food product type. A number of unit operations are performed before freezing on fruits and vegetables destined for freezing preservation that yield high-quality frozen food (Desrosier and Tressler 1977).

Microbiological and Enzyme Considerations to Prevent Spoilage of MPR Fruits and Vegetables

MPR fruits and vegetables with wounded or intact plant tissues, or both, require special manipulation of preservation methods for the purpose of extending storage life and preventing spoilage. These problems can relate to both microbe and enzyme control. In the recent past, conventional wisdom suggested that a refrigeration temperature from $-2.2°$ to $4.4°$ C (Anon. 1989a) would generally control outgrowth of pathogenic and spoilage psychrotrophic types (see Chapter 7). Today, there is considerable evidence that the low temperature or refrigerator temperature treatment or storage of MPR foods is not enough to control some psychrotrophic types. It has been suggested that all refrigerated foods be divided into two categories for labeling purposes and this approach tends to be helpful in attempting to classify MPR fruits and vegetables by preservation method (Anon. 1989). They are as follows (Anon. 1989a):

- "Group A Foods: Highly perishable, packaged [minimally]* processed foods that must be refrigerated for safety reasons." [Most of the vegetable products].
- Group B Foods: Products intended to be refrigerated that do not pose a safety hazard if temperature abused." [Most of the fruit products and properly acidified vegetable products].

"Products that possess all of the following attributes should be considered Group A products that could potentially cause a public health hazard if improperly handled:

1. Product has a pH >4.6; and
2. Water activity >0.85; and
3. Does not receive a thermal process adequate to inactivate food-borne pathogens, which could, through persistence or growth in the product, cause a health hazard under moderate conditions of temperature abuse during storage and distribution; and
4. Has no barrier(s) imparted by either intrinsic factors (e.g., presence of nitrites, salt content, the presence of competitive flora, etc.) or intrinsic factors (e.g., a heat treatment to control pathogens) scientifically demonstrated to eliminate or prevent the growth of foodborne pathogens."

---

* [added by author]

The above suggestions by the Microbiology and Food Safety Committee of the National Food Processing Association (NFPA) (Anon. 1989a) have been drawn up for all refrigerated foods and are helpful in discussing the preservation of MPR fruits and vegetables. Several aspects of these labeling requirements that are not addressed are the twin problems of respiration and enzyme activity which must be considered in successful handling of MPR fruits and vegetable to prevent spoilage and extend shelf-life. This is more fully discussed in the postharvest physiology area (see Chapter 6.)

An interesting approach to inhibit the growth of microorganisms in foods is the development of the "hurdles concept" developed by Leistner and Rodel (1976). Scott (1989) has suggested that it is not productive from a quality standpoint to provide extreme treatment conditions to inhibit the growth of microorganisms in refrigerated foods. She suggests that suitable combinations of growth-limiting factors can be used for preservation, so that no growth can take place, and suggests that this may involve several subinhibitory treatments or preservation methods. Figure 3-1, taken from Scott (1989), diagrammatically presents the "hurdles concept."

In Figure 3-1 it is assumed the products will be properly packaged to prevent the entry of microorganisms and they will be stored at the optimum refrigerated temperature for the specific fruit or vegetable. The examples are only for explanation; however, hurdles will have to be developed for the many individual products and formulas that will be minimally processed and refrigerated. Figure 3-1A shows five hurdles—a_w, pH, E_h, heat treatment, and a preservative—all at the same intensity (size of solid line arc). The preservative finally stops growth of the "weakened" microorganisms. Figure 3-1B shows several hurdles used on a product at different intensities with the microbes again unable to overcome the preservative hurdle. Figure 3-1C shows only two hurdles (a_w and pH) used to preserve a product. Figure 3-1D shows the synergistic effect in combining hurdles to provide greater difficulty for microbial reproduction. Because MPR fruits and vegetables are in large part "living" tissue, treatments to reduce or eliminate enzyme activity should be included in the microbe hurdle concept (Figure 3-2).

In Figure 3-2A, a fruit product has a natural or added acidity to lower the pH to 4.6 or below, which will reduce microbial activity and increase the effectiveness of the added antioxidant. When an antioxidant such as ascorbic acid is added to inhibit PPO, it may not have much effect on the microbial systems present; however, as long

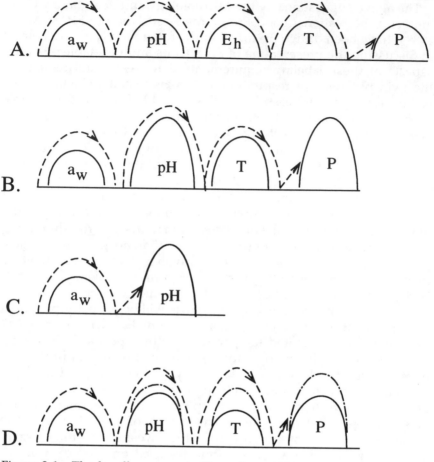

Figure 3-1 The hurdles concept. (From Scott 1989.)

as the ascorbic acid is present in the acid medium little browning
will take place. Finally a light heat treatment is provided to reduce
the level of remaining enzymes and lower the number (count) of
fungi, yeasts, and bacteria present. This product would be packaged
and subject to refrigerated temperatures during storage, distribution, and marketing. This hurdle concept considers two levels of
temperature for microbe and enzyme control, the initial heat treatment for a limited period and then low temperature control at 4.4° C
(Anon. 1990) over an extended but undefined shelf-life period.

In the example shown in Figure 3-2B a vegetable product may
receive a short heat treatment, acidification to provide a more acid

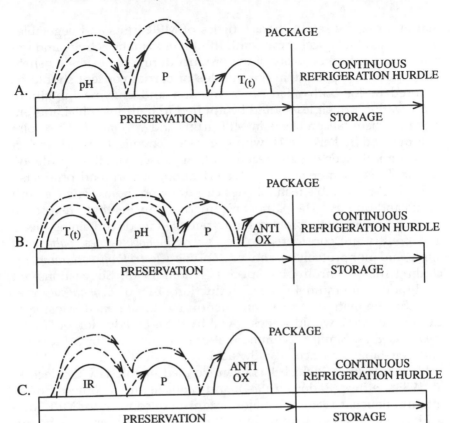

Figure 3-2   Applying the hurdles concept to microbe and enzyme control in MPR fruits and vegetables. Enzymatic browning reaction.

pH, treatment with a preservative to reduce microbial activity, followed by an antioxidant treatment to reduce enzymatic browning, and finally refrigerated storage which would act as the final preservation barrier. If a packaged product is subjected to a modified atmosphere (MA) (Figure 3-2C), a low-dosage radiation of a fruit and vegetable at the prescribed level, treatment with a preservative to reduce microbial activity, and a final treatment to reduce browning a refrigerated storage temperature could complete this preservation sequence. The information in Figure 3-2A–C is illustrative of various preservation treatments. Refrigerated storage temperatures that improve the safety characteristics of MPR fruits and vegetables from a microbiological standpoint, inhibit enzymatic activity and improve or sustain the quality of the product during the extended shelf-life period. It appears that the hurdles or barrier concept should be factored in for both microbe destruction and enzyme inhibition. Preservation principles should be applied to both microbial and enzymatic (chemical) problems in MPR fruits and vegetables. This point is supported by Peri (1991), who suggested chemical hazards in fact are chemical or enzymatic reactions that cause oxidation, proteolysis, lipolysis, isomerization, polymerization, etc. in food products.

Fruit and vegetable technologies can draw on the experience with meats and poultry. The pathogenic microorganisms that present the greatest human safety problems in refrigerated foods containing meats and poultry are considered to be *Listeria monocytogenes, Salmonella* spp., and nonproteolytic and proteolytic *Clostridium botulinum* including the psychrotrophic species (Anon. 1990). Suggestions are made for a minimum 4-decimal reduction (4-D) of *L. monocytogenes* and the elimination of toxin production by *C. botulinum*. Most species of *Salmonella* would be destroyed by the 4-D reduction of *Listeria monocytogenes*. Similar recommendations are needed for MPR fruits and vegetables, particularly low-acid vegetables.

L. monocytogenes, which has been isolated in coleslaw (Schlech et al. 1983), lettuce (Radovich 1984), and cabbage juice (Conner, Brachett, and Beuchat 1986), is a major organism of concern for MPR low-acid vegetables, because many of the hurdles discussed above applied to these foods to control *Listeria* have not been successful (Scott 1989). Unfortunately these have included low-temperature preservation treatments. On the other hand high-temperature studies showed *Listeria* could not be isolated from milk heated to 76.4° to 77.8° C for 15.4 sec (Doyle et al. 1987) whereas Bunning et al. (1986) found a D-value of 1.6 sec at 71.7° C for the freely suspended bacteria in milk. D-values are the time it takes to reduce a microbial population by 90% or the time it takes to make a similar reduction of specific enzyme activity at a defined temperature. The z-values are sometimes called the slope of the thermal resistance curve (Pflug and Esellen 1963). Also read Farber (1989). Heat treatment of this magnitude (to get 70°–75° C center temperatures) for many fruits and vegetables could be deleterious in preserving their like-fresh quality. When considering the possible presence of *L. monocytogenes*, it should be noted that MPR fruits have the best opportunity to provide safe products because of their natural acidities and pH values.

Plant pathogens provide problems for MPR fruits and vegetables, and control of these spoilage organisms must be considered in order to provide high-quality shelf-life. (Chapter 7). Decayed and discolored tissues have to be eliminated from products destined to be minimally processed. The preservation treatments or hurdles applied to fruits and vegetables will be destructive to plant pathogens that have not been removed by peeling, trimming, cutting, etc.

Enzymes are of particular concern in MPR fruit and vegetable preservation. Table 3-1 summarizes the quality defects that may be caused by enzyme activity. The most important enzyme in MPR fruits and vegetables is PPO, which causes browning, usually a very undesirable reaction in terms of appearance. The second in importance from a quality defect standpoint are probably the endogenous and exogenous pectin methylesterases (PEs) and polygalacturonase (PG) which are related to softness, sloughing, and wholeness of fruit and vegetable tissue. The POs, catalases, and lipoxygenases, which are primarily associated with flavor changes, but also can be related to color changes in plant tissue, are also very important. In the freezing preservation of fruits and vegetables, the inhibition of PO, which is one of the most heat-resistent enzymes, is the standard of determining the adequacy of blanch (Desrosier and Tressler 1977).

Heat Preservation

Heat preservation, one of the oldest forms of preservation known to man, has potential to provide hurdles or barriers to reduce microorganisms and inhibit enzyme activity. The major problem in MPR fruits and vegetables is that heat is associated with destruction of flavor, texture, color, and nutritional quality. Heat resistance of *Listeria monocytogenes* appears to be greater after a light heat shock of about 48° C which increased the D-value 2.2-fold at 55° C in nonselective agar (Linton, Pierson, and Bishop 1990). Also, consideration probably should be given to whether heat-stressed spores and vegetative cells could recover better under MPR conditions than the non-heat-stressed organism. Heat may also reduce microorganisms that would be competitive with existing pathogens. This means heat treatments, if used, must be carefully controlled and used sparingly, or not at all, to maintain like-fresh quality.

Modes of Heat Transfer

Steam

Systems that use live steam to treat MPR fruits and vegetables are somewhat difficult to control in terms of the time and exact temperature needed to maintain proper texture and prevent overcooking, yet provide benefits.

Hot water

This commonly used mode of heat treatment has been reported by workers too numerous to mention. Among its many applications, it has been used on fruit and vegetable products as a means to reduce pathogens in fruit and pieces of peeled fresh root vegetables, to reduce endogenous microflora on mushrooms, to reduce microbial levels, and to partially reduce PPO activity (Orr 1990). Losikoff (1990) has used a boiling water blanch of celery to provide thermal inactivation of *L. monocytogenes*.

Hot Air (Gases)

There is little current data available relating to the use of hot gases to reduce microbes and enzymes in MPR fruits and vegetables. Properly used, hot gases might reduce moisture levels in centrifuged products but would have the disadvantage of adding heat to the product.

Ionizing Radiation (Warm); Also See Section on Irradiation

The two types of ionizing radiation (warm) used in the food industry are infrared heating and microwave heating. Practically no information is available regarding the use of this method for preserving MPR fruits and vegetables.

Types of Heat Preservation

One of the best reviews of the use of heat for refrigerated foods comes from the National Advisory Committee on the Microbiological Criteria for Foods (Anon. 1990) for uncured meat or poultry products. They suggest nine heat processes which are divided into three major categories relative to the microbial risks during pre- and postpreservation. These categories could easily be applied to MPR fruits and vegetables.

Category 1. Assembled and Cooked

Products are assembled and packaged. The product is given a final heat treatment to destroy non-spore-forming pathogens and normal spoilage flora. This heat treatment does not kill spore-formers. Category 1 includes sous vide and cook-in-bag products with raw or slightly precooked components assembled and packaged, then cooled.

Category 2. Cooked and Assembled

Ingredients are cooked and then assembled into the final package with no further heat treatment applied after final packaging. The microbial flora can reflect flora originally in the ingredients and those added during packaging and those in the package. All spore-formers could be present.

Category 3. Assembled with Cooked and Raw Ingredients

Components are cooked individually, combined with raw ingredients, then assembled and packaged. Raw vegetables are added prior to final packaging and may introduce pathogens into the product. There may be no further heat treatment prior to distribution.

(Category 4. [Added by author] Assembled with Raw Ingredients

Components such as raw fruits or vegetables are not heat treated but are treated with a preservative and an antioxidant, assembled, and packaged. The products may contain human and plant pathogens, and full or partial enzyme activity. Although this category does not strictly relate to heat preservation it is a category required for MPR fruits and vegetables.)

The following process types (Anon. 1990) are primarily heat preservation methods with packaging and refrigeration included. They are mainly for cooked, uncured meat and poultry products but also have application in the MPR fruit and vegetable field. Actual time and temperature recommendations are not yet available for the many products involved in this compilation. These are not standardized and depend on the food manufacturer or source of the product.

Type 1.   Example: sous vide (Figure 3-3; Table 3-2)

Raw ingredients → Precook (optional) → Formulate → Vacuum package → Pasteurize → Chill* → Distribute

Type 2.   Examples: rolls and roasts

Raw ingredients → Formulate → Vacuum package → Cook → Chill* → Distribute

Type 3.   Examples: roast or fried chicken, other roasts, and uncured sausages.

Raw ingredients → Cook → Chill* → Package → Distribute

Type 4.   Examples: Some uncured luncheon meats and diced meats.

Raw ingredients → Formulate → Cook → Chill* → Slice or dice → Package → Distribute

Type 5.   Examples: Meat and pasta, meat and sauces, dinners, sandwiches, pizza

Raw ingredients → Cook → Chill* → Assemble → Package → Distribute

Type 6.   Examples: Chef salad, chicken salad, and sandwiches or pizza with raw ingredients.

Raw ingredients → Chill* → Formulate → Recook and chill (optional) → Package → Distribute

Type 7.   Examples: Meat pies, quiches, patties, and pates.

Raw ingredients → Formulate → Cook (optional) → Fill into dough → Cook (optional) → Chill* → Package → Distribute

Type 8.   Examples: Uncured jellied meats

Raw ingredients → Cook → Chill* → Add raw ingredients → Final chill → Package → Distribute

Type 9.   Examples: Stews, sauces, and soups

Raw ingredients → Formulate → Cook → Fill while hot → Seal → Hold (optional) → Chill* → Distribute

MPR fruits and vegetables that use mild heat treatments could be projected to fall into some of the heat-treated meats and poultry chilled food examples supplied here. Many of these examples can include like-fresh low-acid vegetables and the less sensitive to microbial problems, like-fresh high-acid fruit products.

* Denotes continuous chilling at the given step with the asterisk and through all subsequent steps to consumption.

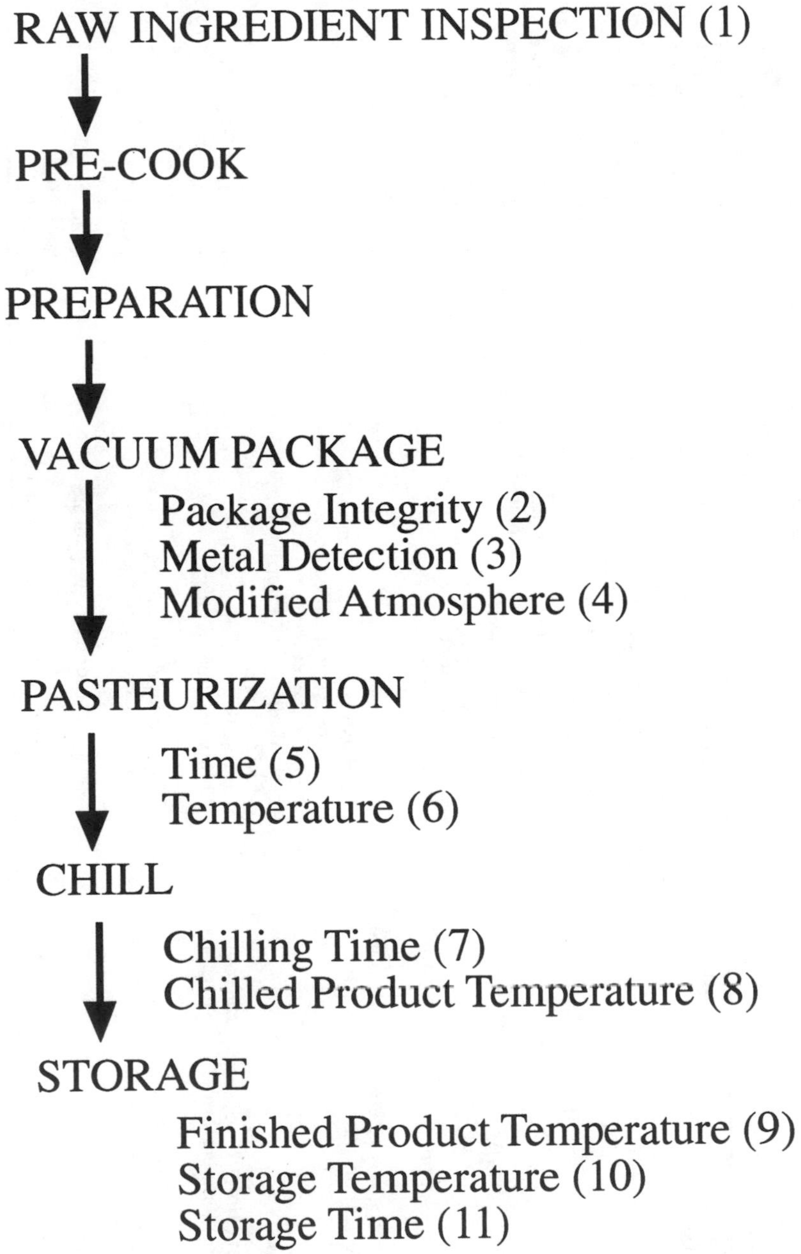

RAW INGREDIENT INSPECTION (1)

↓

PRE-COOK

↓

PREPARATION

↓

VACUUM PACKAGE

Package Integrity (2)
Metal Detection (3)
Modified Atmosphere (4)

↓

PASTEURIZATION

Time (5)
Temperature (6)

↓

CHILL

Chilling Time (7)
Chilled Product Temperature (8)

↓

STORAGE

Finished Product Temperature (9)
Storage Temperature (10)
Storage Time (11)

Figure 3-3   Pasteurized-in-container with sous vide. (From Anon, Chilled Food Association 1990.)

Table 3-2

Critical Control Points for Products Pasteurized in Container with Vacuum (Sous Vide)

No.	Control Point	Potential Hazard	How Monitored	Action to Take for Deviation
1	Raw material inspection	Microbial	Establish specifications.	Notify vendor reject if not within specification.
			Vendor certification and warranty. Inspect shipping vehicle.	
			Measure record temperature of product when received.	Audit quality
			Visual examination of product. Note physical condition of packaging material.	Rework/reject as per PQC/TQC program.
2	Package integrity	Microbial	Seal integrity check	Rework
			Vacuum check	Rework
			Date code check	Rework
3	Metal detection	Metal fragments in product	Metal detector	Reject positive detentions
4	Modified atmosphere	Microbial	Vacuum test	Reject
5, 6	Pasteurization time and temperature	Microbial	Establish correct pasteurization.	Rework or reject
			Measure pasteurization temperatures.	
			Monitor pasteurization times.	
			Periodically check internal temperature at coldest point.	
7	Chilling time	Microbial	Automatic or manual chiller	Rework or reject
8	Chilling temperature	Microbial	Chill water temperature	Hold for QC evaluation
9	Finished product temperature	Microbial	Chlorine level in chilling water	Reject
			Temperature monitoring device	
10	Storage temperature	Microbial	Chart recorder TTIs on packages	Hold for QC evaluation
11	Storage time	Microbial	Date code checks TTIs on packages	Reject

Adapted from Chilled Food Association (Anon. 1990).

For the sake of amplification of the problems in refrigerated (chilled) foods, Type 1 Pasteurized-in-container with vacuum, for example, sous vide, will be presented as an example of heat preservation and critical control points in these types of foods which actually may take place in two distinctive time frames (Figure 3-3; Table 3-2) (Ebert 1990). Precooking can reduce microbes in MPR fruits and vegetables and also provide for inactivation of enzymes. As the second heat treatment, a specific temperature may be used for further reduction of microbes to inactivate enzymes and still allow the fruit and vegetable product to be like-fresh in quality. It is hard to visualize the use of sous vide for MPR fruits or vegetables using heat alone. One scenario may be vegetarian meals where the entire entree may be fruits and vegetables. Another could be the preparation of bulk (sized to consumer requirements) MPR fruits and vegetables that are prepared for the institutional market. The term individually quick-frozen (IQF) foods, which operates on the fluidized bed principle, has long been used in the frozen food industry (Desrosier and Tressler 1977). The same concept could be applied to MPR fruits and vegetables as mixed commodities or as individual commodities such as sliced, diced, or shredded carrots. Schlimme (1990) has suggested the term individually quick chilled (IQC) fruits and vegetables which could be linked with heat or other preservation methods.

In the sous vide process there are two effective heat preservation steps to consider. The first is the precook, which is optional, to slightly soften the tissue and reduce pathogens. The product should still exhibit like-fresh characteristics. Any number of methods may be used for this precook including high-humidity cooking ovens, steriflow retort with racks to hold product, water baths using different temperatures of water, and microwave (especially for pasta). Meats require a center temperature up to 77° C depending on the species. The product should be chilled to 7° C or less as quickly as possible. Then size reduction operations may take place and the product is filled in a package of standard thickness or shape and vacuumized. After vacuumizing the product is pasteurized at temperatures which will kill vegetative cells and further reduce enzyme activity. This includes a 4-D process for *Listeria monocytogenes* or a 7-D process for *Salmonella* (Table 3-3). The initial temperature (IT) for these processes is considered for safety's sake to be 0° C.

There have been numerous studies related to the use of heat to preserve refrigerated fruits and vegetables. Some studies such as the one of Losikoff (1990) have considered diced raw celery and determined the effects of a short boiling water blanch on the thermal

Table 3-3
D-values at Various Pasteurization Temperatures for *Salmonella* and
Listeria

°C	°F	*Salmonella* 7-D Time (min)	*Listeria* 4-D Time (min)
54	130	121	87.8
60	140	12	11.4
66	150	1.2	1.48
71	160	0.12	0.19

inactivation of *Listeria*. Raw diced celery was inoculated with 1×10^7 cells/g of visible *L. monocytogenes*. First, the product was blanched in boiling water in the laboratory for 15 sec (0.25 min) and then for 30 sec (0.50 min). Viable cells were found after the former treatment but none after the latter. In a commercial food processing plant, the general method was used to determine cumulative lethality at reference temperatures of 60° C using a z-value of 5° C and at 70° C and 71.7° C using a z-value of 10° C. The z-values are sometimes called the slope of the resistance curve (Pflug and Esselen 1963). The recommended process for celery of 2 min at 70° C was reached by holding the diced product for 1 min and 20 sec in boiling water (Table 3-3). It appears the heat transfer to the cold spot of the celery is relatively slow under these conditions; however, Losikoff (1990) felt a boiling water blanch could be one of the hurdles imposed on raw diced celery to inactivate *L. monocytogenes*. There was no report on the effect of temperature on texture and flavor quality of the celery.

Enzymes can be inactivated by high temperature except for highly thermostable enzyme systems such as the peroxidases. As is well known, enzyme activity increases in that the reaction rate doubles for every 10° C increase in temperature. Most of the enzymes of interest in MPR fruits and vegetables have optimum temperatures in the 30–50° C temperature range (Svensson 1977). This means short heat treatments in the lower temperature ranges to reduce microbe count may possibly increase the activity of certain undesirable enzymes.

Most thermal inactivation of enzymes of importance in the fruit and vegetable processing field, that is, PO/catalase, PPO, lipoxy-

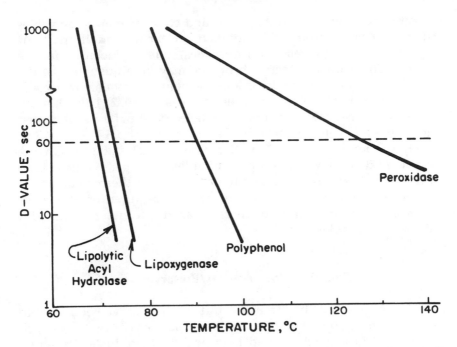

Figure 3-4   Thermal inactivation of the thermostable fraction of potato lipolytic acyl hydrolase, lipoxgenase, polyphenoloxidase, and peroxidase as a function of temperature. (From Svensson 1977.)

genase, PE, and PG follow first-order reaction kinetics. To compare thermal inactivation of enzymes with thermal death time curves for microorganisms, the heat treatment data for enzymes should be reduced to D-values and z-values. This approach will help processing (preservation) specialists to interpret the effect of heat on both enzymes and microbes. Figure 3-4 is illustrative of the thermal inactivation of the thermostable fraction of several potato enzymes (Svensson 1977). It is obvious from this figure that at lower temperatures much longer times are required to reduce enzyme activity by 90% and that PO in potato tissue is much more heat resistant than lipoxygenase or PPO. The z-values for lipoxygenase, PPO, and PO are 3.6° , 7.8° , and 35° C, respectively.

The information in Figure 3-4 illustrates the problems for control of injurious enzymes in MPR fruit and vegetable tissue by heat alone. The D-values (in seconds) are very high at lower temperatures, making it difficult to inactivate enzymes and retain like-fresh quality. Peroxidase, which affects flavor and color of many vegetables and fruits, best illustrates this point. It is clear that additional hurdles for enzymes (as well as for microbes) must be included for the preservation regimen. One such hurdle may be adjustment of the pH of the food away from the isoelectric point of key enzymes causing less heat stability. For example, Svensson (1977) has reported that pea lipoxygenase, which has its isoelectric at pH 5.8 and heated to 65° C has a D-value of 400 min, has a D-value at pH 4.0 and 65° C of only 0.1 min, a tremendous decrease in heat stability. On the other hand there have been reports that decreasing a_w (a method to control microbes) has considerably increased the thermostability of enzymes (Svensson 1977). Much research is required on the interaction of pH, heat, and a_w in thermostability of enzymes in MPR fruits and vegetables.

Chemical Preservation/Preservatives

Chemical compounds both natural and synthetic have been used to control spoilage and maintain quality in low-acid vegetables, acidified low-acid vegetables, and high-acid fruit products. Preservatives that act as antimicrobials best fit the definition of preservation as expressed in this text; however, those preservatives that serve as antioxidants are also very important in MPR fruits and vegetables to prevent browning; reduce discoloration of pigments; and protect against loss of flavor, changes in texture, and loss of nutritional quality.

The preservative action of antimicrobials depends on the type, genus, species, and strain of the microorganism tested. Antimicrobials are also effective at various stages of growth of the endospore into a vegetative cell as shown in Figure 3-5. Efficiency of an antimicrobial also depends to a great extent on environmental factors such as pH, water activity (a_w), temperature, atmosphere, initial microbial load, and low-acid, or high-acid food substrate, each factor acting singly or in combination. If they are varied to their extremes, many of these environmental factors such as a_w, temperature, gaseous atmosphere, etc., can be considered individually as methods of preservation. Some of these treatments were the basis of the hurdles or barrier concept of using less than extreme preservation treatments in a logical sequence to provide like-fresh quality in food products. The isobolograms in Figure 3-6 by Davidson and Parish (1989) suggest that antimicrobial compounds used together can produce three

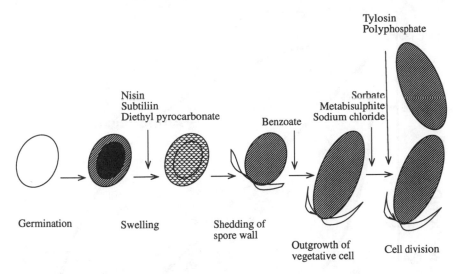

Figure 3-5 Diagrammatic representation of growth of an endospore into vegetative cells showing stages arrested by minimum inhibiting concentrations of some food preservatives. (From Jay 1986.)

types of results: synergism, additive effect, and antagonism. Similar results might be expected by combining heat, pH change, etc. with antimicrobials. It is obvious that combination of preservation methods including the use of antimicrobial combinations must be tested in the specific food product systems before application. In other words, the hurdles provided must at minimum be additive in action (preferably synergistic) and not antagonistic. A great deal of research must be conducted on MPR fruits and vegetables using specific food or food mixtures to determine preservation results of hurdle or treatment variables.

Those preservatives that serve as antioxidants to extend shelf-life and preserve fruits and vegetables are of great interest. As indicated earlier, their efficiency depends on a number of environmental factors such as pH, water activity (a_w), temperature, light, type and activity of the enzyme system, gaseous atmosphere, food substrate, and heavy metal content (Buck 1985). The effectiveness of antioxidants is controlled by environmental conditions for the preservative in the food system, its concentration, and longevity during the storage or shelf-life of the product. Those working with, MPR fruits and vegetables must consider the use of both antimicrobials and antioxidants to provide a safe and high-quality like fresh product over

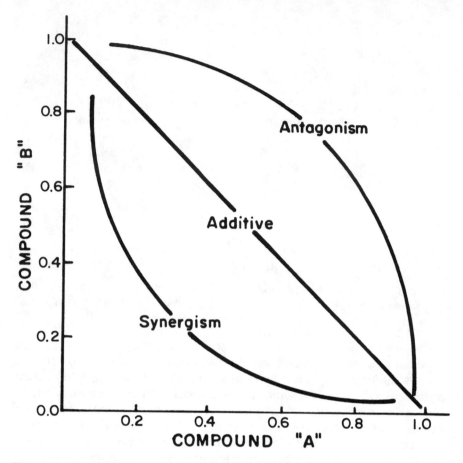

Figure 3-6   Isobolograms displaying the three types of results possible with combinations of antimicrobials. (From Davidson and Parish 1989.)

an extended shelf-life period. This suggests that the preservation hurdles used for MPR fruits and vegetables must test both type and load of microbial flora and key enzymes that could cause quality problems. Some "generally recognized as safe" (GRAS) chemical food preservatives are found in Table 3-4 (Jay 1986b). (Also see Lewis 1989.)

Table 3-4
Summary of Some GRAS Chemical Food Preservatives

Preservatives	Maximum tolerance	Organisms Affected	Foods
Propionic acid/ propionates	0.32%	Molds	Bread, cakes, some cheeses, rope inhibitor in bread dough
Sorbic acid/ sorbates	0.2%	Molds	Hard cheeses, figs, syrups, salad dressings, jellies, cakes
Benzoic acid/ benzoates	0.1%	Yeasts and molds	Margarine, pickle relishes and apple cider, soft drinks, tomato catsup, salad dressings
Parabens[a]	0.1%[b]	Yeasts and molds	Bakery products, soft drinks, pickles, salad dressings
SO_2/sulfites	200–300 ppm	Insects, microorganisms	Molasses, dried fruits, winemaking, lemon juice (not to be used in meats or other foods recognized as sources of thiamine)
Ethylene/propylene oxides[c]	700 ppm	Yeasts, molds, vermin	Fumigant for spices, nuts
Sodium diacetate	0.32%	Molds	Bread
Dehydroacetic acids	65 ppm	Insects	Pesticide on strawberries, squash
Sodium nitrite[c]	120 ppm	Clostridia	Meat-curing preparations
Caprylic acid	—	Molds	Cheese wraps
Ethyl formate	15–200 ppm[d]	Yeasts and molds	Dried fruits, nuts

GRAS (Generally Recognized As Safe) per Section 201 (32)(s) of the U.S. Federal Food, Drug, and Cosmetic Act as amended.
[a]Methyl-, propyl-, and heptyl-esters of p-hydroxybenzoic acid.
[b]Heptyl ester—12 ppm in beers; 20 ppm in noncarbonated and fruit-based beverages.
[c]May be involved in mutagenesis and/or carcinogenesis.
[d]As formic acid.
(From Jay 1986.)

Antimicrobials

Organic Acids and Related Compounds

Organic acids can be naturally present in fruits and vegetables (Table 3-5), accumulate as a result of fermentation, or be added during processing. For a good review and detail relating to antimicrobials occurring naturally in foods see Beuchat and Golden (1989). Acid foods or organic acids added to low-acid foods as a preservation measure are usually considered as acidification in foods destined to be thermally processed. The main objective of this procedure is to adjust the pH of the product below pH 4.6 which is generally accepted as the minimum pH for sporulation and growth of *C. botulinum*. Acidification is a safety measure also used for MPR fruits and vegetables. Some organic acids may act as fungicides or fungistats, whereas others tend to be more effective at inhibiting bacterial growth. Beuchat and Golden (1989) suggest that the mode of action for organic acids can be related to direct pH reduction of the substrate, some reduction of internal pH of the cell due to ionization of the undissociated acid molecule, or disruption of the transport mechanism through the cell membrane. It appears that the antimicrobial effectiveness of organic acids is primarily related to the dissociation constant (pK_a) of the acid. Table 3-6 shows proportion of total acid undissociated at different pH values for some common organic acids (Dziezak 1986). The pK_a values of most organic acids used in foods are somewhere between pH 3 and 5; thus acidification of low-acid foods greatly improves the antimicrobial characteristics of the food. However, this mechanism relies on complete diffusion of the acid throughout the sample and to the center of every food particle involved in acidification.

Citric Acid. Citric acid ($C_6H_8O_7$) is the main organic acid of fruits such as citrus, cranberries, currents, figs, strawberries, etc. and vegetables including beans and tomatoes (Gardner 1966). Citric acid has been shown to inhibit the growth of bacteria (Fabian and Graham 1953), flat-sour bacteria in canned tomato juice (Murdock 1950), and to be more inhibitory to salmonellae in milk than lactic and hydrochloric acids (Subramaniun and Marth 1968). Unfortunately most of the above examples of efficiency of citric acid as an antimicrobial relate to thermally processed products. There have been a number of studies that have suggested the antimicrobial activity of citric acid is due to the chelation of metal ions which are essential for microbial

Table 3-5
Some Natural Acids of Fruits and Vegetables

Fruits	Acids[a]
Apples	*Malic, quinic, a*-ketoglutaric, oxalacetic, citric, pyruvic, fumaric, lactic, and succinic acids
Apricots	*Malic* and *citric* acids
Avocados	*Tartaric* acid
Bananas	*Malic, citric,* tartaric, and traces of acetic and formic acids
Blackberries	*Isocitric, malic,* lactoisocitric, shikimic, quinic, and traces of citric and oxalic acids
Blueberries	*Citric,* malic, glyceric, citramalic, glycolic, succinic, glucuronic, galacturonic, shikimic, quinic, glutamic, and aspartic acids
Boysenberries	*Citric,* malic, and isocitric acids
Cherries	*Malic, citric,* tartaric, succinic, quinic, shikimic, glyceric, and glycolic acids
Cranberries	*Citric,* malic, and benzoic acids
Currants	*Citric, tartaric,* malic, and succinic acids
Elderberries	*Citric,* malic, shikimic, and quinic acids
Figs	*Citric,* malic, and acetic acids
Gooseberries	*Citric,* malic, shikimic, and quinic acids
Grapefruit	*Citric,* tartaric, malic, and oxalic acids
Grapes	*Malic* and *tartaric* (3:2), citric and oxalic acids
Lemons	*Citric,* malic, tartaric, and oxalic acids (no isocitric acid)
Limes	*Citric,* malic, tartaric, and oxalic acids
Orange peel	*Malic, citric,* and oxalic acids
Oranges	*Citric,* malic, and oxalic acids
Peaches	*Malic, citric,* tartaric, and oxalic acids
Pears	*Malic, citric,* tartaric, and oxalic acids
Pineapples	*Citric* and *malic* acids
Plums	*Malic, tartaric,* and oxalic acids
Quinces	*Malic* acid (no citric acid)
Strawberries	*Citric,* malic, shikimic, succinic, glyceric, glycolic, and aspartic acids
Youngberries	*Citric,* malic, and isocitric acids

Table 3-5   (Continued)

Vegetables	Acids[a]
Beans	*Citric, malic,* and small amounts of succinic and fumaric acids
Broccoli	*Malic* and *citric* (3:2) and oxalic and succinic acids
Carrots	*Malic, citric, isocitric,* succinic, and fumaric acids
Mushrooms	*Lactarimic,* cetostearic, fumaric, and allantoic acids
Peas	*Malic* acid
Potatoes	*Malic, citric, oxalic,* phosphoric, and pyroglutamic acids
Rhubarb	*Malic, citric,* and *oxalic* acids
Tomatoes	*Citric, malic, oxalic,* succinic, glycolic, tartaric, phosphoric, hydrochloric, sulfuric, fumaric, pyrrolidinonecarboxylic, and galacturonic acids

[a]Acids that occur in appreciable quantities are shown in italics. The relative amount of each varies widely with the variety, degree of ripeness, and seasonal effects. Complete identification of all the acids present in many of the products is obviously lacking in many instances.
(From Gardner 1966.)

Table 3-6
Proportion of Total Acid Undissociated at Different pH Values

Organic Acids[a]	pH values				
	3	4	5	6	7
Acetic acid	98.5	84.5	34.9	5.1	0.54
Benzoic acid	93.5	59.3	12.8	1.44	0.144
Citric acid	53.0	18.9	0.41	0.006	<0.001
Lactic acid	86.6	39.2	6.05	0.64	0.064
Methyl, ethyl, and propyl parabens[b]	>99.99	99.99	99.96	99.66	96.72
Propionic acid	98.5	87.6	41.7	6.67	0.71
Sorbic acid	97.4	82.0	30.0	4.1	0.48

[a]Values given as percentage.
[b]Parabens, p-hydroxybenzoic acid.
(From Dziezak 1986.)

growth (Beuchat and Golden 1989). Citric acid can be used to prevent browning by chelating copper in PPO. Inactivation of enzymes and potentiation of antioxidants in fruits and vegetables such as ascorbic acid, erythorbic acid, or sodium erythorbate can be achieved by the use of citric acid. Usage levels for citric acid are typically 0.1–0.3% with an antioxidant at 100–200 ppm (Dziezak 1986).

Benzoic Acid (C_6H_5COOH) and Parabens. The earliest reference to benzoic acid was made in 1608 by Blaise de Vigenire in "Traite' du Feu et du Sel," which described its preparation by the sublimation of gum benzon (Smith 1938). Benzoic acid occurs naturally in cranberries, prunes, cinnamon, cloves, raspberries, plums, and other fruits and vegetables. Its sodium salt ($C_7H_5NaO_2$), along with the esters of *p*-hydroxybenzoic acid (parabens), are some of the most important food preservatives. The sodium salt is particularly helpful in products with pH values below 4.6. It can be used in fruit products, fruit drinks, and juices as an antimicrobial. For example, Rushing and Senn (1962) found levels of 0.033–0.066% of sodium benzoate could extend the shelf-life of chilled citrus salads to 5–6 weeks at 4.4° C and 12–16 weeks at 1.11° C. However, it appeared that off-flavor development in the salad occurred before bacterial count had increased significantly. A number of workers have suggested that the undissociated benzoic acid molecule, which appears to be responsible for antimicrobial activity, diffuses through the microbial cell membrane, where it ionizes, causing rather complete acidification of the cell (Beuchat and Golden 1989; Jay 1986a). This acidity in turn has been postulated to interfere with substrate transport and oxidative phosphorylation systems (Freeze, Shaw, and Galliers 1973). Figure 3-5 suggests that the stage of endospore germination after shedding the spore wall is most sensitive to benzoate treatment. The benzoate compounds are most active in the lower pH acid foods such as apple cider, soft drinks, tomato catsup, and the like and not as effective in low-acid vegetables such as corn, peas, beans, lettuce, etc. The pK_a of benzoate is 4.2. This means this acid would be much more effective around a pH of 4.0–5.0. At a pH of 6.0, which is normal for many vegetables, only 1.5% of the benzoate is undissociated (Jay 1986b).

The benzoates are more effective against molds and yeasts rather than bacteria. In acid foods, they can be effective against bacteria in the 50–500 ppm range. In the pH 5.0–6.0 range, at 100–500 ppm, they are effective in inhibiting yeast, whereas at 30–300 ppm they are inhibitory to molds (Jay 1986b). Care has to be taken with the addition of benzoates to acid foods in that they can deliver a "peppery" or a burning taste sensation at levels of about 0.1%.

The useful parabens in food systems—methylparaben (methyl *p*-hydroxybenzoate), propylparaben (propyl *p*-hydroxybenzoate), and heptylparaben (*n*-heptyl-*p*-hydroxybenzoate)—are permitted in the United States whereas the butyl- and ethylparabens are permitted in some other countries (Jay 1986b). Parabens are most effective against molds and yeast and are less effective against bacteria, especially gram-negative bacteria. The pK_a of these compounds is around pH 8.47. Their antimicrobial activity tends to increase with the length of the alkyl chain and extends up to pH 7.0 (Dziezak 1986), which should make these useful in vegetable salads and vegetable soup stocks. Both methyl and propyl parabens are affirmed as GRAS under 21 CFR 184.1490 and 21 CFR 184.1670 (Anon. 1992) respectively and are limited to a combined usage level of 0.1%. The length of the alkyl chain is related to solubility in water which is usually necessary for use on fruits or vegetables. The parabens are available as a free-flowing white powder. The methyl ester imparts a slight odor and taste reminiscent of sodium benzoate, whereas the propyl ester is essentially odorless (Dziezak 1986).

Acetic Acid.   Acetic acid ($C_2H_4O_2$) and its salts Na acetate, Ca acetate, Na diacetate, and Ca diacetate have preservative antimicrobial properties. In addition acetic acid is known for its sequestering ability and its flavoring properties. Most vinegars contain acetic acid at the 4% level. Acetic acid and its salts are GRAS and are effective to a pH of 4.5. Acetic acid itself, which is a product of lactic acid bacteria fermentation or saccharomycete fermentation in such products as pickles, sauerkraut, olives, and cider, may also be added directly to the product. The limiting factor of acetic acid/vinegar addition to foods is the loss of desirable flavors and "bite" from high levels of use.

The main targets of acetic acid are yeast and bacteria and it has less effect on molds. The antimicrobial effect of acetic acid appears to be due to the depression of pH below the optimum growth range of microorganisms and metabolic inhibition by the undissociated molecules. In vegetable, meat, and fish products, 1–2% of the undissociated acid is sufficient to inhibit or kill all nontolerant microbes (Dziezak 1986). Acetic acid is used as a flavoring agent in condiments such as catsup, mayonnaise, and salad dressing. The treatment levels for acetic acid set forth by the International Commission on Microbiological Specifications for Foods (ICMSF) (Christian 1980) indicates 0.1% inhibits the growth of most food poisoning and spore-forming bacteria whereas 0.3% of the undissociated acid is required to inhibit the growth of mycotoxigenic molds.

In studies by Oscroft, Banks, and McPhee (1989) acetic acid showed good antimicrobial properties both at 0.05% and 0.5% wt/vol combinations in a combined heat 95° C acetic acid treatment of cocktails containing *Bacillus* spores. The results were the best when the pre-cooked chilled ready-to-eat meals were cooled to 12° C. Colder refrigerated temperatures should provide even more safety for these meals. Acetic acid/vinegar in dressings and condiments could be helpful in preserving MPR vegetables.

Lactic Acid.   This organic acid ($C_3H_6O_3$) is widely employed as a preservative in foods as a result of the action of lactic acid bacteria and related inhibiting substances other than organic acids (see Doores 1983; Jay 1986a; and Daeschel 1989, for more information). Lactic acid can also be added directly to food and provide antimicrobial properties by depression of pH below growth range and metabolic inhibition of the undissociated acid molecules. It should be emphasized that it is the titratable acidity rather than hydrogen ion concentration (pH) per se that is important in a treatment using an organic acid such as lactic since there is incomplete ionization of the acid even at lower acid pH values.

Banks, Morgan, and Stringer (1989) used lactic acid alone at 0.05% and 0.5% levels to treat 10^6 spores/ml *Bacillus* spp. cocktail heated to 65° C/60 min and stored at 30° , 20° , and 12° C for 42 days. Results indicated the lactic acid treatments were not effective inhibitors in storages of 20° and 30° C. The treatments stored at 12° showed outgrowth at pH 6.0 but no outgrowth at pH 5.7, 5.4, 5.1, 4.8, 4.5, and 4.2. The results were similar in experiments carried out with 10^4 spore/ml and 10^2 spore/ml. Similar experiments were conducted by Oscroft, Banks, and McPhee (1989) using a thermally stressed (95° C/15 min) cocktail of *Bacillus* spp. at 10^2, 10^4, and 10^6 spores/ml in trypticase soy broth (TSB). The treated samples were incubated for 42 days at 12° , 20° , and 30° C. The control treatment had lower counts than the Banks, Morgan, and Stringer (1989) experiments and there was outgrowth at 12° C storage in the pH 6.0 and 5.7 treatments but none at pH 5.4, 5.1, 4.8, 4.5, and 4.2. These are similar results to the heat treatments for a longer time at a lower temperature of 65° C. The integrated sterilizing (IS) values for these heat treatments were not reported.

Table 3-7
Effect of pH on Sorbic Acid Dissociation

pH	Undissociated (%)
7.00	0.6
6.00	6.0
5.80	7.0
5.00	37.0
4.75 (pK_a)	50.0
4.40	70.0
4.00	86.0
3.70	93.0
3.00	98.0

(From Liewen and Marth 1985.)

Propionic acid (CN$_3$CH$_2$COOH) and its salts.   This acid and its sodium and calcium salts are primarily used to prevent mold growth in breads, bakery products, cheeses, and other foods. The antimicrobial action of propionates is similar to that of benzoate in the undissociated form. The pK_a of propionate is 4.87 and at a pH of 4.0, 88% of the compound is undissociated whereas at a pH of 6.0 only 6.7% remains undissociated (Jay 1986b). Because these compounds do not have a tendency toward dissociation they are useful in low-acid foods. Dziezak (1986) suggested 0.2–0.4% levels of propionates to retard mold growth on syrups, blanched apple slices, figs, cherries, blackberries, peas, and lima beans. The compound seems to act as a fungistat rather than a fungicide according to Jay (1986b).

Sorbic Acid (CH$_3$CH=CHCH=CHCOOH) and its salts.   Sorbic acid is a monocarboxylic acid and its potassium salt forms (both GRAS status) are used to preserve foods. According to Liewen and Marth (1985), a German chemist, A.W. Hoffmans, first isolated sorbic acid from the pressed unripened berry of the rowan or mountain ash tree in 1959. For further information on sorbic acid, see review of Liewen and Marth (1985).

With use of the sorbates it is also the undissociated molecule that provides antimicrobial properties. Table 3-7 shows the effect of pH on sorbic acid dissociation and its pK_a of 4.75 (Sofos and Busta 1980). It appears that the upper pH limits for sorbates to be effective as antimicrobial agents are around 6.0–6.5 whereas for propionate and benzoates they are 5.0–5.5 and 4.0–4.5, respectively (Liewen and Marth 1985). This provides a basis for the traditional uses of sor-

Table 3-8
Typical Concentration (%) of Sorbic Acid Used in Various Food Products

Cheeses	0.2–0.30
Beverages	0.03–0.10
Cakes and pies	0.05–0.10
Dried fruits	0.02–0.05
Margarine (unsalted)	0.05–0.10
Mayonnaise	0.10
Fermented vegetables	0.05–0.20
Jams and jellies	0.05
Fish	0.03–0.15
Semimoist pet food	0.1–0.3
Wine	0.02–0.04
Fruit juices	0.05–0.20

(From Liewen and Marth 1985.)

bates in cottage cheese, baked goods, beverages, syrups, fruit juices, wines, jellies, jams, salads, pickles, margarine, and dried sausages. Work has also explored the use of sorbate in fresh produce, fresh fish and poultry, and yeast-raised and baked goods (Robach 1980).

Table 3-8 (Liewen and Marth 1985) shows the suggested concentration of sorbic acid for a number of foods. As indicated earlier, a number of environmental factors including more acid pH, lower a_w, lower temperature, higher CO_2, the type and number of microbial flora, and food components all have important effects on the efficiency of sorbate and should be considered in its use on a specific food product.

Robinson and Hills (1959) worked with preserving apple juice (cider), peach slices, and fruit salad (pineapple and citrus slices) that were subjected to temperatures of 37.8° C–54.4° C for 5 min in the presence of sodium sorbate. The apple juice, peach slices, and fruit salad had a final concentration of sodium sorbate of 0.06%, 0.048%, and 0.12% by weight on the basis of 16 ounces net contents, respectively. These treatments greatly increased the storage life of these products at storage temperatures of 22.8° C and 10° C. In the cider study 0.06% sorbate with a 37.8° C heat treatment for 5 min destroyed 50% of the initial yeasts, molds, and bacteria in the cider as well as improved storage life to 14 days at room temperature. At 48.9° C there was a 99% reduction in microbial counts and storage life was increased to 23 days at 21.1° C. Similar results were shown with peach slices and fruit salad, with peach slices showing a 92-day shelf-life before gas formation in most treatments. The 10° C storage temperature gave slightly better results than the 22.8° C storage samples. Although the flavor of these samples was rated as good, refrigerated/chilled temperatures would have improved the results of this work. Interactions of sorbates with other preservatives and other preservation methods are also discussed later in this chapter.

Malic, Succinic, and Tartaric Acids.   Malic acid ($C_4H_6O_5$) was reported by Gardner (1966) in the following fruits: apples, apricots, bananas, cherries, grapes, orange peel, peaches, pears, plums, quinces; and in vegetables: broccoli, carrots, peas, potatoes, and rhubarb. In his somewhat short list, malic acid is reported in all fruits and vegetables except avocados and mushrooms (Table 3-5) (Gardner, 1966).

Succinic acid ($C_4H_6O_4$) and succinic anhydride ($C_4H_4O_3$) are white crystals, and powder and white crystals, respectively. Succinic acid is found in a number of fruits and vegetables (Table 3-5), and in asparagus, rhubarb, and sugar beets as well according to Beuchat and Golden (1989).

Tartaric acid ($C_4H_6O_6$), which is a white crystal and imparts a bitter tart flavor sensation, is present in a number of fruits and tomatoes (Table 3-5).

The antimicrobial activity of these natural organic acids appears to be the result of a decrease in pH. Yeasts and some bacteria are target populations. Because they have not been studied in any detail for use on MPR fruits and vegetables, they should be considered in products where they are naturally present and possibly in others.

Indirect Antimicrobials

This category of antimicrobials is summarized by primary use and most susceptible organisms in Table 3-9 taken from Jay (1986b).

Medium-Chain Fatty Acids

Medium-chain fatty acids, that is, those containing 12–18 carbon atoms, have been known since the early part of this century to exhibit antimicrobial properties (Branen, Davidson, and Katz 1980). This is an additional benefit of these compounds which are used primarily as emulsifying agents in foods. Some organisms may be killed by

Table 3-9
Some GRAS Indirectly Antimicrobial Chemicals Used in Foods

Compound	Primary Use	Most Susceptible Organisms
Butylated hydroxyanisole (BHA)	Antioxidant	Bacteria, some fungi
Butylated hydroxytoluene (BHT)	Antioxidant	Bacteria, viruses, fungi
t-butylhydroxyquinoline (TBHQ)	Antioxidant	Bacteria, fungi
Propyl gallate (PG)	Antioxidant	Bacteria
Nordihydroguaiaretic acid	Antioxidant	Bacteria
Ethylenediamine tetraacetic acid (EDTA)	Sequestrant/stabilizer	Bacteria
Sodium citrate	Buffer/sequestrant	Bacteria
Lauric acid	Defoaming agent	Gram-positive bacteria
Monolaurin	Emulsifier	Gram-positive bacteria, yeasts
Diacetyl	Flavoring	Gram-negative bacteria, fungi
d- and *l*-Carvone	Flavoring	Fungi, gram-positive bacteria
Phenylacetaldehyde	Flavoring	Fungi, gram-positive bacteria
Menthol	Flavoring	Bacteria, fungi
Vanillin, ethyl vanillin	Flavoring	Fungi
Spices/spice oils	Flavoring	Bacteria, fungi

(From Jay 1986.)

fatty acids but the antimicrobial action of fatty acids is more static than cidal (Neiman 1954). The undissociated form of the fatty acid molecule is thought to be responsible for antimicrobial activity against yeasts and gram-positive bacteria. Therefore compounds will react in the same manner as organic acids to changes in pH. One would expect greater antimicrobial activity as the pH is lowered. Concentrations needed for inhibition usually are in the 10–1,000 mg/ml range (Branen, Davidson, and Katz 1980).

The gram-negative bacteria and molds seem to be less susceptible than gram-positive bacteria to the antimicrobial properties of the various fatty acids. For control of gram-positive bacteria, the most effective chain length for saturated fatty acids is 12 carbons; the most effective monounsaturated fatty acid is $C_{16:1}$ (palmitic) and the best polyunsaturated is $C_{18:12}$ (linoleic) (Beuchat and Golden 1989). Kabara (1983) has reviewed the antimicrobial activity of fatty acids. Also see Kabara (1981) for food-grade chemicals to use in designing food preservative systems.

For use in MPR foods, medium-chain fatty acids could be most helpful in fruits and vegetables that are slightly acidic and do not yield well to other preservatives. In addition, there are other factors aside from pH and acidity that control effectiveness of these compounds. Neiman (1954) has found that antagonists such as starch, cholesterol, and serum albumen reduce antimicrobial action of fatty acids. The effectiveness of these compounds may also rest on their solubility or lack of solubility in water. To assist in solving this problem, fatty acids could be added to dressings or condiments and should be considered as a method to extend shelf-life of MPR fruits and vegetables. Other preservation hurdles might also be included in such a system to improve the effectiveness of fatty acids.

Fatty Acid Esters of Polyhydric Acids

Fatty acid esters of sucrose and other polyhydric alcohols are used primarily as emulsifiers but they also provide antimicrobial properties. They can be manufactured or occur naturally in plants (Beuchat and Golden 1989). Monolaurin, a glycerol monoester, is a satisfactory compound to be used against gram-positive organisms or yeasts. Combining monolaurin with other food additives such as citric acid, polyphosphoric acid, EDTA, and BHT or with other physical food preservation hurdles such as refrigeration or heating could increase the effectiveness of monolaurin against the more difficult to control gram-negative organisms (Branen, Davidson, and Katz 1980). Lipid esters will have to be tested in food products to gain insights on their functionality in a specific situation. For more information concerning these preservatives see the above listed references and Jay (1986b) and Kato (1981).

Other Indirect Antimicrobials

According to Jay (1986b), many other compounds including those found in Table 3-9 have some antimicrobial properties. (Also see Marth 1966.) The literature does not cover these compounds for use in MPR fruits and vegetables but applications should be sought where capability and functional properties could be used to advantage. This would be especially true with spices and flavoring agents used in MPR fruits and vegetables. Beuchat and Golden (1989) have covered in detail other natural antimicrobials such as pigments and related compounds, humulones and lupulones, hydroxycinnanic acid derivative, oleuropein, caffeine, theophylline and theobromine, and phytoalexins, and their article should be read for more detail than can be provided here.

Sugar and Salt

Sugars such as sucrose, glucose, fructose, etc. exert antimicrobial properties at concentrations much higher than are normally used in MPR fruits or vegetables. Some yeasts and molds can grow in sugar solutions of 60% sucrose which could rarely be used in MPR products (Jay 1986b).

Salts may be used in MPR vegetables but at relatively low levels. Conner, Brachett, and Beuchat (1986) found NaCl concentrations in cabbage juice at 7.2% caused a decrease in strains of *L.monocytogenes*, Scott A, and LCDC 81861. The levels of salt in MPR vegetables should be studied to determine if salt concentration alone could lower microbial activity. In most instances it would be expected that the levels of sugar or salt added to MPR fruits and vegetables alone would not be effective antimicrobial agents; however, they might be linked with other preservative hurdles and provide antimicrobial protection. See also the section on water activity (a_w) for more information.

Antibiotics

A great number of antibiotics are mentioned in the literature as antimicrobials. They include nisin, natamycin, tetracylines, subtilin, and tylosin. Nisin produced by *Streptococcus lactis* is usually referred to as an antibiotic but probably should be classified as a bacteriocin because it has no therapeutic value in human or veterinary medicine, feedstuffs, or growth promotion (Banks, Morgan, and Stringer 1989). Nicin and natamycin have been approved for food use in many countries and recently nisin has been approved in the United States by the Food and Drug Administration (USFDA) for use in processed cheese spreads. The tetracyclines, that is, chlortetracycline and oxytetracycline, have been studied widely for their use in fresh foods, and natamycin has been suggested as a food fungistat (Jay 1986b).

Jay (1986b) has summarized the considerations one should make in deciding on the use of antibiotics on foods or MPR fruits and vegetables. These were developed because of the general resistance of consumers to the use of antibiotics in foods to preserve them. See below:

1. "The antibiotic agent should kill, not inhibit the flora, and should ideally decompose into innocuous products, or be destroyed on cooking for products that require cooking.
2. The antibiotic should not be inactivated by food components or products of microbial metabolism.
3. The antibiotic should not readily stimulate the appearance of resistant strains.
4. The antibiotic should not be used in foods if used therapeutically or as an animal feed additive."

Nisin along with subtilin, and tylosin have been used as adjuncts to the use of heat in canning many vegetables. The concept includes giving canned low-acid foods the typical F_0 3-min or "bot cook" heat treatment and then the added antibiotic will prevent more economic or pathogenic spoilage by attacking the more heat-resistant thermopiles. F_0 is the time in minutes required to destroy a stated number of organisms with a known z at temperature T.

MPR fruits and vegetables may need a mild pasteurization temperature but this will not prevent the outgrowth of the *Bacillus* and *Clostridum* species if temperature abuse should occur. Banks, Morgan, and Stringer (1989) have studied pasteurization temperatures in conjunction with use of pH, acidity control, and preservatives. Nisin was used in *Bacillus* spore cocktails at levels of 0,125, 250, and 5,000 IU ml^{-1}. Addition of nisin alone to the heating medium did prevent germination and outgrowth of spores. As the inoculum concentration increased to 10^6 spores/ml^{-1}, the efficacy of nisin decreased and as the pH was decreased from 6.0 to 4.2, the effectiveness of nisin increased.

According to Wagner and Moberg (1989), to ensure successful application of nisin as a preservative the food should be acidic in nature to provide stability of the antimicrobial during processing and storage and the spoilage organism to be controlled should be gram-positive, nisin-sensitive, and not contain nisinase. If nicin is depleted from the food system its protection could be lost.

It appears nisin could be helpful in mildly heated refrigerated fruits and vegetables where heating could induce germination and outgrowth of spores. This might reduce the potential for growth of psychrotrophic and mesophilic aerobic spore-formers and their resultant spoilage of food. Little research has been conducted on the use of antibiotics to provide antimicrobial activity in MPR fruits and vegetables and it is an area that should be investigated.

Although gas—controlled atmosphere (CA) and modified atmosphere (MA)—treatments in storages or through packaging provide antimicrobial protection and can logically be covered under antimicrobials, special emphasis for this area in MPR fruits and vegetables is presented in the section on gas preservation in this chapter.

Antioxidants

The U.S. Food and Drug Administration (FDA) in 21 Code of Federal Regulators (CFR) 170.3(0)(3) (Anon. 1992) has defined antioxidants as substances used to preserve food by retarding deterioration rancidity or discoloration due to oxidation. In MPR fruits and vegetables there are several types of oxidative reactions in which electrons are removed from atoms or molecules to lead to a reduced form. These reactions cause browning reactions; discoloration of endogenous pigments; loss or changes of product flavor or odor; changes in texture; and loss of nutritional value from destruction of vitamin A, C, D, or E and essential fatty acids such as linoleic acid. These changes are important in most MPR fruits and vegetables. Special problems arise in seed crops and lipid-containing vegetables such as avocado leading to the possible development of rancid off-flavors and toxic oxidation products (Dziezak 1986).

As seen in Figure 3-7 there are four categories of chemical structures used to stabilize foods. They are (1) the free-radical interceptors such as BHA, BHT, etc., which are usually used for oil- and lipid-containing foods and are very insoluble in H_2O; (2) the reducing agents such as ascorbic acid and isomer erythorbic acid and related compounds which are used extensively to transfer hydrogen ions; (3) chelating agents such as citric acid and EDTA; and (4) the "secondary" antioxidants including dilauryl acid, thiodipropionate, and thiodipropionic acid.

The most important compounds used in stabilizing MPR fruits and vegetables are reducing agents and certain GRAS chelating agents that are not actually antioxidants but are important in preventing

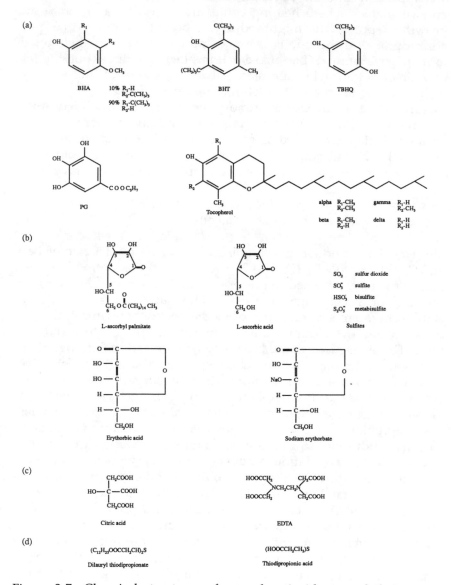

Figure 3-7   Chemical structures of several antioxidants and their synergists: (a) free-radical interceptors, (b) reducing agents, (c) chelating agents,
and (d) secondary antioxidants. (From Dziezak 1986.)

oxidative reactions in fruits and vegetables. With the recent restrictions of the use of sulfites on fruits and vegetables to be served raw or sold raw to consumers or presented to customers as fresh (21 CFR 182.3739, 182.3766, 182.3862, 182.3798, 182.3637, and 182.3616) (Anon. 1992), there can be little doubt these regulations relate to like-fresh MPR foods. Much research is being conducted to find suitable substitutes for sulfites for all fresh and MPR fruits and vegetables. The most promising substitutes may be combinations of the ascorbic acid derivatives with citric or other organic acids.

L-Ascorbic Acid

L-ascorbic acid (vitamin C) and its various neutral salts and other derivatives have been leading GRAS antioxidants for use on fruits and vegetables and their juices to prevent browning and other oxidative reactions (Bauernfeind and Pinkert 1970). Sapers et al. (1989a) have recently reported on a number of ascorbic acid derivatives, PPO inhibitors, and complexing agents used to control enzymatic browning. The L-ascorbic acid isomer erythorbic acid is covered later in this section. In its removal of oxygen from food, ascorbic acid is oxidized to form dehydroascorbic acid. Ascorbic acid is usually added together with citric acid which tends to maintain more acid pH levels and also acts as a chelating agent on such enzymes as copper-containing PPO (Whitaker 1972a). Ascorbic acid is a moderately strong reducing compound, is acidic in nature, forms neutral salts with bases, and is very water soluble. The product may be added to foods as tablets or wafers, dry premixes, liquid sprays, or as a pure compound. It is important to add the ascorbic acid as late as possible during processing or preservation to maintain highest levels during the shelf-life of the food commodity. If the goal is to maintain a vitamin C level in fruit and vegetable juices of about 30 mg/8 fl. oz. then 3 oz. of crystalline ascorbic acid need to be added to 100 gallons of juices (Bauernfeind and Pinkert 1970). Potter (1968) suggested that levels of ascorbic acid dissolved in a sugar syrup should be 0.05%– 0.2% and given adequate time to penetrate could keep peaches from darkening for 2 years at 0° F. Sapers, Garzarella, and Pilizota (1990), working with the problem of penetration of ascorbic acid, erythorbic acid, or their sodium salts in combination with citric acid found apple plugs and potato plugs were best infiltered with 34 kPa and 108 kPa pressure, respectively. Storage life was increased 3–7 days for apple plugs and dice and 2–4 days for potato plug under refrigerated temperatures of 4° C. Because low levels such as 100 ppm of ascorbic acid may induce proxidative effects, levels such as 2,000 ppm are suggested to prevent these reactions (Cort 1982).

Erythorbic Acid

Erythorbic acid and its salt, sodium erythorbate, are GRAS and are strong reducing agents; they act as oxygen scavengers, thus reducing molecular oxygen. Erythorbic acid is the D isomer of ascorbic acid but has no vitamin C activity. Most research suggests L-ascorbic acid and erythorbic acid have about equal antioxidant properties; thus L-ascorbic acid might be used only where vitamin C addition is a necessity. At today's prices (1992) L-ascorbic acid is about five times more expensive than erythorbic acid.

The use of erythorbic acid with citric acid has been often suggested as a substitute for sulfites. This combination is used at retail to inhibit oxidative rancidity and discoloration in salad vegetables, cole slaw, apples, and frozen seafood. Erythorbic acid or sodium erythorbate can suppress browning reactions in frozen fruits and should be helpful in MPR fruits.

See Sapers et al. (1989a), Sapers et al. (1989b), and Sapers, Garzarella, and Pilizota (1990) for information on use of ascorbic acids and their derivatives to prevent browning reactions in fruits and vegetables. The 1989b article covers some uses of ascorbic acid-2-phosphate, ascorbic acid-2-triphosphate, and ascorbic acid-6 fatty acid ester as novel browning inhibitors. These substances have not yet been approved by the USFDA.

Sulfites

Sulfites are increasingly under fire for use in raw fruits and vegetables. As indicated earlier in this section, sulfites are no longer GRAS for fruits and vegetables served raw, sold raw, or presented to the consumer as raw. Foods containing a detectable level of a sulfiting agent defined as 10 ppm, regardless of source, must declare the sulfite and its content on the ingredient label (21 CFR Part 182.3862) (Anon. 1992). It is likely that more and more regulatory restrictions will be applied to the use of sulfites in foods globally because of the sulfite allergies in a significant portion of our population. They are not recommended for MPR fruits and vegetables.

Chelating Agents

As seen in Figure 3-7 chelating agents are not antioxidants but work as synergists with antioxidant preservatives. They complex with prooxidative agents such as prooxidative copper and iron ions through an unshared pair of electrons in their molecular structures which provides the complexing or chelating action. The best known chelating agents for use on fruits and vegetables that are GRAS are citric acid and EDTA. Sapers et al. (1989b) reports on papers describing *non-GRAS* chelating agents such as cyanide, diethyldithiocarbonate, 2-mercaptobenzothiazole, and azide which inhibit PPO by interacting with its prosthetic group and polyvinylpyisolidone which bonds the phenolic substances, preventing their conversion to quinones.

Friedman (1991) has been testing an acidic polyphosphate, Sporix, on precut apples, potatoes, broccoli florets, snow pea pods, and other fruits and vegetables. It is soluble in water and has a pH of 2.0. The recommended dip for these commodities is a 0.5% solution. Sporix–ascorbic acid combinations were synergists in reducing browning in the juice of Granny Smith apples and the cut surface of Red Delicious and Winesap apples (Sapers et al. 1989b). According to Friedman (1991) the compound is allowed on fruits and vegetables in Taiwan, Korea, and Japan and is being considered in the United States by USFDA.

Citric Acid

Citric acid (covered earlier) is also a chelating agent that is GRAS and used synergistically with ascorbic or erythorbic acids and their neutral salts to chelate prooxidants which might cause rancidity and inactivate enzymes such as PPO that cause browning reactions. Suggested usage levels for citric acid are typically 0.1–0.3% with the appropriate antioxidant at 100–200 ppm (Dziezak 1986). Citric acid can also be used as a chelating agent in many other foods.

EDTA

EDTA is another chelating agent permitted as a chemical preservative. The major compounds approved as additives by FDA are calcium disodium EDTA (21 CFR 172.120) and disodium EDTA (21 CFR 172.135) (Anon. 1992). The former compound can be used in potato salad (100 ppm), pickled cabbage (220 ppm), pickled cucumbers (220 ppm), nonstandardized dressings (750 ppm), salad dressing and sauce (75 ppm), as well as in many other food products. The intended usage of calcium disodium EDTA is to promote color, flavor, and texture retention and as a preservative. Disodium EDTA may be used as a preservative at 75 ppm in nonstandardized dressing, French dressing, mayonnaise, salad dressing, and sauces. It might be expected that sauces, dressings, and the like would be added to MPR fruit and vegetable salads. Highly stable complexes are formed by the sequestering action of the EDTA compounds on iron, copper, and calcium. The maximum chelating efficiency occurs at the higher pH values where the carboxyl groups are dissociated (Dziezak 1986).

Miscellaneous Chemical Preservatives

Dehydroacetic Acid

Dehydroacetic acid ($C_7H_6O_4$) (21 CFR 172.130) (Anon. 1992), a pyranose structured compound, or its sodium salt may be used as a preservative for cut or peeled squash to control molds. The use levels should be no more than 65 ppm of the acid remaining on or in the squash. This compound can also be used on other fruits and vegetables in Mexico and other countries.

Chlorine Compounds (Cl_2)

These compounds are normally used in connection with washing MPR fruits and vegetables and are sometimes the primary preservation agent. (See Chapter 2 for details.)

Antifungal Agents for Fruits and Vegetables

This area is not covered in depth because most postharvest dips have been stopped in Europe and the United States and there are very stringent rules on application time before harvest; however, Benomyl, a fungicide in foods for human consumption such as raisins and concentrated tomato products, is allowed up to levels of 50 ppm (CFR 21 193.30), (Anon. 1992), as a result of application to the growing of grapes and tomatoes in the United States. Thiobendazole, an important fungicide, is allowed a tolerance of 3 ppm in or on milled wheat fractions (except flour) resulting from applications to growing wheat. Other antifungal agents should be checked out in consultation with regulatory authorities even though they are normally added to the skin or peel of the fruit or vegetable. MPR fruits and vegetables should have much lower levels than fresh or raw products that are not partially processed.

Combinations of Chemical Preservatives

Chemical preservatives/antimicrobials in combination are currently utilized in the food industry and this area has been addressed by Davidson and Parish (1989), Scott (1989), Banks, Morgan, and Stringer (1989), Oscroft, Banks, and McPhee (1989), and Aguilera and Parada (1991). A good example of combination treatment in the food industry is the combination of potassium sorbate and sulfur dioxide to preserve sparkling wines. Data showing additive synergistic or antagonist results from combinations of preservatives (Figure 3-6) have not been studied in detail for MPR fruits and vegetables although there have been studies such as those of Banks, Morgan, and Stringer (1989) investigating heat and chemical preservatives to improve stabilized "pasteurized/chilled" recipe dishes. Most of the preservative interaction studies appear to have used microbial "cocktails" studies on fish, meats, poultry, and dairy products. These studies have centered on type E *C. botulinum, S. aureus, Salmonella typhimurium, L. monocytogenes,* and *Yersenia enterocolitica* control in the above mentioned substrates, using salt concentrations with sodium nitrite and phenolic antioxidants with sorbates (Scott 1989). Restaino, Komatsu, and Syracuse (1982) studied the synergistic antimicrobial effects between potassium sorbate and lactic, citric, phosphoric, or hydrochloric acids on growth of *Yersinia enterocolitica, Salmonella pseudomonas,* and lactic acid bacteria in trypticase soy broth and APT broth. They found organic acids, specifically citric and lactic, potentiate the antimicrobial action of potassium sorbate. There need to be many additional combination studies of chemical preservatives for MPR fruits and vegetables.

Gas and Controlled/Modified Atmosphere Preservation

The use of gases, vapors, and controlled/modified atmosphere for preservation does not include packaging factors (Chapter 4) and the gas mass transfer (Chapter 5) taking place in the tissues of MPR foods. With fresh fruits and vegetables voluminous research information is found to reduce O_2 levels, increase CO_2 levels, and reduce ethylene as methods to improve storage and shelf-life. A symposium chaired by Blanpied (1987) gives a good summary of the postharvest work conducted in this area until 1987.

However, this chapter necessarily covers mainly the antimicrobial and antioxidant properties of gaseous substances used with packaging to extend shelf-life of MPR fruits and vegetables. The area is receiving much attention by research laboratories and industry as a way to preserve MPR fruits and vegetables.

One of the earlier workers to study gas exchange and the use of bactericidal and enzymicidal gases to keep fruits and vegetables like-fresh and extend storage life was Kramer et al. (1980). This preservation and shelf-life extension technique consisted of replacement of intratissue gases in particulate raw foods with one or more gases, in appropriate sequence. The idea was to stabilize the product and extend the like-fresh shelf-life of the foods at ambient or refrigerated temperatures. Kramer et al. (1980) felt the new preservation method was an extension of CA/MA storage used for fresh products. However, there are several differences between normal CA/MA storages and the gas-exchange process. The atmosphere changes are slower in normal CA/MA storages, usually days or minutes, as compared to gas-exchange; times of treatment are relatively short, and additional gases such as carbon monoxide (CO), ethylene oxide, (EO), and SO_2 were used in the gas exchange system as compared with N_2, O_2, and CO_2 modifications used in CA/MA storages. Also, only the edible portion or a minimally processed portion of the fruit or vegetable is treated in the gas-exchange method. Emphasis in the gas-exchange method is placed on antimicrobial properties of the gases and their efficacy in inhibiting enzyme activity. These are also the objectives in the preservation of MPR fruits and vegetables.

Some of the problems with the gas-exchange treatment were related to the gases selected for use. Such gases as EO should be used in a very low a_w atmosphere and unfortunately its by-products are ethylene glycol (EG) and ethylene chlorohydrin (ECH), which show mutagenicity at certain concentrations. FDA regulations 21 CFR Part 193.20 (Anon. 1992) state there should not be over a 50 ppm residue of EO in whole and ground spices. The content of carbon monoxide (CO), a product of combustion gases (21 CFR 193.65) (Anon. 1992), should not be over 4.5% by volume in gas treatments. The use of CO is banned in France.

The concept of using gas-exchange preservation treatments on MPR fruits and vegetables has merits if safe and suitable bactericidal and enzymicidal gas can be found or linked with other preservation hurdles.

The most important gases and vapors to be discussed in detail are CO, CO_2, EO, propylene oxide (PO), SO_2, and ozone. Propane, helium, N_2, combustion gases 21 CFR, 184.1655, 184.1355, 184.1540, and 193.65 (Anon. 1992) respectively will not be covered. Antimicrobial effectiveness of a gas can be related to the food substrate, other processing and preservation methods, and the microorganisms and enzymes present.

Carbon Monoxide

As indicated earlier there are safety problems with the use of this gas. CO at the 1% level has been shown to inhibit yeasts and molds and prevent postharvest decay in fruits and vegetables (Aharoni and Stadelbacher 1973). However, treatments of apple and potato plugs with pure CO were not able to reduce counts of *Escherichia coli* ATCC II 229, a standardized suspension of *Clostridium botulinium* 62A, and *Staphylococcus aureus* ATCC 6538 (Kaffezakis, Palmer, and Kramer 1969). These workers also studied the enzymicidal activity of CO and showed CO was effective is slowing down PPO activity (Figure 3-8). In a two-step gas treatment with SO_2 followed by CO, potato strips after 60 days at room temperature showed 93.7% and 99.9% of the PO and PPO inactivated (Kramer et al. 1980).

Carbon Dioxide

This gas has antimicrobial properties that kill or inhibit various microorganisms and that depend on the gas concentration, temperature of incubation, age of the cells used, and the a_w of the microbial medium. Most work has been conducted on meat and meat products, and these results showed a 10% level of CO_2 usually gives about 50% inhibition on the basis of total counts after a given incubation time (Wagner and Moberg 1989). Huxsoll and Bolen (1989) have recently reviewed CA and MA storage of MPR foods. Table 3-10 shows the effects of SO_2, CO_2, and temperature on peroxidase, PPO, and PE. It appears that there is less effect of these gases on the texture-related enzymes such as PPE than PPO (Kramer et al.

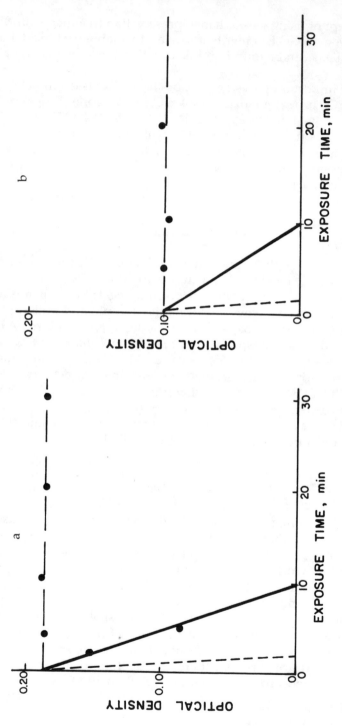

Figure 3-8 Polyphenoloxidase activity following exposure to carbon monoxide (———), ethylene oxide (———), or sulfur dioxide gas (---): (a) potato plugs, (b) apple plugs. (From Kaffezakis et al. 1969.)

1980). The same results for PG were reported by Puri (1980). It is likely the enzymicidal properties shown in Table 3-10 are mainly due to SO_2 since CO_2 was used as a flushing and carrier gas but such results could not be determined from the data supplied.

Sulfur Dioxide

SO_2 (discussed earlier under sulfites in the section on antioxidants is also well known to be effective against molds, yeasts, and bacteria (Dziezak 1986). In the fruit and vegetable realm it has been used to control microorganisms on soft fruits, fruit juices, wines, pickles, leafy greens, and the like. However, the sulfite compounds have been banned on fruits and vegetables to be sold or consumed (21 CFR 182.3862) (Anon. 1992). Nonetheless, earlier Kramer et al. (1980) reported good results with SO_2 combined with CO_2 (Table 3-10) but because the great sensitivity of a small part of the population to SO_2 we should assume more and more pressure will be brought to bear to reduce all uses of SO_2. Therefore, finding alternatives to SO_2 use on fruits and vegetables is an important research area in the development of MPR fruits and vegetables (Sapers et al. 1989a, Sapers, Garzarella, and Pilizota 1990).

Ethylene Oxide

Ethylene oxide (C_2H_4O) (21 CFR Part 193.200) (Anon. 1992) has been used primarily to reduce microbial contamination and insect infestation in dried foods such as spices with maximum allowed levels at 50 ppm. There have been concerns that the toxicity of this compound or its reaction products, particularly in a_w situations ≤ 0.80. See Table 3-11 for effectiveness of this gas on several microorganisms at relative low a_w. Attempts to use this gas at higher a_w on fresh apple and potato plugs containing *E. coli*, *S. aureas*, and *C. botulinium* showed EO was not as effective as SO_2 as an antimicrobial (Figure 3-9) (Kaffezakis, Palmer, and Kramer 1969). As an enzyme inhibitor, the gas appears to have little effect on PPO activity (Figure 3-8).

Propylene Oxide

Propylene oxide (C_3H_6O), which exists as a gas, has not been studied to the same extent as EO. Its effectiveness is increased by higher

Table 3-10
Results of SO$_2$ Followed by CO$_2$ Treatment[a] of Potato Strips, Stored Under CO$_3$ at 21° C and 4° C for 45 Days

Determination	Results	
	21° C	4° C
Aerobic count/g	10	0
Anaerobic count/g	0	80
Color, visual	Slightly white	Normal
Color, Hunter La.b	85.9. 1.7. 14.2	84.3. 2.8. 13.1
Time until color change, h	>5	>5
pH	5.1	5.2
Soluble solids, %	4.5	3.5
Texture, lbf/100 g	787	717
Odor (sniff)	Normal	Normal
Free liquid, ml/100 g	9.4	12.2
Total SO$_2$, ppm	104	328
Free SO$_2$, ppm	0	0
Peroxidase inactivation, %[b]	79.2	87.4
Polyphenoloxidase inactivation, %[b]	100.0	100.0
Pectinesterase inactivation, %[b]	54.6	62.4

[a]The product was prepared as follows:
  Pretreatment:
    Treated with 100% SO$_2$, 5 min, 5 psi
    Evacuated, 5 min, 26 in Hg
    Flushed with 100% CO$_2$, 10 min
  Peeling: Steam
  Treatment:
    Evacuated, 5 min, 25 in Hg
    Vacuum broken with 10% SO$_2$ in CO$_2$, 5 sec, vacuum reduced to 20 in Hg
    Evacuated, 5 min, 25 in Hg
    Vacuum broken with 100% CO$_2$, 15 sec, vacuum reduced to 0 in Hg
[b]Percent reduction from activity before treatment.
(From Kramer et al. 1980.)

temperatures and concentrations and lower a_w. Bacteria are more resistant to this gas than molds and yeasts. There have been few reports of toxicity of this compound and its reaction products and most applications have been to dried foods such as starch, cocoa, gums, spices, and processed nutmeats (Wagner and Moberg 1989). Propylene oxide CFR 21 Part 380 (Anon. 1992) is a food additive permitted in the United States up to levels of as high as 700 ppm in glace fruits and dried prunes. All other allowed products—cocoa,

Table 3-11
D-values for Ethylene Oxide Sterilant of Some Foodborne Microorganisms

Organism	D^a	Concentration	Temperature[b]	Condition
C. botulinum 62A	11.5	700 mg/L	40	47% RH
C. botulinum 62A	7.4	700 mg/L	40	23% RH
C. sporogenes ATCC 7955	3.25	500 mg/L	54.4	40% RH
B. coagulans	7.0	700 mg/L	40	33% RH
B. coagulans	3.07	700 mg/L	60	33% RH
B. stearothermophilus ATCC 7953	2.63	500 mg/L	54.4	40% RH
L. brevis	5.88	700 mg/L	30	33% RH
M. radiodurans	3.00	500 mg/L	54.4	40% RH

[a] In minutes.
[b] °C.
(From Jay 1986.)

gums, processed nutmeats (except peanuts), processed spices, and starch—can have maximum levels of 300 ppm.

Ozone

Bacteria are more susceptible to ozone (O_3) (21 CFR 184.1563) (Anon. 1992) than yeasts and molds, with bacterial spores 10–15 times more resistant than vegetative cells. It appears that ozone attacks many vital constituents of microbial cells but actual cause of death is not known (Wagner and Moberg 1989). It is usually used to sterilize bottled water. U.S. Good Manufacturing Practices GMP's allow maximum residual level at time of bottling of 0.4 mg of ozone/L of bottled water. Its use in fruit and vegetable juices has been limited because of the oxidative properties of the gas.

Other Vapors

Acetaldehyde vapors have been used to control postharvest pathogens of fruits and vegetables, and vapors from 0.25% to 20% applied for 0.50–120 min at room temperature killed tested organisms. The

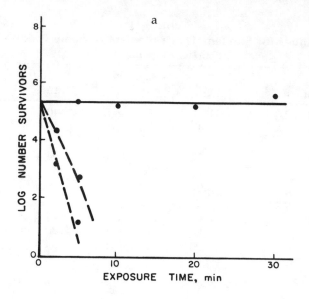

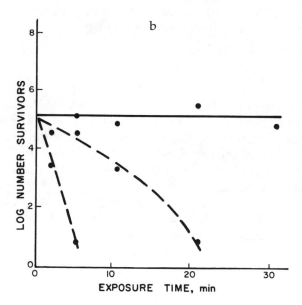

Figure 3-9 Survivor curves for microorganisms exposed to carbon monoxide (——) (CO), ethylene oxide (— —), (C_2HO), or sulfur dioxide (----)
(SO_2) gas: (a) *E. coli* on apple plugs, (b) *S. aureus* on apple plugs.

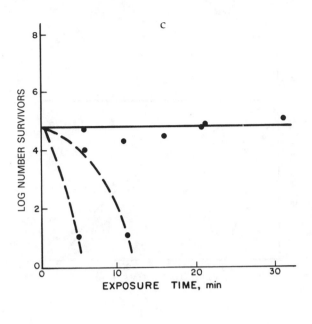

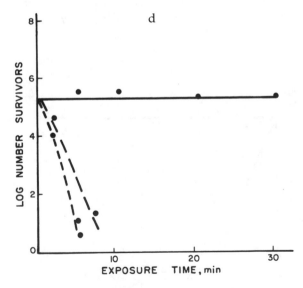

Figure 3-9 Continued   (c) *C. botulinum* on apple plugs, (d) *E. coli* on potato plugs.

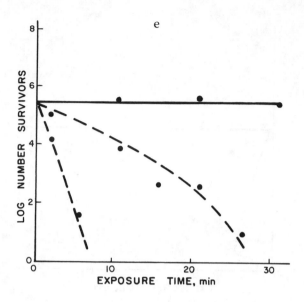

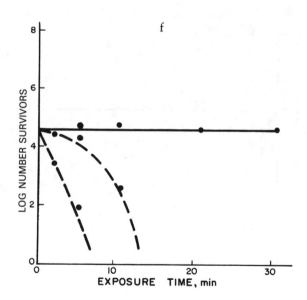

Figure 3-9 Continued   (e) *S. aureus* on potato plugs, (f) *C. botulinum* on potato plugs. (From Kaffezakis et al. 1969.)

organisms that cause postharvest decay in order of most sensitivity to acetaldehyde to least sensitivity were *Erwinia carotovora, Pseudomanas fluorescens, Botrytis cinerea, Monilinia fructicola, Rhizopus stolonifer,* and *Penicillium expansum.* Low levels of acetaldehyde can control pathogens in strawberries without injuring the product (Stadelbacher and Aharoni 1971).

Ethanol (C_2H_5OH) vapors have been used in preservation because of their desiccant and denaturant properties (Jay 1986b).

Cold Preservation

The cold preservation/refrigeration/chilled storage during distribution and retailing is a necessary and required step in MPR fruits and vegetables. This is based on the idea that refrigerated temperatures slow down most microbial growth and are effective to reduce enzyme activity. Freezing of foods as indicated earlier, although effective in reducing microbial and enzyme activity, may change some of the like-fresh qualities of the fruit or vegetable.

Most of the metabolic reactions of plant or human pathogens in fruit and vegetable tissue are enzyme catalyzed. The concern in MPR fruits and vegetables of enzyme activity make cold temperatures (the refrigerated chain) an absolute necessity for these products. The rate of enzyme-catalyzed reactions is controlled to a great extent by temperature. With every rise in temperature of 10° C (in the biological important ranges) there is a twofold increase in rate of reaction. This is known as the temperature coefficient (Q_{10}). On the other hand every 10° C reduction in temperature gives a similar decrease in the rate of biological activity. This means that the refrigeration hurdle is broad based and is a continuing factor in the preservation of MPR fruits and vegetables. As discussed in Chapters 7 and 9, the low temperature growing psychrotrophs are destructive microbes in refrigerated foods as compared with mesophiles and thermophiles.

In the past, temperatures below about 6° C were considered safe from food poisoning bacteria. However, with the advent of MPR foods exhibiting fairly long shelf-life, much more attention has been given to microorganisms that grow below about 6° C such as *C. botulinium* type E and nonproteolytic B and F strains, strains of *V. parahaemolyticus,* and *Y. entercolitica* (Jay 1986a). See also Chapters 7 and 9 for information regarding the above organisms and strains of hydrophila that are associated with gastroenteritis. Another foodborne disease caused by *L. monocytogenes,* a facultative anaerobe, has also been associated with low temperatures of 1° C up to 45° C with optimum at 30° –37° C and has become a major safety problem in MPR fruits and vegetables.

For fruits and vegetables there is a great deal of variation in ideal refrigerated temperatures. Some workers such as Jay (1986a) prefer to call temperatures between 10° and 15° C chill temperatures and temperatures between 0°–2° and 5°–7° C refrigeration temperatures. Since the composite Appendix Tables IIIA, IIIB, and IIIC (Anon. 1989a) give ideal temperature values from −1.7° to 21.1° C it is not possible to draw a distinct line between refrigerated and chilled temperatures because it depends to a great extent on the commodity studied. Chill-sensitive fruits that are sliced, diced, etc., such as citrus fruits and vegetables such as cucumbers and tomatoes, are considered to be MPR fruits or vegetables by definition.

Appendix Tables IIIA, IIIB, and IIIC (Anon. 1989a) do not attempt to predict shelf-life and safety for the commodities listed because of the minimal processing that may take place and could make the usual storage period different than that published data for intact items. Shelf-life and safety data for MPR fruits and vegetables have not yet been suitably developed in the public domain.

The preservation method required for all MPR fruits and vegetables that is emphasized throughout this text (Figure 1-2) has been refrigeration. A major problem associated with MPR fruits and vegetables is the possibility of temperature abuse during the time interval after preservation and packaging during distribution, transportation, storage, retailing, or wholesaling before use by the ultimate consumer. MPR fruits and vegetables are normally classified as extended shelf-life foods (ESL) and under best conditions should have a time–temperature indicator (TTI). The field has been studied extensively with mathematical analysis of the relationships between TIIs and chemical and sensory quantity attributes and the remaining shelf-life of food products (Taovkis and Labuza 1989; Wells and Singh 1988, etc.) The Anon (1991a) reference lists 23 recent patents, 21 commercial indicators (cold chain monitoring, partial and full history), and about 50 references that cover TTI devices for refrigerated and frozen foods. The field is much too extensive to cover in this section on cold preservation. One system described by LaGrenade, Schlimme, and Fields (1986) consists of (1) indicator labels printed in a bar code format that contain polymer compounds that change color as a result of accumulated temperature exposure; (2) a hand-held microcomputer with optical wand for reading the indicator label; and (3) software for data analysis and telecommunications. The accumulated time–temperature readings for fruit juices, vegetable juice, and fruit punch showed good correlations with objective and subjective color and flavor changes in these products at 3° C. These techniques are especially useful for manufacturers, and for storage and transportation operators and perhaps the consumer to track location and extent of temperature abuse in MPR products (Fields and Prusik 1986). For more information on TTIs also see Anon. (1991b) and Labuza and Breene (1989).

Preservation Using Irradiation

The term "irradiation of food" refers primarily to electromagnetic radiation. The electromagnetic spectrum can be separated on the basis of wavelength with the shortest wavelengths considered the most damaging to biological systems (Figure 3-10) (Jay 1986c).

Infrared Heating

This type of direct heating of food shown in Figure 3-10 located on the electromagnetic spectrum above 8,000 Å units is characterized by low penetration but can produce rapid surface cooking of the food which is highly undesirable in MPR fruits and vegetables unless carefully controlled. Brennan et al. (1976) suggested the results of infrared treatment can result in rapid sealing and browning of the outer layers. The process if used properly would tend to seal in volatile flavors and water which could be lost in preparation operations such as peeling, dicing, etc. This sort of heating would have to be combined with other forms of heat, for example, to get heat transfer to the center of the piece or be combined with other types of preservation hurdles for application to MPR foods. Heat has to be carefully managed to preserve the like-fresh quality of MPR fruits and vegetables.

Microwave

Microwave energy, which causes intermolecular friction, yields a heating effect and lies on the electromagnetic spectrum between the

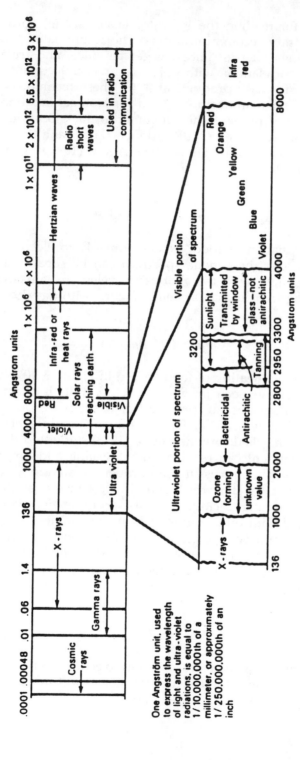

Figure 3-10   Spectrum charts. (From Jay 1986.)

infrared and the radiofrequency section (Figure 3-10). The use of in-depth heat treatment in MPR fruits and vegetables alone is limited because of possible effects on the like-fresh quality required in these types of foods. Microwave energy could be used in providing mild heat treatments in a hurdles system with other preservation methods. The cost of this type of heating as compared with steam, hot water, and the like would have to be considered.

Ultraviolet Light

Ultraviolet (UV) light, which has the most effective wavelength of about 2,600 Å (Figure 3-10), is nonionizing and is primarily absorbed by proteins which eventually causes cell death. Poor penetration of UV light limits its uses to surface treatment of food products (particularly meats and bakery products) before packaging and to processing surface and storages. It is more likely to be used in storage rooms to prevent surface mold growth on room surfaces and products.

Ionizing Radiation

There are a number of forms of ionizing energy that are approved for foods which are derived from radionuclide and machine sources. The only radionuclide sources permitted are cobalt-60 and cesium-137, both of which emit gamma rays and have good penetrating ability. There are many different types of electron beam generators or electron accelerators that produce x-rays or electron beams. X-rays have some physical characteristics similar to those of gamma rays, but the electron beams are somewhat different (Anon. 1989b). All of these treatments can be called "cold sterilization" if the levels of treatment are high enough, since very little heat is produced (Desrosier and Rosenstock (1960). These preservation methods have been selected for their *inability* to produce significant radioactivity in treated foods. For complete details for food processing applications for ionizing energy see Anon. (1989b) which summarizes much of the research of the late Dr. Eugen Wierbicki, his colleagues, and a host of experts.

A great deal of research has been conducted relating to the use of ionizing radiation for postharvest handling of fresh fruits and vegetables. An excellent review of this area has been published by

Table 3-12
Relative Tolerance of Fresh Fruits and Vegetables to Ionizing-Radiation Stress at Doses < 1 kGy

Relative Tolerance	Commodities
High	Apple, cherry, date, guava, longan, mango, muskmelon, nectarine, papaya, peach, rambutan, raspberry, strawberry, tamarillo, tomato
Moderate	Apricot, banana, cherimoya, fig, grapefruit, kumquat, loquat, lychee, orange, passion fruit, pear, pineapple, plum, tangelo, tangerine
Low	Avocado, cucumber, grape, green bean, lemon, lime, olive, pepper, sapodilla, soursop, summer squash, leafy vegetables, broccoli, cauliflower

(From Kader 1986.)

Kader (1986). Treatment of fresh fruits and vegetables with up to 1 kGy (100 k rad) was approved by the USFDA in 1986. Of course, this is lower than the treatments to inactivate most enzymes which range from 1,100,000 to 100,000,000 rads (Jay 1986c). According to Kader (1986) 1,152 reports on ionizing energy use on fruits and vegetables have been published in the last 30 years. The research to date suggests that ionizing energy has potential for some fresh fruits and vegetables but also has potential limitations. Kader (1986) suggests that this form of preservation should be considered as a supplement to refrigeration or some other postharvest procedure and this idea fully supports the use of the hurdle or barrier concept for preservation/extension of shelf-life.

The major biological problem in using ionizing energy on fruits and vegetables is that they are particularly sensitive to stress of all kinds (Kader 1986) and the unit operations used to prepare MPR fruits and vegetables would only increase these problems. The cutting, slicing, dicing, and shredding increase the respiration and ethylene production of MPR fruits and vegetables; therefore considerable research has yet to be conducted to determine those commodities that can benefit from ionizing energy. It would be expected that the same relative tolerance to ionizing-radiation stress that is found for intact fresh fruits and vegetables would also be found for MPR fruits and vegetables though these forms may be less tolerant (Table 3-12). From the table it is apparent that fruits

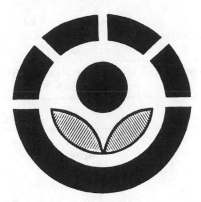

Figure 3-11   Logo to be used on irradiated foods. (From Kader 1986.)

are much more tolerant to ionizing radiation than vegetables such as broccoli, leafy greens, cucumbers, and the like.

In addition there are many other factors that affect the radiation processing quality of MPR fruits or vegetables and they include production area and cultivar, season and climate, quality of irrigation water, maturity at harvest, maturity and quality at time of processing, processing and preservation hurdles, and postharvest handling including careful control of refrigeration. Much of this information has not been developed for MPR fruits and vegetables treated by ionizing energy or combined preservation methods.

There is a social problem associated with use of ionizing energy to preserve MPR fruits and vegetables and it relates to the safety issue brought to consumers' attention by anti-irradiation advocacy groups. It should be emphasized that most food scientists agree that food irradiation can prolong the shelf-life of many foods and does not cause safety or health problems. Kantor (1989) in his article, "The great food irradiation controversy," covers in succinct form the advantages and disadvantages of using ionizing radiation and some of the consumer issues. Kantor (1989) feels there may be an uncertain future for irradiation that has to be faced by both industry and the government. There is an apparent reluctance by industry to use the irradiation logo shown in Figure 3-11 (Kader 1986).

In the *Packer*, which is a national weekly business newspaper of the fruit and vegetable industries, Waterfield (1991) has reported public opposition to the use of irradiated produce and the lack of retail initiative has severely hampered marketing of irradiated fresh fruits and vegetables, but they have not entirely vanished from the

124 Robert C. Wiley

Table 3-13
Irradiation: The Consumer's View
From Waterfield 1991.

In a 1990 survey of consumers who were asked to try irradiated and non-irradiated strawberries, here's how the irradiated produce fared:

Appearance		Color	
Worse	14.6%	Worse	8.8
Same	42.2%	Same	58.4%
Better	42.2%	Better	32.2%
Do not know	1.1%	Do not know	0.5%

Freshness		Storage Life	
Worse	12.7%	Worse	17.9%
Same	43.8%	Same	27.8%
Better	41.4%	Better	40.0%
Do not know	2.1%	Do not know	14.3%

Taste		Nutrition	
Worse	20.4%	Worse	2.2%
Same	41.9%	Same	17.6%
Better	27.6%	Better	4.4%
Do not know	10.1%	Do not know	75.8%

Firmness		Overall Quality	
Worse	18.9%	Pleased with Irradiated strawberries	80.1%
Same	41.9%		
Better	38.8%	Pleased with nonirradiated strawberries	67.2%
Do not know	0.5%		

scene. Table 3-13 gives a relatively recent viewpoint of consumer's reactions to irradiated and nonirradiated strawberries. It appears that consumers are about equally divided on the question of whether irradiated strawberries are higher in quality and data also imply considerable education is required relating to the nutritional quality of the treated and untreated strawberries.

There is considerable reluctance by the industry to gamble with ionizing energy as a hurdle to preserve MPR fruits and vegetables because of consumer doubts concerning its safety; however, a commercial concern in Mulberry, Florida is continuing to irradiate fruits and vegetables to reduce the use of chemicals and pesticides and reduce spoilage (Waterfield 1991). One anti-irradiation advocacy group has reported a consumer survey that showed 93% of the respondents expressed concern about irradiation, with 59% saying they are either "extremely" or "very" concerned (Anon. 1991a).

The issue seems to boil down to market-driven and safety aspects of irradiated MPR fruits and vegetables. Research and utilization of ionizing energy as hurdles for MPR fruits and vegetables seem to rest on suitable and stable markets for these products. This controversy must be satisfactorily resolved in the future.

Reduction of Water Activity (a_w)

This preservation method is well known and is based on the desiccation of food to a_w levels that will not support the growth of vegetative microbial cells. According to Jay (1986a) the approximate minimum a_w for the growth of the major groups of microorganisms is 0.9 for most spoilage bacteria, 0.88 for most spoilage yeast, and 0.80 for most spoilage molds. Many MPR fruits and vegetables have an a_w of 0.98 or above and are therefore very sensitive to reduction in a_w as a means of controlling microbial and enzyme activity. This means the use of reduction of a_w as a preservation measure for MPR fruits and vegetables must be carefully controlled to preserve the like-fresh quality demanded of the product.

This method is primarily involved in removing moisture from the food product by some sort of dehydration or by adding an ingredient with a high osmotic pressure which will form a complex with the water in the product (Huxsoll and Bolin 1989). If reduction of a_w is used as the sole preservation method for fruits and vegetables the process will dehydrate them. Although this system is considered to be a conventional hurdle in many food products, the use of a_w probably does not hold promise for MPR fruits and vegetables because of possible loss of the like-fresh character. Huxsoll and Bolin (1989) suggested a_w reduction by application of osmotic agents will result in products with undesirable flavor characteristics such as too sweet or too salty because high concentrations of sugars and salts are needed for osmotic dehydration.

The use of a_w reduction coupled with other preservation methods has been well covered by Scott (1989) and Lazar (1968). The former author has covered preservatives, pH, heat, and other interactions with a_w reduction, whereas the latter author utilized a_w reduction with freezing. So far little application and little reporting of a_w reduction as a single preservation method has been used for MPR fruits and vegetables because of troublesome quality problems in the like-fresh characteristics of the products, primarily crispness and turgidity. It is not likely that this method of preservation will find much use with MPR fruits and vegetables as defined by most workers.

Oxidation–Reduction Potential

The oxygen tension/atmosphere surrounding a food, whether it is aerobic or anaerobic or variations thereof, has a great effect on the growth of microorganisms. This type of preservation relates closely to controlled (CA) and modified atmosphere packaging (MAP) (Chapters 4 and 5), and various types of gas preservation (this chapter). These preservation methods may be included with other hurdles to preserve/maintain the like-fresh quality of MPR fruits and vegetables.

Oxidation will occur in atoms or groups of atoms when electrons are removed, whereas reduction occurs with the addition of electrons to a different atom or group of atoms, both reactions being simultaneous (Lindsay 1985). Oxidation can also be accomplished by the addition of oxygen to atoms or group of atoms.

The element or compound that loses electrons is generally considered to be oxidized whereas the elements/substrates that gain electrons become reduced. In these cases a substance that easily gives up electrons is a satisfactory reducing agent, whereas the one that easily takes up electrons is a satisfactory oxidizing agent (Jay 1986a).

As electrons are transferred from one compound to another, a potential difference is developed between the two reactive compounds and this is known as oxidation–reduction potential which is expressed by the symbol E_h. The potential difference can be measured instrumentally and expressed as positive, negative, or neutral millivolts (mV). (Christian 1980). A substance that becomes more highly oxidized will have a more positive electrical potential whereas the substance that becomes more reduced will have a more negative electrical potential. In MPR fruit processing it is important to maintain reducing (more anaerobic) conditions that are less favorable for aerobic growing conditions for molds and yeasts, which are major problems in these products. However, this opens the threat of C.

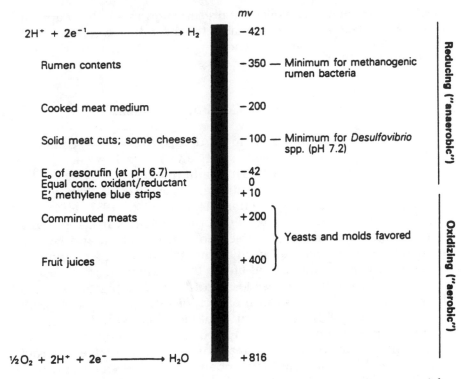

Figure 3-12 Schematic representation of oxidation–reduction potentials relative to the growth of certain microorganisms. (From Jay 1986.)

botulinium under strongly anaerobic conditions with highly negative E_h values in most vegetable products that have a pH < 4.6. Figure 3-12 shows the oxidation–reduction potentials for growth of several types of microorganisms and the foods in which they will reproduce (Jay 1986a). Those compounds that tend to maintain reducing conditions in fruits and vegetables are ascorbic acid and reducing sugars. Oxygen of course would oxidize a system and tend to maintain aerobic conditions in the food or package but may also increase respiration. For more on oxidation–reduction see Jay (1986a).

The oxidoreductases tend to catalyze both oxidation and reduction of substrates (Whitaker 1972b). However, most of these enzymes catalyze oxidation of the substrate and these include PPO (*o*-diphenol activity), PPO (hydroxylation reaction), catalase, PO, and lipoxygenase which collectively or individually affect color and flavor of MPR fruits and vegetables and intact fruits and vegetables as well if not properly controlled by preservation methods. It appears that a great deal of research remains to be conducted relative to O/R, control of microorganisms, and enzymes to preserve and extend shelf-life of MPR fruits and vegetables.

Preservation by Combined Methods

Recently a symposium was held to discuss the use of combined preservation methods to provide safety and satisfactory shelf-life for foods (Aguilera and Parada 1991). The hurdle technology suggested included heating, a_w control, chilling, pH control, O/R potential, preservatives, and competitive flora (Leistner 1978, 1987, 1991). The hurdles concept must be carefully applied to MPR fruits and vegetables and the issue is still subject-to much research and governmental regulation. Selected hurdles must maintain safety and like-fresh quality, and extend shelf-life of the product.

In Ibero American countries losses of fruits and vegetables range between 35% and 40% because of lack of satisfactory preservation facilities. Welte (1991) reports that combined method techniques that seem to imply mainly a_w and pH reduction for products such as pineapples, papayas, bananas, mangos, peaches, potatoes, carrots, etc. can prolong shelf-life longer than 1 year and still retain their like-fresh characteristics. The preservation parameters given were $0.92 < a_w < 0.97 \ a_w$, and pH control to 3.5. The use of minimal processes combined with proper packaging was shown to be much more complicated than those used for fresh intact nonprocessed fruits and vegetables. One unique application to extend storage life of oranges whose rinds are chill sensitive is to peel the fruit and store in a 5% O_2, 5% CO_2, and 90% N_2 gas mixture at 0° C. The peeled fruit was equal to the control in sensory and other quality characteristics. This is a good example of a combination preservation method of low temperature and modified gaseous atmospheres to improve shelf-life quality (Mannapperuma and Singh 1990).

Earlier sections of this chapter have introduced the concepts of one or more preservation methods in combination or combinations of preservation steps within a major preservation category such as combined chemical preservatives and multiple heat treatments at different stages of the processing and packaging cycle. Scott (1989) has reported the interaction of factors to control the microbial spoilage in refrigerated foods not specifically MPR fruits and vegetables. One is directed to her article which more specifically covers interactions of various preservation systems including water activity (a_w), pH, preservatives, temperature during storage, and modified atmosphere packaging. In the latter case, a warning should be re-emphasized that vacuum packaging utilizing MAP has the potential with minor temperature abuse to induce the growth and production of *C. botulinum* toxin.

Scott (1989) comments that there is information available on some interactions of preservation methods found in the literature and reported earlier in this chapter but there is a great need for studies of multiple variables (more than two) which might involve pH, a_w, preservatives, strains of pathogen, storage temperature, etc. This makes for very complicated experiments and it appears at the present time much of the work that is being conducted on preservation by combined methods is proprietary and found only in research institutes and industry laboratories.

The use of multiple preservation methods for MPR fruits and vegetables is even more complex because enzymes or living biological plant systems have to be dealt with as well as microorganisms, both pathogens and spoilage types, to extend shelf-life and provide like-fresh quality. This is a difficult task and challenge to the food industry in the years to come.

References

Aguilera, J.M. and E. Parada. 1991. Symposium: Food Preservation by Combined Methods Abstracts 609-613. Inst. of Food Tech. Meeting, June 1–5, 1991, Dallas, TX.

Aharoni, Y. and G.J. Stadelbacher. 1973. The toxicity of acetaldehyde vapors to post-harvest pathogens of fruits and vegetables. *Phytopathology* **63**:544–545.

Anon. 1987. *Webster's New Collegiate Dictionary*. Merriam-Webster, Springfield, MA.

Anon. 1989a. Guidelines for the development, production, distribution, and handling of refrigerated foods, 63 pp. Washington, DC: National Food Processors Association.

Anon. 1989b. Ionizing Energy in Food Processing and Pest Control: II Applications, 98 pp. Task Force Report. No. 115. Ames, IA: Council for Agricultural Science and Technology.

Anon. 1990. Refrigerated foods containing, cooked, uncured meat or poultry products that are packaged for extended refrigerated shelf-life and that are ready-to-eat or prepared with little or no additional heat treatment, 20 pp. Washington, DC: National Advising Committee on Microbiological Criteria for Foods.

Anon. 1991a. Just say no! In "Food Section," p. 5. *Washington Post* Wednesday May 29, 1991.

Anon. 1991b. Time–temperature indicators and integrators. New Technologies Bull. 4 July 1991, 22 pp. Campden Food and Drink Association, Chippen Campden, Gloucestershire GL55, 6LD England.

Anon. 1992. *Code of Federal Regulations, Food and Drugs* 21 Parts 170–199. Washington, DC: Office of the Federal Register National Archives and Records Administration.

Appert, N. 1810. The art of preserving animal and vegetable substances for many years. In *Introduction to Thermal Processing of Foods*, S.A. Goldblith, M.A. Joselyn, and J.T.R. Nickerson (eds.), pp. 2–147 (1985). Westport, CT: Avi Publishing now van Nostrand Reinhold.

Banks, J.G., S. Morgan, and M.F. Stringer. 1989. Inhibition of pasteurized bacillus spores by combination of nitrite, nisin, pH and organic acids. Techn. Memo No. 520, 71 pp. Chipping Campden, Gloucestershire GL55 6LD, England. Campden Food and Drink Research Association.

Bauernfeind, J.C. and D.M. Pinkert. 1970. Food processing with added ascorbic acid. *Adv. Food Res.* **18**:220–315.

Beuchat, L.R. and D.A. Golden. 1989. Antimicrobials occurring naturally in foods. *Food Technol.* **43**(1):134–142.

Blanpied, G.D. 1987. Symposium on factors that influence commodity response to controlled atmosphere storage. *HortSci* **22**:762–794.

Branen, A.L., P.M. Davidson, and B. Katz. 1980. Antimicrobial properties of phenolic antioxidants and lipids. *Food Technol.* **34**(5):42–53, 63.

Brennan, J.G., J.R. Butters, N.D. Cowell, and A.E.V. Lilly. 1976. Heat processing I. In *Food Engineering Operations*, pp. 237–239. London: Applied Science.

Buck, D.F., 1985. Antioxidant application. *The Mfg. Confectioner* June, p. 45.

Bunning, V.K., R.G. Crawford, J.G. Bradshaw, J.T. Peeler, J.T. Tierney, and R.M. Twedt. 1986. Thermal resistance of intracellular *Listeria monocytogenes* cells suspended in raw bovine milk. *Appl. Environ. Microbiol.* **52**:1398–1402.

Christian, J.H.B. 1980. In *Microbial Ecology of Foods*, Vol. 1, pp. 50–70. International Commission on Microbiological Specifications for Foods. New York: Academic Press.

Conner, D.E., R.E. Brackett, and L.R. Beuchat. 1986. Effect of temperature, sodium chloride and pH on growth of *Listeria monocytogenes* in cabbage juice. *Appl. Environ. Microbiol.* **52**:59–63.

Cort, W.M. 1982. Antioxidant properties of ascorbic acid in foods. In *Advances in Chemistry Series, No. 200, Ascorbic Acid Chemistry, Metabolism and Uses*, P.A. Seib and B.M. Tolbert (eds.), Chapter 22. Washington, DC: American Chemical Society.

Daeschel, M.A. 1989. Antimicrobial substances from lactic acid bacteria for use as food preservatives. *Food Technol.* **43**(1):164–166.

Davidson, P.M. and M.E. Parish. 1989. Methods for testing the efficacy of food antimicrobials. *Food Technol.* **43**(1):148–155.

Desrosier, N.W. and D.K. Tressler (eds.) 1977. *Fundamentals of Food Freezing*, 29 pp. Westport, CT: Avi Publishing, now Van Nostrand Reinhold.

Desrosier, N.W. and H.M. Rosenstock. 1960. *Radiation Technology in Food, Agriculture and Biology*. Westport, CT: Avi Publishing, now van Nostrand Reinhold.

Doyle, M.P., K.A. Glass, J.T. Beery, G.A. Garcia, D.J. Pollard, and R.D. Schultz. 1987. Survival of *Listeria monocytogenes* in milk during high-temperature short-time pasteurization. *Appl. Environ. Microbiol.* **53**:1433–1438.

Doores, S. 1983. Organic acids. In *Antimicrobials in Foods*, A.L. Branen and P.M. Davidson (eds.), pp. 75–109. New York: Marcel Dekker.

Dziezak, J.D. 1986. Preservative systems in foods, antioxidants and antimicrobial agents. *Food Technol.* **40**(9):94–136.

Ebert, A. 1990. Personal Communication, Chilled Food Association.

Fabian, F.W. and H.T. Graham. 1953. Viability of thermophilic bacteria in the presence of varying concentrations of acids, sodium chloride, and sugars. *Food Technol.* **7**:212–217.

Farber, J.M. 1989. Thermal resistance of *Listeria monocytogenes* in foods. *Int. J. Food Microb.* **8**:285–291.

Fields, S.C. and T. Prusik. 1986. Shelf like estimation of beverage and food products using bar code time–temperature indicator levels. In *The Shelf Life of Foods and Beverages*, pp. 85–96. Amsterdam: Elsevier.

Freeze, E., C.W. Shaw, and E. Galliers. 1973. Function of lipophilic acids as antimicrobial food additives. *Nature* **241**:321–322.

Friedman, S. 1991. Personal Communication, International Sourcing, Inc., South Ridgewood, NJ.

Gardner, W.H. 1966. Food Acidulants. Allied Chem. Corp. Bull., p. 44 New York: Allied Chemical Corp.

Huxsoll, C.C. and H.R. Bolen. 1989. Processing and distribution alternatives for minimally processed fruits and vegetables. *Food Technol.* **43**(2):124–128.

Jay, J.M. 1986a. Intrinsic and extrinsic parameters of foods that affect microbial growth. In *Modern Food Microbiology*, pp. 40–47. New York: Van Nostrand Reinhold.

Jay, J.M. 1986b. Food preservation with chemicals. In *Modern Food Microbiology*, pp. 259–296. New York: Van Nostrand Reinhold.

Jay, J.M. 1986c. Food preservation with irradiation. In *Modern Food Microbiology*, p. 298. New York: Van Nostrand Reinhold.

Kabara, J.J. 1981. Food-grade chemicals for use in designing food preservative systems. *J. Food Prot.* **44**:633–667.

Kabara, J.J. 1983. Medium chain fatty acids and esters. In *Antimicrobials in Foods*, A.L. Branen and P.M. Davidson (eds.), 109 p. New York: Marcel Dekker.

Kader, A.A. 1986. Potential application of ionizing radiation in postharvest handling of fresh fruits and vegetables. *Food Technol.* **40**(6):117–121.

Kaffezakis, J.G., S.J. Palmer, and A. Kramer. 1969. Microbiology of fresh apple and potato plugs preserved by gas exchange. *J. Food Sci.* **34**:426–429.

Kantor, M.A. 1989. The great food irradiation controversy. *Prof. San. Manag.* **17**:29–30.

Kato, N. 1981. Antimicrobial activity of fatty acids and their esters against film-forming yeast in soy sauce. *J. Food Safety* **3**:121–126.

Kramer, A., T.S. Solomos, F. Wheaton, A. Puri, S. Sirivicha, Y. Lotem, M. Fowke, and L. Ehrman, 1980. A gas exchange process for extending the shelf life of raw foods. *Food Technol.* **34**(7):65–74.

132   *Robert C. Wiley*

Labuza, T.P. and W.M. Breene. 1989. Applications of "active packaging" for improvement of shelf-life and nutritional quality of fresh and extended shelf-life food. *J. Food Proc. Pres.* **13**:1–69.

LaGrenade, C., D.V. Schlimme, and S.C. Fields. 1986. Computerized monitoring systems. Results of studies on shelf life of aseptic juices and puddings. In *Proceedings of the Fourth International Conference and Exhibition on Aseptic Packaging*, pp. 291–295, Princeton, NJ: Schotland Business Research.

Lazar, M.E. 1968. Dehydrofreezing of fruits and vegetables. In *Freezing Preservation of Foods*, 4th edit., Vol. 3, D.K. Tressler, W.B. Van Arsdel, and M.J. Copley (eds.), p. 347. Westport CT: Avi, now Van Nostrand Reinhold.

Leistner, L. 1978. Microbiology of ready to serve foods. *Fleishwirtschaft* **58**:2088–2111.

Leistner, L. 1987. Shelf-stable products and intermediate moisture foods based on meat. In *Water Activity: Theory and Applications to Food*, L.B. Rockland and L.R. Beuchat (eds.), pp. 295–327. New York: Marcel Dekker.

Leistner, L. 1991. Food preservation by combined methods. Abstract. 603 Inst. of Food Tech. Meeting. June 1–5, 1991, Dallas, TX.

Leistner, L. and W. Rodel. 1976. The stability of intermediate moisture foods with respect to microorganisms. In *Intermediate Moisture Foods*, R. Davies, G.G. Birch, and K.J. Parker (eds.), pp. 120–130. London: Applied Science.

Lewis, R.J. 1989. *Food Additives Handbook*. New York: Van Nostrand Reinhold.

Liewen, M.B. and E.H. Marth. 1985. Growth and inhibition of microorganisms in the presence of sorbic acid: a review. *J. Food Prot.* **48**:364–375.

Lindsay, R.C. 1985. Food Additives. In *Food Chemistry*. O.R. Fennima (ed.), pp. 643–644. New York: Marcel Dekker.

Linton, R.H., M.D. Pierson, and J.R. Bishop. 1990. Increased heat resistance of *Listeria monocytogenes* due to heat shock response. 1990 IFT Annual Meeting Abstract No. 445, p. 188.

Losikoff, M.B. 1990. The efficacy of a boiling water blanch on the inactivation of *Listeria monocytogenes* in diced celery. M.S. Thesis, University of Maryland, College Park, MD, 59 pp.

Mannapperuma, J.D. and R.P. Singh. 1990. Modified atmosphere storage of peeled oranges. Inst. of Food Tech. Meeting, June 16–20, 1990. Abstract 765, p. 250.

Marth, E.H. 1966. Antibiotics in foods—naturally occurring, developed, and added. *Residue Rev.* **12**:65–161.

Murdock, D.I. 1950. Inhibitory action of citric acid on tomato juice flat-sour organisms. *Food Res.* **15**:107–113.

Neiman, C. 1954. Influence of trace amounts of fatty acids on the growth of microorganisms. *Bacteriol. Rev.* **18**:147–152.

Orr, A. 1990. In *Vegetable Preservation*. DNA Plant Tech. Corp. U.S. Patent 4,919,948.

Oscroft, C.A., J.G. Banks, and S. McPhee. 1989. Inhibition of thermally-stressed bacillus by combinations of nisen, pH, and organic acids. Tech Memo No. 541, 33 pp. Chipping Campden, Gloucestershire GL55 6LD, England, Campden Food and Drink Research Association.

Peri, C. 1991. PACCP: Process analysis critical control point in food technology. *Ital. J. Food Sci.* **3**:5–10.

Pflug, I.J. and W.B. Esselen. 1963. Food processing by heat sterilization. In *Food Processing Operations*. M.A. Joslyn and J.L. Heid (eds.), 411 pp. Westport, CT: Avi Publishing, now Van Nostrand Reinhold.

Potter, N.N. 1968. *Food Science*. Westport, CT: Avi Publishing, now Van Nostrand Reinhold.

Puri, A. 1980. Biochemical changes in potatoes preserved by gas exchange. Ph.D. Dissertation, University of Maryland, College Park, MD, 120 pp.

Radovich, B. 1984. Listeriosis research present situation and perspective. *Akademiai Kiado* (Budapest), pp. 73–74.

Restaino, L., K.K. Komatsu, and M.J. Syracuse. 1982. Effects of acids on potassium sorbate inhibition of food-related microorganisms in culture media. *J. Food Sci.* 47:134–138, 143.

Robach, N.C. 1980. Use of preservatives to control microorganisms in food. *Food Technol.* 34(10):81–84.

Robinson, J.F. and C.H. Hills. 1959. Preservation of fruit products by sodium sorbate and mild heat. *Food Technol.* 13:251–253.

Rolle, R.S. and G.W. Chism III. 1987. Physiological consequences of minimally processed fruits and vegetables. *J. Food Quality* 10:157–177.

Rushing, N.B. and V.J. Senn. 1962. Effect of preservation and storage temperatures on shelf life of chilled citrus salads. *Food Technol.* 16:77–79.

Sapers, G.W., F.W. Douglas, Jr., A. Bilyk, A.-F. Hsu, H.W. Dower, L. Garzarella, and M. Kozempel. 1989a. Enzymatic browning in Atlantic potatoes and related cultivars. *J. Food Sci.* 54:362–365.

Sapers, G.M., K.B. Hicks, J.G. Philips, L. Garzarella, D.L. Pondish, R.M. Matulaitis, T.J. McCormack, S.M. Sondey, P.A. Seib, and Y.S. El-Ataway. 1989b. Control of enzymatic browning in apple with ascorbic acid derivatives, polyphenol oxidase inhibitors, and complexing agents. *J. Food Sci.* 54:997–1002.

Sapers, G.M., L. Garzarella, and V. Pilizota. 1990. Application of browning inhibitors to cut apple and potato by vacuum and pressure infiltration. *J. Food Sci.* 55:1049–1053.

Schlech, W.F., P.M. Lavigne, R.A. Bortolussi, A.C. Allen, E.V. Haldane, A.J. Wort, A.W. Hightower, S.E. Johnson, S.H. King, E.S. Nichols, and C.V. Broome. 1983. Epidemic listeriosis—evidence for transmission by food. *N. Engl. J. Med.* 308:203–206.

Schlimme, D.V. 1990. Personal Communication, University of Maryland, College Park, MD.

Scott, V.N. 1989. Interaction of factors to control microbial spoilage of refrigerated foods. *J. Food Prot.* 52:431–435.

Smith, E.E. 1938. The use of sodium benzoate in preserving food products. *Western Canner and Packer*, October 1938 (Reprint).

Sofos, J.N. and F.F. Busta. 1980. Alternatives to the use of nitrate as an antibotulinal agent. *Food Technol.* 34(5):244–251.

Stadelbacher, G.J. and Y. Aharoni. 1971. Acetaldehyde vapor treatment to control postharvest decay in strawberries. *Horticult. Sci.* 63:280 (abstr.)

Subramaniun, C.S. and E.H. Marth. 1968. Multiplication of *Salmonella typhimurium* in skim milk with and without added hydrochloric, lactic and citric acids. *J. Milk Food Technol.* **31**:321–326.

Svensson, Svante. 1977. Inactivation of enzymes during thermal processing. In *Physical, Chemical, and Biological Changes in Food Caused by Thermal Processing*, T. Hoyem and O. Kvale, (eds.), p. 202 London: Applied Science.

Taovkis, P.S. and T.P. Labuza. 1989. Applicability of time–temperature indicators as shelf life monitors of food products. *J. Food Sci.* **54**:783–788.

Wagner, M.K. and L.J. Moberg. 1989. Present and future use of traditional antimicrobials. *Food Technol.* **43**(1):143–146.

Waterfield, L. 1991. Lining up our kilorads. *The Packer* **98**(9):1A–2A.

Wells, J.H. and R.P. Singh. 1988. A kinetic approach to food quality prediction sing full-history time-temperature indicators. *J. Food Sci.* **53**:1866–1871, 1893.

Welte, J. 1991. Fruit preservation by combined methods. Abstract. 612 Inst. of Food Tech. Meeting. June 1–5, 1991, Dallas, TX.

Whitaker, J.R. 1972a. Polyphenol oxidase. In *Principles of Enzymology for the Food Sciences*, pp. 571–582. New York: Marcel Dekker.

Whitaker, J.R. 1972b. Introduction to the oxidoreductases. In *Principles of Enzymology for the Food Sciences*, pp. 545–548. New York: Marcel Dekker.

4

Packaging of Minimally Processed Fruits and Vegetables

Donald V. Schlimme and Michael L. Rooney

Introduction

A food package must protect and contain the product from the place and time of manufacture to the point of consumption (IFT 1991). Packaging of fresh produce using polymeric films has been practiced for several decades to contain and protect fruits and vegetables from environmental contaminants. Moreover, perforated polymeric packaging film has long been used successfully to reduce moisture loss from produce during storage, shipment, and display by reducing the magnitude of the moisture vapor deficit between the produce and its immediate in-package environment. In more current times, unperforated polymeric film packages have been used to minimize moisture loss and reduce respiration rate of produce commodities; most recently minimally processed fruits and vegetables have been packaged in polymeric film in an effort to maintain product quality while extending shelf-life.

135

The use of polymeric packaging material to establish a modified atmosphere around produce commodities and minimally processed refrigerated (MPR) products can achieve a degree of product "preservation." Indeed, the use of sealed, unperforated, polymeric packaging with carefully selected gaseous permeability characteristics in conjunction with appropriate prepackaging cooling/preparation and sanitation treatments is a major tool utilized to achieve adequate shelf-life for both unprocessed produce and minimally processed fruits and vegetables.

As recently as 1970 it was reported by Brody (1970) that "radishes are the only produce packaged in impermeable packages," that is, packaged in unperforated polymeric films, and that "packaged, mixed salad vegetables or cole slaw cabbage are often (packed) in a three-side sealed polyethylene pouch." Since 1970 considerable research has been conducted to elucidate and expand the use of permeable polymeric packaging for both produce commodities and MPR products. This chapter reviews MPR products packaging requirements as they are influenced by factors that mediate product quality retention and shelf-life extension, including pertinent physical and chemical characteristics of potential packaging plastics; passive and active alteration of in-package gas and moisture vapor concentrations; packaging materials selection and package design considerations; packaging safety considerations in terms of migration of chemicals from packaging materials to food; and finally transport packaging.

Requirements of a Package or Packaging Materials

According to Gibbons (1973), Kelsey (1978), Crosby (1981), Kumar and Balasubrahmanyam (1984), Myers (1989), Institute of Food Technologists (1991), and many others the functions of a food package include:

1. To prevent loss through leakage, spillage, or pilferage
2. To protect contents from external physical, mechanical, and biological forces throughout storage, transport, and marketing
3. To preserve contents and prevent or retard direct and indirect chemical decomposition or diminution of contained-product quality
4. To facilitate ease of filling and closure and provide satisfactory closure integrity

5. To withstand thermal conditions to which it will be subjected in both production and postproduction service
6. To provide acceptable appearance, color, texture, design, and labeling potential
7. To meet all regulatory criteria with regard to materials of construction
8. To provide for minimum or acceptable level of contained-product/package material interaction

It is necessary for food packaging materials to fulfill numerous functions; however, the primary role of food packaging is to contain a product while retarding or preventing loss of product quality, and to provide protection against environmental contaminants and facilitate transport, handling, storage, and marketing. Therefore, food packaging involves both the art and the science of preparing foodstuffs for storage, transport, and sale (Crosby 1981). Thus, major requirements of a food packaging material encompass at least several of the following factors: control of moisture transfer, control of gas transfer, protection from external physical or mechanical damage and biologic contamination, tolerance of routine storage environments without undue loss of functionality, adequate machinability and closure characteristics, compliance with regulatory requirements and guidelines, compatibility and utility with the product up to and even including its preparation for consumption, and cost effectiveness.

Parameters of Produce Quality Loss

Both fresh and minimally processed fruits and vegetables (see Chapter 1 for a definition of minimally processed fruits and vegetables) are living tissue undergoing catabolic metabolism including respiration (Institute of Food Technologists 1990). Furthermore, postharvest processing operations are essentially limited to those that take place prior to blanching (but may include mild, preblanch heating) or preservation treatments which are covered in Chapter 3. Thus, enzyme systems remain functional, and abundant microflora are present (Saddik, El-Sherbeeny, and Bryan 1985) on produce at the time it is packaged prior to storage or distribution. For example, King et al. (1991) reported the average microbe count per gram on the outer leaves and central portion of iceberg lettuce heads in a grocery store as 5.93 and 3.62 $\log_{10}$, respectively; 97.3% of the bacterial population was gram-negative rods with *Pseudomonas, Serratia,* and *Erwinia* species predominating with smaller numbers of yeasts ($2.77-4.27 \log_{10}$) and only occasional mold.

Degradation of postharvest produce quality is primarily a function of respiration and the onset and progression of ripening (in climacteric fruit) and eventual subsequent tissue senescence as energy stores are depleted in both climacteric and nonclimacteric commodities (Kader 1980), water loss via transpiration (Ben-Yehoshua 1985; Ben-Yehoshua et al. 1983; Bhowmilk and Sebris 1988; Kader 1986) decay and rot from the growth of plant pathogen storage microbes (Brecht 1980, El-Goorani and Sommer 1981), and mechanical damage during shipment (Shewfelt 1987; Wills et al. 1989). All four of these degradative processes function in concert to provide for a relentless loss of produce sensory and nutritional quality which is initiated immediately subsequent to harvest. It is important to recognize that minimal processing, in large measure, exacerbates this quality loss by increasing respiration rate (Myers 1989), increasing the rate of moisture loss via increasing cut surface area, and increasing the availability of released cellular nutrients for microflora utilization and growth (King and Bolin 1989). Moreover, as the tissue ripens/matures and begins to become senescent, its resistance to plant pathogen invasion/infection declines (El-Goorani and Sommer 1981; Rolle and Chism 1987).

Mechanical damage to produce that occurs during harvest and in postharvest handling operations inevitably results in some bruising and abrasion, scuffing, and skin/periderm damage which contributes to subsequent quality loss from induction of wound ethylene evolution which further increases respiration rate and accelerates the onset of senescence (Rolle and Chism 1987). Such damage, along with tissue damage due to slicing, cutting, trimming, and the like, allows cellular constituents including enzyme/substrates to intermix and induce discoloration reactions (O'Beirne 1990) as well as tissue softening (Rosen and Kader 1989).

Methods Available for Control of Produce Quality

Up to May 1985 approximately 4,000 research reports have been published on modified atmosphere (MA) (Kader, Zagory, and Kerbel 1989). In general, methods and treatments that decrease aerobic respiration rate (without inducing anaerobic respiration), decrease microbial populations or retard microbial growth rate, retard moisture loss from produce tissue, minimize mechanical damage to tissue, inhibit or retard enzyme-catalyzed softening and discoloration reactions, and delay ripening/maturation/senescence are employed to extend the shelf-life of fresh and minimally processed fruits and vegetables.

These methods include the following:

1. Decreasing produce temperature to a level just above the freezing point of the tissue or just above the threshold chill injury temperature of "chill sensitive" produce

2. Decreasing the concentration of oxygen in the atmosphere surrounding the produce to a point somewhat above the threshold where anaerobic respiration is initiated, that is, the "extinction-point" (Veeraju and Karel 1966)

3. Increasing the concentration of CO_2 in the atmosphere surrounding the produce to a level somewhat below the threshold level where physiological tissue injury or anaerobiosis is induced

4. Decreasing the concentration of ethylene in the produce tissue or in the atmosphere surrounding the produce

5. Maintaining relative humidity (RH) in the atmosphere or microenvironment surrounding the produce at levels that minimize tissue moisture loss but do not result in condensation of liquid water on the produce or inside package surface

6. Treating the produce with chemicals, additives, surface waxes, or radiation to reduce microbial populations, undesirable oxidation reactions, moisture loss, shrivel, discoloration, and softening and to delay the onset of senescence

7. Providing a concentration of CO in the atmosphere surrounding the produce sufficient to suppress microbial growth

8. Washing produce in potable water to reduce the magnitude of microbial load and remove cellular constituents discharged from cut/ruptured cells

Utilization of permeable polymeric films to achieve modification of package atmospheric gases concentration offers ample potential to extend produce shelf-life. When fresh or minimally processed fruits and vegetables are sealed inside plastic film packages of relatively low gas permeability, O_2 concentration decreases and CO_2 concentration increases as a consequence of tissue respiration. Eventually O_2 concentration is reduced to a level that induces tissue anoxia while there is a concomitant increase in CO_2 which intensifies the anaerobic environment in the package atmosphere. This results in anaerobic respiration in the produce which rapidly destroys produce quality via tissue breakdown, accumulation of ethanol and acetaldehyde, and development of off-flavor. In anaerobic respiration glucose is converted to pyruvate via the Embden–Meyerhof–Parnas (EMP) pathway. Pyruvate is then metabolized into acetaldehyde and ethanol (Wills et al. 1989). This undesirable consequence of plastic film packaging of fresh or minimally processed produce can be circumvented by the use of polymeric films which demonstrate reasonably high permeability to O_2 and CO_2. Conversely, using a plastic package that demonstrates very high permeability to O_2 and CO_2 can result in an internal package atmosphere high in O_2 (above 8%) and low in CO_2 (below 1–2%) that has minimal or, at best, only moderate potential to retard respiration and extend shelf-life. Unfortunately, the use of plastic packaging materials to achieve an *ideal* concentration of both O_2 and CO_2 within the sealed package is not yet possible for all produce commodities.

Modified Atmosphere Packaging of Fresh and Minimally Processed Produce

Utilization of polymeric film or other plastic materials such as semirigid trays of appropriate permeability to provide an internal package atmosphere concentration of O_2 and CO_2 that results in substantial reduction of produce respiration rate without inducing significant produce anaerobiosis is considered a major aspect of modified atmosphere packaging (MAP).

After lowering produce temperature, MAP (along with controlled atmosphere or CA storage) is considered to be the second most effective method for extending the shelf-life of fresh and minimally processed produce. According to O'Beirne (1990), lowering produce temperature reduces respiration by a factor of 2–3 ($Q_{10} = 2$–3) and use of an appropriate MA package can bring about an additional reduction in respiration rate as great as fourfold. However, it is recognized that MAP is not a replacement for proper temperature control (Hotchkiss 1988), and temperature modification is the most important factor in controlling respiration (Shewfelt 1986). MAP, in fact, is often included as one of the integral or crucial steps in the sequence of preservation or "processing" events that characterize minimally processed produce (Huxsoll and Bolin 1989). According to Ronk, Carson, and Thompson (1989) the quality and safety of refrigerated foods hinge on proper processing, appropriate packaging, and proper storage. MAP of produce is a dynamic process wherein the sealed package interacts with contained product (usually under careful temperature control) to ultimately provide for an equilibrium internal package gaseous atmosphere that will reduce product respiration rate, sensitivity to ethylene, and transpirational moisture loss as well as extend the lag phase of microbial growth and increase microflora generation time (Hotchkiss 1988).

There are two modes of MAP—passive and active (Zagory and Kader 1988). Passive MAP involves placing produce in a gas-permeable package, sealing the package, and then allowing produce respiration to reduce O_2 and increase CO_2 concentrations inside the package to a desired steady-state equilibrium. Active MAP involves placing produce in a gas-permeable package, evacuating the package atmosphere, and replacing it by flushing the unsealed package with a preselected mixture of O_2, CO_2, and N_2 gases (Smith, Ramaswamy, and Simpson 1990) followed by rapid sealing of the package. The flushing gas composition is usually selected to provide optimum levels of O_2 and CO_2 (with a balance of N_2) to immediately diminish the aerobic respiration rate of the particular produce, produce mixture, or MPR product being packaged. Active MAP may also include the utilization of absorbers or adsorbers inside the sealed package to scavenge O_2, CO_2, C_2H_4 (Kader, Zagory, and Kerbel 1989), and water vapor as well as the use of antimicrobial agents such as CO.

Factors that Affect MAP-Induced Atmosphere Within Sealed MA Packages of Produce

MA package selection and design has as its goal the achievement of a balance between the enclosed produce or MPR product respiration rate and film permeability to attain and maintain an acceptable equilibrium atmosphere within the package, that is, a MA that will delay ripening/maturation/senescence, and thereby extend product shelf-life. Achievement of this goal is dependent on a knowledge of several product and package parameters including:

Product factors

1. Respiration rate of the produce or MPR at the selected storage temperature

2. Respiratory quotient of the produce or MPR at the selected storage temperature

3. Quantity (mass) of the product to be placed inside the MA package

4. Oxygen and CO_2 concentrations necessary to approximately achieve optimum reduction of product aerobic respiration rate

Packaging film factors

1. Permeability of available polymeric packaging materials to O_2, CO_2, and water vapor at the selected storage temperature per unit thickness of packaging material

2. Effect of relative humidity on film permeability to O_2 and CO_2 (Hardenburg 1975)

3. Total surface area of the sealed package

4. Seal integrity of the package

5. Abuse resistance of the packaging film

Other factors

1. Free volume inside the package

2. Air velocity and relative humidity around the package

Polymeric Film Permeability

Permeability is defined as transmission of a penetrant through a resisting material (Kader, Zagory, and Kerbel 1989, 13). The permeability process in polymeric packaging materials is accomplished by activated diffusion where penetrant molecules dissolve in the film matrix and diffuse through it in response to a concentration gradient (Kester and Fennema 1986). The permeability coefficient (P) of polymeric films to a gas according to Crank (1975) is:

$$P = \frac{Jx}{A(p_1 - p_2)}$$

where

J = volumetric rate of gas flow through the film (at steady state)
A = area of permeable surface
x = thickness of the polymeric film
p_1 = gas partial pressure on side 1 of the film

p_2 = gas partial pressure on side 2 of the film

$p_1 > p_2$

The permeability coefficient includes the term (x) which provides a factor to account for film thickness. It is common practice to refer to permeability in terms of transmission rate of a given film as it is supplied. The film thickness must then be specified in order to allow comparison of gas and water vapor transmission rates among various thickness specifications for films of identical chemistry.

Respiring produce and MPR products utilize considerable oxygen, and plastic films that are suitable for use with fresh and minimally processed produce need to have relatively high O_2 permeability coefficients in order to avoid development of an anoxic atmosphere within the package. The diffusion of gases such as oxygen and carbon dioxide depends on the size, shape, and polarity of the penetrating molecule, and crystallinity, degree of crosslinking, and polymer chain segmental motion within the film matrix (Kader, Zagory, and Kerbel 1989; Kester and Fennema 1986). Giacin and Miltz (1983) provide an excellent presentation of the mathematical aspects of permeability of plastic packaging materials.

Table 4-1 presents gas transmission rates for several polymeric films that might be selected for use in MA packaging of fresh and minimally processed fruits and vegetables. In most instances rather wide ranges for gas transmission rates of polymer films are reported because of, among other factors, testing procedure variability; for example, moisture vapor transmission rate results obtained by one procedure on several specimens from the same sample of film may differ by as much as 10% from their average (ASTM 1987). In addition, the permeation characteristics of a given plastic film are approximately proportional to film thickness (Gibbons 1973), which also is variable within manufacturing tolerance limits. Moreover, during the production of plastic resins additives such as plasticizers, stabilizers, impact modifiers, fillers, lubricants, and antifog agents can be introduced to provide tailor-made materials for specific applications (Henkel 1973) and these additives can affect permeability characteristics. In addition, copolymers are also used during the manufacture of plastic resins which often affect finished product gas permeability characteristics; for example, an ethylene chain resin containing <5% vinyl acetate is defined as "polyethylene" (or as modified polyethylene) and the presence of the copolymer alters gas permeability of the film vis-a-vis polyethylene film without a copolymer.

Table 4-1
Permeability Characteristics of Several Plastic Films with Potential for Use as MAP of Fresh and Minimally Processed Produce.[a]

Film Type	Transmission Rates[b,c]		
	O_2	CO_2	H_2O Vapor
Low-density polyethylene (LDPE)	3,900–13,000	7,700–77,000	6–23.2
Linear low density polyethylene (LLDPE)	7,000–9,300	—	16–31
Medium-density polyethylene (MDPE)	2,600–8,293	7,700–38,750	8–15
High-density polyethylene (HDPE)	520–4,000	3,900–10,000	4–10
Polypropylene (PP)	1,300–6,400	7,700–21,000	4–10.8
Polyvinylchloride (PVC)	620–2,248	4,263–8,138	
Polyvinylchloride (PVC), plasticized	77–7,500	770–55,000	>8
Polystyrene (PS)	2,000–7,700	10,000–26,000	108.5–155
Ethylene vinyl acetate copolymer (12% VA)	8,000–13,000	35,000–53,000	60
Ionomer	3,500–7,500	9,700–17,800	22–30
Rubber hydrochloride (Pliofilm)[d]	130–1,300	520–5,200	>8
Polyvinylidine chloride (PVDC)[e]	8–26	59	1.5–5

[a]Values used to develop this table were obtained from numerous reference sources including: Anon. 1979; Anon. 1982; Ballantyne 1986; Ballantyne, Stark, and Selman 1988; Brydson 1982; Crosby 1981; Davies 1987; Gibbons 1973; Gopal 1984; Hall, Hardenburg, and Pantastico 1975; Jenkins and Harrington 1991; Kader, Zagory, and Kerbel 1989; Labuza and Breene 1989; Miles and Briston 1979; O'Beirne 1990; Sacharow 1976; Zagory and Kader 1988.

[b]O_2 and CO_2 transmission rates are expressed in terms of $cm^3 \ m^{-2} \ day^{-1}$ at 1 atm pressure differential for film 0.0254 mm (1 mil) thick at 22–25°C at various or unreported RH.

[c]H_2O vapor transmission rates are expressed in terms of $g \ m^{-2} \ day^{-1}$ at 37.8°C and 90% RH.

[d]Pliofilm is the registered trademark of a commercial film material no longer used for MAP of fresh produce.

[e]PVDC is a polyvinylidene chloride film that is considered to be a good gas and moisture barrier and is included as a contrast to the other films which have much lower gas barrier characteristics; PVDC cannot be used for MAP of fresh produce because of the low O_2 and high CO_2 concentrations generated in the package atmosphere, that is, due to its very low permeability to O_2 and CO_2.

Copolymerization of ethylene monomer with an octene monomer results in formation of linear low density polyethylene (LLDPE). Copolymerization of ethylene monomer with a low amount ($<5\%$) of vinyl acetate monomer reduces final copolymer crystallinity, thereby increasing flexibility and permeability and reducing hardness (Duncan 1987). Conversely, increasing polymer crystallinity decreases permeability to gases and vapors (Sacharow 1976). Thus, a vast array of formulation/manufacturing variables as well as permeability measurement anomalies result in published permeability data being quite variable for any given class or type of polymeric packaging film. Standard procedures for testing film permeability to gases and moisture vapor are published (ASTM 1986, 1987). Additional detail related to measuring permeability of films to gases is provided by Giacin et al. (1984), Demorest (1989), and Rooney (1989). A tabular listing of the properties of polymeric films which includes water vapor transmission rate (WVTR) and gas transmission data is found in Anon. (1984).

Polymeric Films Used for MA Packaging of MPR Products

Some Basic Definitions

Polymers are a class of organic chemicals that have long, high molecular weight (up to 10^6) molecules capable of being synthesized from or depolymerized into numbers of chemically identifiable, simple recurring units termed monomers (Oswin 1975). More specifically, plastics (including films used for MA packaging) are formulations containing one or more high molecular weight polymers in combination with various additives such as plasticizers, fillers, stabilizers, etc. (Barmore 1991). They are synthetic materials produced by the application of heat and pressure and while solid in the finished state are at some stage of their manufacture made liquid and capable of being formed into various shapes (Sacharow 1976).

A plastic film is a planar flexible material having a thickness of 0.254 mm or less (Sacharow 1976), that is, thick enough to be self-supporting but thin enough to be flexed, folded, or creased without cracking; the upper limit of thickness for a film is vague but usually lies between 75 and 150 µm (approximately 0.075 and 0.150 mm) (Oswin 1975). More recently an upper thickness limit of 380 µm has been suggested (Jenkins and Harrington 1991).

Thermoplastic polymers are those that, when heated to a proper temperature, become soft and become hard again only on cooling. In most cases, the cycle of heating to soften and cooling to harden or cure may be repeated time and time again (Henkel 1973; Sacharow 1976). Polymers undergo some degradation under extrusion conditions and usually require addition of stabilizers or antioxidants even for first-time extrusion. Additional antioxidant can be required when scrap material is reextruded. Polypropylene is particularly readily oxidized compared with polyethylene. Polyvinylchloride is subject to decomposition to form hydrogen chloride and requires the use of extruders made from highly corrosion-resistant steel. Most plastics used to manufacture food packaging film are thermoplastics (Crosby 1981). The most convenient polymers for film making are those thermoplastics that have glass-transition temperatures below 0° C, melting temperatures above 100° C, and decomposition temperatures at least 50° C higher than the melting temperature (Oswin 1975). Polystyrene (PS), polyvinylchloride (PVC), polypropylene (PP), ethylene–vinyl acetate (EVA), nylon, ionomers, and acrylics are all thermoplastics (Henkel 1973). Most thermoplastics can be regarded chemically as derivatives of ethylene ($CH_2{=}CH_2$). They are often referred to as (1) vinyl plastics since they all contain the vinyl grouping ($CH_2{=}CHX$), or (2) polyolefins since their monomers are only unsaturated hydrocarbons (Jenkins and Harrington 1991).

Film manufacture consists of processing any thermoplastic by melting, usually under heat and pressure in an enclosed Archimedean screw; feeding the melt to and through a shaping orifice, such as a circular or slit die, at a metered rate; cooling; and removing to a wind-up station (Oswin 1975; Sacharow 1976). As the molten plastic leaves the die during extrusion it can be formed into a film in several ways. Frequently film is blown with compressed air as it leaves a circular die, giving a tubular bubble that has the required film thickness. The film can often be oriented as it is blown either uniaxially (by as little as ×2) or biaxially to a total size increase of as much as ×80 in both directions (Jenkins and Harrington 1991).

The basic physics of stress-induced orientation of plastic films is well described by Benning (1983). In short, when a plastic is above its glass transition temperature (T_g) applied stress causes polymer chains to unfold, disentangle, and straighten and slip past adjacent chains. Then, rapid cooling to a temperature below T_g results in freezing this structure into the film as it is taken up onto rolls. This uniaxial orientation leads to increased strength in the strain direction but not in the transverse direction. Biaxial orientation increases strength in both directions and this two-directional orientation can be balanced in terms of magnitude or degree. Thus, a soft polyolefin-like polyethylene can be transformed into a stronger, harsher film by biaxial orientation. Moreover, orientation of a plastic film alters its permeability to gases and water vapor (Oswin 1975).

Heat-shrinkable films take advantage of part of this "frozen" orientation on reheating (Benning 1983) and decrease in size as, for example, in the shrink wrapping of individual fruits. So long as the film is not heated above the temperature at which orientation occurred it retains its oriented dimensions. However, if the film is heated above orientation temperature, the phenomenon of "plastic memory" exerts itself, molecules seek to return to their former unoriented state, and the film shrinks (Griffin, Sacharow, and Brody 1985).

Film can be cast through a slit die when closer thickness tolerances are required and can be readily oriented in the machine direction by control of the speed of the drive and take-up rolls and by other treatments. Biaxial orientation of cast film is achieved by tentering in an oven in which the heated film is stretched in the transverse direction by a series of "grips" exerting stress on the edge of the film (Benning 1983). After orientation, films are often annealed and heat set. The tentering process can result in waste film at the edges, compared with oriented blown film, but offers higher film production speeds and easier control of film thickness (Benning 1983).

Copolymerization is a process whereby more than one type of monomer is reacted to form a chain macromolecule that contains both monomers in approximately equivalent proportion to the original monomer proportion. Conversely, a homopolymer plastic is formed by the polymerization of a single monomer. Coextrusion is a process in which two or more plastic films from two or more extruders are forced through concentric dies to give a film bubble consisting of two or more layers. The coextruded films produced offer better control of gas and water vapor permeability and improved performance properties such as better heat-sealability or "slip" (Jenkins and Harrington 1991).

The term resin invariably means the pure polymer produced by either polycondensation or polyaddition reaction of monomers using heat, pressure, and catalysts (Sacharow 1976).

Family of Ethylenic Thermoplastics

Figure 4-1 is a representation of monomers, taken from Crosby (1981), used to manufacture ethylenic thermoplastics and demonstrates their chemical relationship to the ethylene monomer.

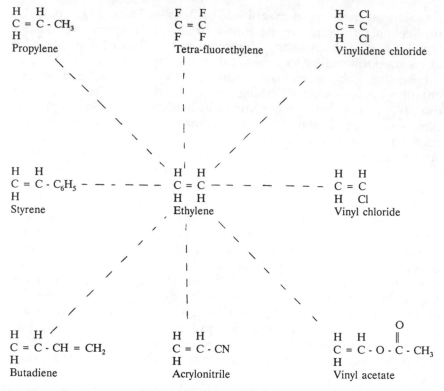

Figure 4-1 Monomers used to manufacture ethylenic thermoplastics (From Crosby 1981.)

Principal MA Plastic Packaging for Potential Use with Minimally Processed Fruits and Vegetables

Various plastic films have been used as packages for fresh fruit and vegetables including low-density polyethylene (LDPE), high-density polyethylene (HDPE), thin-gauge polypropylene (PP), polystyrene (PS), various grades of polyvinyl chloride (PVC), and rubber hydrochloride (Pliofilm) (Ben-Yehoshua et al. 1983; Kader, Zagory, and Kerbel 1989; Kumar and Balasubrahmanyam 1984; O'Beirne 1990). Ethylene vinyl acetate (EVA) and ionomers also have potential to be utilized for packaging both fresh and minimally processed fruits and vegetables (O'Beirne 1990).

According to Radian Corporation (1986) the United States market for plastics utilized for packaging in 1980 was 4,546,800 tons and comprised 28.4% of the United States plastics market. Of this quantity LDPE, HDPE, PS, PP, and PVC were 45.8, 20.5, 13.5, 7.2, and 4.4%, respectively. Obviously only a fraction of this amount was used for MA packages for fresh and minimally processed produce. According to Rice (1989) approximately 500–600 million MA packages per year were utilized in the United States retail market in the late 1980s. In contrast she estimated the number of MA packages in the European retail marketplace to be about 3 billion.

The United States loses about 6 billion pounds (2.7 billion kg) of produce a year to spoilage (Rice 1989). According to Labuza and Breene (1989) produce waste in the United States exceeds 15–20% from field to home. Expanded use of MAP techniques for fresh fruits and vegetables could contribute to significant reductions in such losses. Furthermore, the use of MAP for cut produce will likely continue to grow both for food service and supermarkets (O'Beirne 1990; Rice 1989).

The major thermoplastic materials with potential for use in MA packaging are characterized below using information obtained from an array of sources (Anon. 1979; Anon. 1991; Baijal 1982; Brydson 1982; Crompton 1979; Crosby 1981; Datta 1984; Davies 1987; Duncan 1987; Gopal 1984; Henkel 1973; James 1984; Kader, Zagory, and Kerbel 1989; Labuza and Breene 1989; Miles and Briston 1979; O'Beirne 1990; Oswin 1975; Peters 1987; Radian Corp. 1986; Sacharow 1976; Sacharow and Griffin 1973; Swett 1987; Theis 1987; Thompson 1987; Tomanek and Meyer 1987).

Polybutylene

Polybutylene refers to a group of polymers comprised primarily of poly-1-butene. It is produced by the polymerization of the 1-butene monomer ($CH_2{=}CH{-}CH_2{-}CH_3$) using a catalyst under high pressure at 65° C to provide the polymer:

$$\left[\begin{array}{c} CH_2{-}CH \\ | \\ CH_2 \quad {-}CH_3 \end{array} \rule{2cm}{0pt} \right]_n \begin{array}{c} {-}CH_2{-}CH_2 \\ | \\ CH_2{-}CH_3 \end{array}$$

Polybutylene can also include 1-pentene, propylene, and ethylene as comonomers. Polybutylene has good tear strength and puncture resistance and is used for food and meat packaging. When orientated it offers a range of stiffness and toughness characteristics useful in shrink packaging and as an inflatable dunnage for shipping a wide range of goods.

Low-Density Polyethylene

LDPE is a branched-chain polymer produced by polymerization of the ethylene monomer (CH_2=CH_2) and has a molecular weight range of 14,000–1,400,000. Most LDPE is produced by high pressure (1,000–3,000 atm) addition polymerization at 150–350° C using a radical initiator such as oxygen or an unstable peroxide to yield a resin having density ranging from 0.910 to 0.935 g cm^{-3}. LDPE with densities between 0.926 and 0.940 g cm^{-3} may be referred to as medium-density polyethylene (MDPE). The United States LDPE film market in 1990 was 1,361,000 tons. Permeability data are presented in Table 4-1.

LDPE resin produced using the best catalysts has no more than one side chain per 500 ethylene units (Oswin 1975). This chain branching disturbs the regularity of the arrangement of atoms and hence produces a low degree of crystallinity (55–70%) which results in greater permeability to gases and vapors than the less branched, more crystalline HDPE (Crompton 1979). LDPE can be tailored to serve a wide range of functions. For example, LDPE pallet stretch wrap has a carefully chosen wide molecular weight range to provide both strength and cling. LDPE can be made shrinkable by blending it with HDPE or by radiation induced crosslinking.

Polyethylene, containing particles of a variety of inorganic filler materials, is marketed in Japan as a freshness preservative film (Katsura 1989). One of the effects of using mineral fillers is to perforate the PE, allowing for increased transmission rate of CO_2 while sacrificing fine control of O_2 concentration. Future developments in this area may well focus on gaining such control.

High-Density Polyethylene

HDPE has a very ordered linear structure with little branching such that the polymer is highly crystalline (75–90%). It thus has greater tensile strength, hardness, and stiffness than LDPE but has less impact strength and less permeability to gases and vapors and much reduced clarity. HDPE has a density greater than 0.940 g cm^{-3} with a typical density range of 0.955–0.970 g cm^{-3} and an average molecular weight of 125,000 (range of 90,000–175,000). In addition, two specialty grades of HDPE are produced: high molecular weight HDPE (HMW-HDPE) and ultra-high molecular weight HDPE (UHMWPE) with molecular weight ranges of 200,000–500,000 and >3,000,000, respectively. They are similar to HDPE but have greater abrasion

resistance and impact strength. MDPE copolymers (formed by adding 1-butene or 1-hexene or polypropylene to the HDPE polymerization reactor) increase branching along the PE carbon backbone
and thereby reduce crystallinity and increase gas permeability. The
United States HDPE film market in 1990 was 295,000 tons.

HDPE is produced from the ethylene monomer ($CH_2=CH_2$) using
a coordination catalyst and temperatures of 70°–250° C and pressures typically less than 102 atm. HDPE has the formula
$CH_3-(-CH_2-CH_2-)-_n$ H. Coextrusion of HDPE layers a few mi-
crometers thick with other plastic films gives finished films with
properties that allow side-specific applications. At the same time
finished film gas and water vapor permeability can be varied. Permeability data are presented in Table 4-1.

Polypropylene

PP is produced by the polymerization of the monomer propylene
($CH_2=CH-CH_3$) in a reactor, at between 5 and 40 atm pressure and
50°–90° C temperature, with a catalyst and <1% hydrocarbon solvent. A highly crystalline (65–70%) form of PP (isotactic form where
pendant methyl groups are all on the same side of the carbon backbone) is the useful form of the homopolymer whose formula is:

$$CH_2=\overset{\displaystyle CH_3}{\underset{\displaystyle |}{C}}\left[CH_2-\overset{\displaystyle CH_3}{\underset{\displaystyle |}{CH}}-CH_2-\overset{\displaystyle CH_3}{\underset{\displaystyle |}{CH}}-CH_2-\overset{\displaystyle CH_3}{\underset{\displaystyle |}{CH}}\right]_n$$

The homopolymer has a density of 0.900–0.905 g cm^{-3}. Ethylene,
used as a comonomer, improves low-temperature performance and
widens the heat-sealing temperature range. In 1990 268,000 tons of
PP film (both oriented and unoriented) were used in the United States.

Orientation produces a film (OPP) with a lower permeability to
gases and water vapor than unoriented, blown film (PP) and cast
film (see Table 4-1). PP is widely used as a coextrusion with biaxially
oriented PP (BOPP) as a center film layer between lower melting
point copolymers on either side. This allows for heat sealing without shrinkage. Blown film processes are better for thin films (< ca.
15 μm thick), whereas tenter-frame orientation is better for thicker
films (especially above 25 μm). The permeability of oriented and
unoriented PP film to gases and water vapor is presented in Table
4-1.

Polyvinyl Chloride

PVC is manufactured from the polymerization of vinyl chloride monomer ($CH_2{=}CHCl$) by four different polymerization technologies. In 1981 83% of the United States market used PVC manufactured by the process of suspension polymerization, and 125,000 metric tons of PVC film were marketed. Typical operating parameters for PVC production by the suspension process are a temperature of 45°–55° C and the use of water, monomer, suspension stabilizer, emulsifier, and an initiator in the reactor to produce PVC homopolymer $-\!(\!-CH_2-CHCl-\!)\!-_n$ with substantially amorphous structure (atactic) and a density of about 1.4 g cm^{-3}. Plasticized PVC has a density of 1.16–1.35 g cm^{-3}.

Any of numerous plasticizers are used for film production in order to minimize brittleness; stabilizers and lubricants are also added during resin production. Such compounding and processing can provide polymers with intermediate barrier properties that are capable of being used to produce film packages for fresh produce. Due to the proximity of PVC's decomposition and processing temperatures, the addition of 1–2% heat stabilizer is necessary in order to minimize subsequent HCl evolution. Thin, biaxially oriented PVC film is used for shrink-wrapping fruit and vegetables, and is sometimes copolymerized with vinyl acetate monomer to provide a softer film. In low molecular weight resins, internal porosity is of critical concern due to potential monomer migration in food contact applications. PVC used for food packaging must be made in equipment capable of removing traces of monomer to <1 ppm. In 1990 the United States market for PVC film for packaging was 143,000 tons. Gas and water vapor permeabilities of PVC film are presented in Table 4-1.

Polystyrene

PS is produced by the polymerization of the styrene monomer ($CH_2{=}CH\ C_6H_5$) to give general purpose polystyrene (GPPS) which is a pure homopolymer $[-\!(\!-CH_2-CHC_6H_5-CH_2-CHC_6H_5-\!)\!-_n]$. The absence of comonomers or modifiers, such as rubber, makes GPPS brittle. Impact polystyrene (IPS) is produced by the addition of either polybutadiene or styrene–butadiene rubber to the styrene monomer. These remain as discrete particles dispersed in the finished polymer resin. This lowers tensile strength, hardness, and the softening point and overcomes the brittleness of GPPS. When biaxially oriented, tangled IPS molecules (MW 54,000–416,000) are stretched and arranged in planar form, giving a heat shrinkable PS characterized by high clarity and permeability to vapors and gases. In 1990 98,000 tons of oriented PS film were used in the United States. The rubber content of IPS ranges from 3.4 to 14.5%, with density ranging from 1.02 to 1.05 g cm^{-3}. The permeability of IPS film to gases and water vapor is presented in Table 4-1.

PS is foamed by inclusion of volatile materials such as hexane which form bubbles on extrusion to give strong, expanded PS which has excellent cushioning properties and is used to manufacture nonreturnable trays or boxes for produce. In Europe expanded PS boxes are used for shipping grapes, cherries, and tomatoes. Large boxes can be made using 40 kg m^{-3} density PS that can be reused for more than one shipping trip. Superior protection, as compared to conventional corrugated shipping cases with paper pulp interleaves, can be achieved by using expanded PS interleaves. For produce such as apples and tomatoes the cushioning properties of expanded PS sheet can reduce bruising in shipment, especially when individual fruit are prevented from moving in expanded PS trays by shrink-wrapping (Miles and Briston 1979).

Ethylene–Vinyl Acetate Copolymers

EVA is similar to LDPE in many characteristics; it is greater in clarity and has high flexibility and impact resistance. The vinyl acetate (VA) monomer (CH_2=CH—O—$COCH_3$) can be polymerized using a free radical initiator to produce polyvinyl acetate

$$\left[\begin{array}{c} -CH_2-CH- \\ | \\ O-C-CH_3 \\ \| \\ O \end{array} \right]_n$$

in a reactor at 70°–90° C, but the VA homopolymer is not used as a packaging film. However, when ethylene is copolymerized with vinyl acetate (VA) a family of copolymers is formed that have a range of applications in food packaging because strength increases with VA content. Concurrently, the film becomes more elastic and blocking increases. The clarity of the EVA film which results from decreased crystallinity (as compared to LDPE) must therefore be sacrificed by the addition of antiblocking agents and slip additives at high VA levels. EVA plastic films with VA levels from 6 to 18% are used as tie layers for coextrusion with the low VA levels being found in self-supporting films. EVA (12% VA) is a highly branched, random copolymer with reduced crystallinity. The permeability of EVA to O_2 and CO_2 is in the approximate same range as LDPE when VA level is 12%, but the WVTR is much higher than that of LDPE (see Table 4-1). Increased strength and excellent cling properties make EVA a good material for stretch wrapping of unit loads such as palletized shipping cases. In 1990, 304,000 tons of EVA film was used in the United States market.

Rubber Hydrochloride—Pliofilm®

Rubber hydrochloride was introduced commercially in 1934. This development is considered to be a milestone in the flexible packaging industry, because it marks the development of the first noncellulosic, transparent thermoplastic film (Sacharow 1976). Plasticized varieties of rubber hydrochloride film have moisture vapor and gas transmission rates that depend on the amount of plasticizer used, that is, as plasticizer concentration increases, permeability to vapor and gases also increases. Pliofilm is rather impermeable to gases (see Table 4-1) and in early research with produce it was found that Pliofilm could not be successfully used due to the development of anaerobic conditions within the package that could be circumvented only by perforating the film. Pliofilm is no longer used to package produce (Kader, Zagory, and Kerbel 1989).

Ionomer

Acid copolymer resins are thermoplastic polymers manufactured by copolymerization of ethylene monomer with a vinyl monomer having an acid residue such as methacrylic acid

$$(CH_2{=}\ \overset{\displaystyle CH_3}{\underset{\displaystyle |}{C}}{-}COOH)$$

(Miles and Briston 1979). They are used primarily as tie layers in coextrusions where some of the acid groups are neutralized to form salts with metallic ions and the polymer chains become crosslinked by ionic attraction. As a consequence, ionomers provide excellent hot-tack at heat sealing and allow for packages that resist puncture (Jenkins and Harrington 1991). The structure of a typical ionomer may be represented as:

$$\left[CH_2-CH_2\right]_m \left[\begin{array}{c} CH_3 \\ | \\ CH_2-C \\ | \\ C=O \\ | \\ O(-) \end{array}\right]_n$$

$\dashrightarrow Me^*$

$$\left[CH_2-CH_2\right]_m \left[\begin{array}{c} O(-) \\ | \\ C=O \\ | \\ CH_2-C \\ | \\ CH_3 \end{array}\right]_n$$

*a metal cation with either one or two positive charges, for instance Na^+ or Zn^{2+}; not all carboxylic acid moieties are neutralized and therefore ionic bonding is incomplete

DuPont's "Surlyn A", developed in 1964, is an example of a typical acid copolymer or ionomer. Packaging films made of ionomer have good sealability, oil and fat resistance, high transparency, and excellent toughness (Henkel 1973; Miles and Briston 1979). The permeability of ionomer to O_2, CO_2, and water vapor is presented in Table 4-1.

Linear Low Density Polyethylene

LLDPE is a copolymer of ethylene with butene, hexene, or octene, and it combines the properties of HDPE and LDPE. The presence of the comonomers confers a more highly crystalline structure than that present in LDPE but with a controlled number of short branches. LLDPE is prepared in the presence of a Ziegler catalyst at pressures of ca. 20 atm.

The properties of the resulting copolymer (which has a density akin to that of LDPE) are a consequence of its higher degree of crystallinity. It is tougher and used at lower thickness than LDPE. LLDPE provides strong heat seals and has gained a large share of the market of other polyolefins. In 1990 the United States film market for LLDPE was 562,000 tons. The structure of a butene-derived LLDPE is represented as:

$$\left[\begin{array}{c} CH_2-CH_2 \\ | \\ CH_2CH_3 \end{array}\right]_m \left[CH_2-CH_2\right]_n$$

Substantially enhanced (up to 300%) impact and tear strength are obtained if hexene or octene are used as comonomers instead of butene. Physical properties such as haze and gloss can be inferior to those of LDPE but can be offset by blending with LDPE. The permeability of LLDPE to O_2 and water vapor is presented in Table 4-1.

Relationship of O_2 and CO_2 Permeability for MAP of Fresh and Minimally Processed Produce

It is important that packaging films used for MAP of fresh and MPR produce have a relatively high ratio of CO_2 to O_2 permeability, in order to allow O_2 concentration to decrease without excessive accumulation of CO_2 inside the package (Kader, Zagory, and Kerbel 1989). Although gas permeabilities of polymers used for produce MAP show substantial variation, the ratio of permeability of CO_2 to O_2 usually lies between 4 and 6 (Mannapperuma and Singh 1990). Most polymeric films have higher permeability to CO_2 than O_2, in part because the solubility of CO_2 in the polymer is greater (Kader, Zagory, and Kerbel 1989). According to Labuza and Breene (1989) and Zagory and Kader (1988), CO_2 permeation rate of most polymeric films used for MAP of MPR products generally is three to five times greater than O_2 permeation rate in order to minimize equilibrium CO_2 concentration inside the package.

It is also generally agreed that reduced O_2 concentration below 21% in the package environment has little effect on produce respiration rate until a concentration of 12% is attained (Kader, Zagory, and Kerbel 1989). These authors also point out that O_2 concentration has to be lowered to 8% to have a significant effect on fruit ripening. In practice, the O_2 content in a MA produce package is usually reduced from 21% to 2–5% and there is potential that CO_2 will increase from 0.03% to as high as 16–19% (Zagory and Kader 1988). While most produce commodities can tolerate minimum environmental O_2 concentrations of 2–5% without quality loss due to anoxia, maximum tolerable CO_2 concentrations for many fresh produce commodities are in the 2–5% range. Physiological damage to many fresh produce items such as cauliflower, lettuce, celery, kiwifruit, cabbage, radish, sweet pepper, banana, and carrot can occur at CO_2 concentrations in excess of 2–6% (Kader, Zagory, and Kerbel 1989; Zagory and Kader 1988). According to Barmore (1991) packages of chopped produce in the United States rarely have equilibrium CO_2 concentrations <10% unless the O_2 transmission rate of the packaging film is rather high. Thus, it is sometimes necessary to utilize package parameters for minimally processed (chopped) produce that provide a compromise equilibrium atmosphere somewhat higher in O_2 concentration than optimum in order to avoid excessive CO_2 concentrations.

Active MA Packaging to Alter Package Atmosphere O_2, CO_2, and C_2H_2 Concentration

Kader, Zagory, and Kerbel (1989), and Zagory and Kader (1988) indicate that sealed packets of absorbents/adsorbents (O_2, CO_2, and C_2H_4 scavenging materials) can be placed inside MA packages just prior to heat sealing. Package selection should emphasize achievement of an optimum steady-state O_2 concentration in the MA produce package, which for most products will be between 2 and 5%. If this package proves to induce an excessive concentration of package atmosphere CO_2 then, in addition to making adjustments to film area or thickness and slightly altering produce weight or free volume in the package, a CO_2 absorbing material might be used to achieve the appropriate internal concentration of CO_2. Some of the absorbents currently being used to remove excess CO_2 that could be used in a CO_2-permeable packet placed inside a MAP include $Ca(OH)_2$, activated charcoal, and magnesium oxide. The amount of CO_2 absorbent used would be dependent on the level of excess CO_2 present, the desired level of CO_2, and the duration of shelf-life sought.

Inasmuch as C_2H_4 stimulates respiration rate and onset of senescence of both climacteric and nonclimacteric fruits and vegetables (Wills et al. 1989) at atmospheric concentrations as low as 1–10 ppm (Watada 1986), ethylene absorbers can also be used to exert an active effect on MAP produce shelf-life (Smith, Geeson, and Stow 1987; Watada, Abe, and Yamauchi 1990). According to Kader, Zagory, and Kerbel (1989) some materials that could be used for C_2H_4 absorption within polymeric film packages include potassium permanganate and builder clay powder; Watada, Abe, and Yamauchi (1990) suggest the use of charcoal with palladium chloride. Of course these materials would have to be sealed inside ethylene-permeable packets placed inside the sealed MA package. It is noteworthy that ethylene adsorption in MAP may not be required because the effect of C_2H_4 to trigger increased respiratory metabolism of produce is substantially diminished, if not eliminated, in low (2–5%) O_2 atmospheres (Kanellis, Solomos, and Mattoo 1989; Nakhasi, Schlimme, and Solomos 1991).

Assuming an adequate selection of film type and thickness for a given quantity of a specific MPR product in a properly sized package has occurred, there is limited need to consider the use of an O_2 absorber/adsorber inside the MA package.

Active MA Packaging to Elevate Package Atmosphere CO Concentration

Active MA packaging of fresh and minimally processed produce includes drawing a mild vacuum on the packaged produce and relieving the vacuum with a gas flush just prior to heat sealing the package. Usually, the gas flush is a mixture of O_2, CO_2, and N_2, but carbon monoxide (CO) can also be included in the flushing gas mixture. CO is extremely toxic to animals and humans and because of safety concerns is highly regulated in Europe. However, it also has the ability to suppress microflora growth, especially the growth of psychrotrophs (Wagner and Moberg 1989). El-Goorani and Sommer (1981) have reviewed the literature relative to the effects of CO on packaged produce. They also studied the effect of 9% CO atmospheres on 18 postharvest pathogens (at 5.5° C and 12.5° C) and found that 10 test fungi differed greatly in response to CO with the mean percentage of growth in air plus CO ranging from 20 to 100% of that in air alone. They also found that the effect of CO was greater if the atmosphere was low in O_2. The mean percentage of growth in 9% CO plus 2.3% O_2 was 4.8–89.5% of that in air.

In comparison with air, 9% CO added to 2.3% O_2 and 5% CO_2 reduced rot development in strawberries by 80–90%. Although CO at concentrations of approximately 10% are fungistatic, CO does not completely stop fungal growth. Moreover, several researchers have shown that CO can mimic the biological effects of C_2H_4; thus, commercial use of MAP containing CO may be restricted to commodities or products relatively insensitive to C_2H_4 (El-Goorani and Sommer 1981). It should also be recognized that CO concentrations attained by gas flushing just prior to sealing MA packages will decline with time at a rate proportional to permeability of the MA package to CO.

Moisture Vapor Transmission Rate for MAP of Fresh and Minimally Processed Produce

Importance of Moisture Vapor Control for MAP

The relative humidity (RH) inside a MA package is of major importance in achieving optimum shelf-life and storage quality for fresh and minimally processed produce. Most MAP films used for fresh produce have low permeability to water vapor (Kader, Zagory, and Kerbel 1989). At a RH below about 85–90% excess moisture loss from produce can result in wilting of leafy produce and shrivel of many fruit and vegetable bulky tissues. On the other hand extremely high RH of nearly 100% within the MA package can result (under appropriate internal/external temperature conditions) in the condensation of liquid water on the inside surface of the film and then in the transfer of liquid water to the surface of contained produce. Moreover, high RH within the package may also cause loss of produce quality via increased discoloration and decreased vitamin concentration (Gosselin and Mondy 1989). Development of produce rot/decay by accelerated growth or transfer of plant pathogens within a moisture-saturated package environment can rapidly destroy produce quality and negate the beneficial effects of low O_2–elevated CO_2 concentrations on produce ripening/maturation/senescence (Frazier and Westhoff 1988). A major problem associated with MA jumble packaging of large quantities (7–12 kg) of unripe (mature green or breaker) tomatoes is development of considerable condensation on the inside film package surface which, when transferred to the surface of fruit, can increase microflora populations and spread decay (McGlasson 1991). Addition of an antifogging component to the polymeric film during its manufacture does not reduce the quantity of moisture condensate on the inside package film surface during storage; rather it causes the condensed water to "sheet" over the inside film surface and ultimately can result in the formation of water "puddles" in the bottom of the package. Careful control of temperature to minimize fluctuation during storage and distribution minimizes the quantity of moisture condensation inside the MA package.

According to Barmore (1987) most of the plastic films used to package produce are monolayer films where the CO_2 permeation rate averages three to five times greater than the O_2 transmission rate. However, he points out that there is no simple relationship between O_2 and moisture vapor transmission rates through plastic films as there is for O_2 and CO_2 transmissions rates. The trend in newer films for MAP is to use multilayer construction (Barmore 1991); this is readily achieved by coextrusion or by use of an adhesive layer between films.

Because the control of RH within MA packages of fresh and minimally processed produce offers substantial potential to minimize the growth and spread of plant pathogens and thereby extend shelf-life, selection of films that have moderate to high permeability to moisture vapor at typical produce storage temperatures as well as appropriate O_2 and CO_2 transmission rates should be considered for use with fresh and minimally processed produce.

Active MA Packaging to Control Package Atmosphere RH

The use of compounds such as $CaSiO_4$, KCl, NaCl, xylitol, and sorbitol (Kader, Zagory, and, Kerbel 1989) to provide equilibrium RH in the atmosphere of a closed system between 95 and 97% might be a potential means of exerting some control on the RH of MAP internal package atmosphere. If such a salt or saturated salt slurry was sealed inside a relatively small plastic packet that was highly permeable to water vapor but impermeable to liquid water, and the packet was placed inside the MA package with the produce prior to sealing, perhaps an equilibrium RH < 100% but > about 95% could be developed inside the MA package during refrigerated storage. Such an "intermediate" RH would retard moisture loss from the produce and also minimize condensation of liquid moisture droplets on the inside film surface and the surface of the produce (McGlasson 1991; Solomos 1991). Studies using 85 g dry NaCl sealed inside Tyvec® packettes placed inside 1.5-kg MA packages of fresh peaches have been successfully used to eliminate or substantially reduce water condensation on the inside surface of MA film packages for periods of up to 40 days at 1° C (Schlimme 1991).

Tyvec® is a commercially available heat-sealable packaging material that could be used to contain the water vapor absorbent material inasmuch as it has a WVTR of 684 g m^{-2} 24 h^{-1} and is impermeable to liquid water (Idol 1991). Selection of the appropriate salt or humectant must necessarily be compatible with safety issues and regulatory concerns. Use of a water vapor absorbent with USFDA "generally recognized as safe" (GRAS) status would be prudent if not mandatory.

Selection of MA Packaging Materials

In order to select appropriate packaging materials and a packaging configuration for MAP of fresh or minimally processed fruits and vegetables a considerable amount of knowledge is necessary. As much information as possible must be accumulated about the finished product, including stage of maturity at harvest, cultivar(s) to be utilized, chill injury temperature threshold, sensitivity to C_2H_4 at low O_2 and high CO_2 levels, rate of O_2 consumption and CO_2 and C_2H_4 production at the target storage temperature, low O_2 and elevated CO_2 concentration sensitivity threshold, amount (mass) of product per package, and the shelf-life duration sought. Although some of this information is available in the literature and from packaging material suppliers, much is unavailable—especially that dealing with minimally processed produce items and mixtures of items.

Additional information required is related to package material and use criteria, including package type or style (rigid or semirigid or flexible); desired package dimensions, type of filler/sealer to be used, type and style of shipping container to be used, formability/machinability of plastic film and its clarity, abuse and impact performance specifications, as well as its permeability to O_2, CO_2, and water vapor at the target storage temperature and its seal integrity characteristics and regulatory status.

It is apparent that determining the optimal atmosphere/packaging material requirements for MAP for a mixed vegetable salad, for example, is a complex task. In an effort to make this task somewhat analytical, coherent, and methodical, various researchers have worked to develop mathematical models to aid package selection and design (Kader, Zagory, and Kerbel 1989; Labuza and Breene 1989; Zagory and Kader 1988). Abundant information related to these mathematical models can be obtained by consulting those references enumerated by Zagory and Kader (1988) in a summary of factors included in mathematical models for fruit and vegetable MAP (see Table 4-2). Mannapperuma and Singh (1990) also presented a useful mathematical model system that can be utilized to design MA packages for produce.

Many of the mathematical models assume postclimacteric or nonclimacteric produce, equilibrium conditions, and a respiratory quotient (RQ) equal to one; but even in air RQ for different commodities can be 1 ± 0.3 and may be affected by environmental gas concentrations (Kader, Zagory, and Kerbel 1989). Finally, reduced O_2 and elevated CO_2 levels in the steady-state package atmosphere may act additively to lower the respiration rate below that achieved by modification of either gas concentration alone, but few models have incorporated the effect of CO_2 concentration on respiration (Kader, Zagory, and Kerbel 1989). Thus, although mathematical models may be employed to select MA package design criteria for fresh and minimally processed produce, empirical testing of selected packaging is absolutely essential for ultimate successful use of MAP.

Table 4-2
Summary of Factors Included in Mathematical Models of MAP of Fruits and Vegetables in Flexible Plastic Films

Factors	\(1^a\)	\(2^b\)	\(3^c\)	\(4^d\)	\(5^e\)	\(6^f\)	\(7^g\)	\(8^h\)	\(9^i\)
				Proposed Models					
Effect of O_2 on respiration	−	−	+	+	−	+	+	−	+
Effect of CO_2 on respiration	−	−	−	+	−	−	+	−	+
Injurious gas levels	−	−	−	−	−	−	−	−	−
Product diffusion resistance	−	−	−	−	−	−	−	−	+
Respiratory quotient	−	−	−	−	+	−	−	−	−
Film permeability	+	+	+	+	+	+	+	+	+
Temperature	+	+	−	−	−	−	−	−	−
Optimal atmosphere	−	−	−	−	+	−	−	−	+
Change over time	−	+	−	−	−	+	+	+	+
Package area	+	+	+	+	+	+	+	+	+
Package headspace	+	+	−	−	−	+	+	+	+

[a] Tolle (1971).
[b] Lakin (1987).
[c] Jurin and Karel (1963).
[d] Veeraju and Karel (1966).
[e] Marcellin (1974).
[f] Henig and Gilbert (1975).
[g] Hayakawa et al. (1975).
[h] Deily and Rizvi (1981).
[i] Mannapperuma et al. (1988).
(From Zagory and Kader 1988.)

An example that demonstrates some of the problems associated with MA package design/selection taken from Wilbrandt (1991) follows:

Whole peeled "baby" carrots utilized 0.57 cm^3 g^{-1} 24 h^{-1} O_2 at 4.4° C; a 453.6-g sample utilized 258.6 cm^3 of O_2 per day. Flexible pouch test package dimensions were 15.2 × 22.9 cm with 696.2 cm^2 of sealed package surface area. Theoretical film O_2 permeability needed was calculated to be not more than 3,714.5 cm^3 24 h^{-1} m^{-2} at 4.4° C. Three initial atmospheres were selected for testing, viz.:

1. Air (passive MAP)
2. 5% O_2:3% CO_2:92% N_2 (active MAP)

3. 5% O_2:3% CO_2:1% CO:91% N_2 (active MAP)

Based on film permeability requirements, three polymeric films were selected for testing: (1) commercial film JR 127 with O_2 permeability of 3,797.5 cm^3 24 h^{-1} m^{-2} at 4.4° C and a WVTR of 17.1 g 24 h^{-1} m^{-2}; (2) commercial film C E301 with O_2 permeability of 3,999 cm^3 24 h^{-1} m^{-2} at 4.4° C and a WVTR of 10.1 g 24 h^{-1} m^{-2}, and (3) a 3% VA EVA film with O_2 permeability of 3,596 cm^3 24 h ^{1} m^{-2} at 4.4° C and a WVTR of 24.8 g 24 h^{-1} m^{-2}. More than 25 packages of each polymeric film/initial atmosphere variable were produced and stored at 4.4° C. Test packages and contents were evaluated for internal atmosphere gas composition, taste, and odor at regular intervals over storage duration. Passive MAP carrots achieved an equilibrium atmosphere within 24 h. After 24 h all three atmospheres in all three film types had O_2 and CO_2 concentrations around 5% and 3%, respectively, and carrots packed in the atmosphere containing 1% CO demonstrated a slight off-odor and flavor. However, beyond 24 h of storage the atmospheric O_2 concentration in the active MAP commercial film C E301 fell to approach the anaerobic level and CO_2 concentration increased to approach 15%. The passive modified atmosphere in the C E301 film demonstrated the same response after 120 h of storage. Carrots in the C E301 package evidenced anaerobiosis by the appearance of off-flavor and off-odor. Carrots in the JR 127 film (both active and passive initial atmosphere) maintained acceptable quality throughout storage; O_2 concentration did not fall below 5%, CO_2 concentration did not increase above 5%, and product quality was acceptable for the duration of storage. The 3% VA EVA film provided acceptable but erratic results in terms of equilibrium gas concentrations that the investigator suggested was caused by nonuniformity of the amount of VA present in the film. JR 127 film was selected for use with an active MA of 5% O_2:3% CO_2:92% N_2; a high-quality storage life of 15 days at 4.4° C was achieved.

It is noteworthy that the C E301 film had a slightly greater O_2 permeability than the JR 127 film but still provided an anaerobic atmosphere. The investigator speculated that high RH inside the C E301 MA package may have significantly decreased film permeability to both O_2 and CO_2, whereas high RH inside the JR 127 film did not significantly affect film permeability.

Circumstances such as those presented by Wilbrandt (1991) emphasize that use of mathematical models for MA package selection must be reinforced by a substantial amount of empirical experimentation prior to selecting optimum MA packaging systems. It is also noteworthy that the experimental studies described by Wilbrandt (1991) did not include secondary (shipping case) packaging nor apparently did any actual or simulated shipping tests occur. Such studies may have altered test results due to handling/shipping induced mechanical damage to the package film or the carrots which could compromise film integrity and alter carrot tissue metabolism (Rolle and Chism 1987).

Nonplastic Components of MA Plastic Packaging Material

General Considerations

All food packaging plastics contain some nonpolymeric components at levels ranging from <1 ppm in some plastics to several percent in others such as PVC. These components have implications for the physical characteristics of the finished plastics including gas permeability, clarity, strength, softness, formability, and the like. They also present some degree of concern relative to food safety due to the potential for migration of these relatively low molecular weight components from the package to foodstuffs during storage and distribution. Crompton (1979) presented a comprehensive review of this subject and the following information is in large measure taken from his publication.

The nonpolymeric components of MA packaging plastics are of three categories: polymerization residues, processing aids, and end-product additives.

Polymerization residues include low molecular weight polymer oligomers, catalyst remnants, and polymerization solvents. Processing aids include such materials as thermal antioxidants, heat stabilizers, and slip additives. End-product additives encompass a very wide range of substances including impact improvers, plasticizers, and antistatic agents. Detailed study of a single batch of PP disclosed the presence of substances falling under all three of these nonpolymeric component categories.

Important Nonpolymeric Components of MA Packaging Plastics

Residual and Unreacted Starting Materials

Many polymers contain unreacted monomer or low molecular weight polymer (oligomers) in amounts up to several percent. PE, for example, contains waxy low molecular weight oligomers (usually less than 1%) and up to 1% (vol/vol) of unreacted monomer. PP may contain traces of dimer (C_6H_{12}) and tetramer ($C_{12}H_{24}$).

Polymerization Medium

Polyolefins polymerized by the Ziegler–Nutta low-pressure method have traces of inert paraffinic solvent (from C_4 to C_{18}) present.

Catalyst Decomposition Agents

Alcohols and alkali metal salts used to decompose and neutralize polymerization catalysts can be present in low-pressure polyolefins.

Chemicals Added During Polymerization

Up to 10% mineral oil (to impart flexibility to IPS during manufacture by copolymerization of styrene and synthetic rubbers) can be present.

Processing Aids

Antiblock agent (principally silica) is present at the 0.1–0.5% level, and antisplit agents (usually natural or synthetic rubber) to prevent spontaneous fibrillation of oriented PP film are present at concentrations up to 10%. Antistatic agents (usually glycol or quaternary ammonium salt derivatives) such as lauric diethanolamide are present in the formulation of polyolefins. Lubricants are used to reduce viscosity of the molten polymer and include C_{12}–C_{30} hydrocarbons at a several percent level. Calcium sterate at 0.05–0.30% is added as an external lubricant. Plasticizers are added to plastics to be used for food contact at levels seldom in excess of 5%. Polymeric high molecular weight plasticizers are often used in food contact plastics because they have low rates of migration and lower solubility in foods.

End-Product Additives

Colorants such as titanium dioxide (0.01–1%) and carbon black (0.2–2%) are added to molten plastic. Impact improvers are added to overcome brittleness in PS and PP, and include hydrocarbon oils, waxes, and rubbers. Plasticizers are incorporated into the more rigid plastics such as PVC.

Safety Considerations Relevant to MAP of Fresh and Minimally Processed Produce

In general, there are two safety concerns related to MAP of fruits and vegetables. One important safety consideration is related to the potential for migration of harmful/toxic chemicals from the packaging material in immediate contact with food into the food. Of overriding concern as a safety consideration is the potential for foodborne human pathogens to grow relatively undetected in produce during refrigerated distribution, or storage (Ronk, Carson, and Thompson 1989). Chapter 8 includes information relevant to microbiological safety concerns; thus, only safety concerns related to migration of chemicals from packaging to foods are covered in this chapter.

Migration of Adulterants from Plastic Packages to Produce

Polymerized constituents of plastic packaging materials, due to very high molecular weight and great insolubility in aqueous systems, are unlikely to be transferred to contained foodstuffs during storage and distribution (Crompton 1979). However, because all plastic packaging materials contain nonpolymeric components, there is potential for some of these to transfer from the plastic package to foodstuffs via migration. The amount, transferability, and toxicity of the nonpolymeric components of plastic packaging have potential consumer health and safety implications unless the material complies with governmental (FDA) regulations (Russell 1991).

The U.S. Federal Food, Drug and Cosmetic Act delineates the use of food additives in the United States. Constituents of plastics that may migrate into foodstuffs are termed "indirect additives" (Breder 1988). Unless an additive (either direct or indirect) has "prior sanctioned" or GRAS status, it must be shown that it cannot reasonably be expected to become a "component" of a food before it can legally be utilized in food contact plastics. In order to determine whether a constituent of plastic satisfies this latter condition, the plastic manufacturer must establish the toxicity and extraction behavior of the constituent from the plastic in contact with specified food simulants. The analytical limits of usage are established by the toxicological properties of the constituent and the chemical nature of the specific foods for which the plastic is to be used as a food-contact package material.

The European Community (EC) is preparing to enact regulations requiring application from manufacturers for each plastic constituent to be approved even if it had previously been approved by one or more member states. This process is likely to take several years or more and the implications of this delay for food packagers exporting product to the EC are not clear at this time. One possible outcome is that a significantly smaller range of additives will be approved in the near future and then the range will be extended over time.

Many FDA regulations (FDA 1988a, 1988b) are related to chemicals present in food packaging materials (as additives or unavoidable contaminants) and to use of certain chemicals, for example, polychlorinated biphenyls (PCBs), in establishments manufacturing food-packaging materials [see Chapter 21 Code of Federal Regulations (CFR) 109.15]. Regulations (FDA 1988a) that relate to indirect food additives associated with polymers are published in Chapter 21 CFR Part 177 Subpart B. As an example, Chapter 21 CFR Part 177 Subpart B 177.1350 pertains to substances for use as basic components of single and repeated use food contact surfaces with specific relation to EVA copolymers. This regulation identifies or defines EVA and gives details related to the use of optional substances in the resin such as xanthan gum [Part 177.1350(a)(5)] at a level not to exceed 1% by weight. Additional details related to use of irradiation [Part 177.1350(d)(1-3)] with electron beans to produce molecular crosslinking of polymer chains are also included in this regulation.

Compliance with all facets of FDA regulations governing indirect additives to foods from food contact plastics is essential for all MA polymeric packages for fresh and minimally processed produce. Polymeric packaging suppliers must be able to certify or guarantee to the food processor/packager that their packaging materials comply with all relevant FDA regulations in order that the food processor has confidence that his packaging materials are safe and present no health hazard from toxic materials migration to the foodstuffs.

Packaging Requirements for Shipping and Distribution of Fresh and Minimally Processed MAP Produce

Packaging is a key component of the handling and distribution of fresh and minimally processed fruits and vegetables. Centers of consumption of fresh produce are often remote from production areas (Huxsoll and Bolin 1989); produce packaging, ever since fresh produce has been traded, has been practiced in order to facilitate assembly into convenient units for handling and to protect the produce during distribution (Wills et al. 1989). Modern packaging of fresh produce must meet a wide range of requirements, which according to Wills et al. (1989) include:

1. Provide sufficient mechanical strength to protect contents during handling, transport, and while stacked.

2. Allow freedom from (or adherence to governmental regulatory limits for) chemicals that can transfer to produce and be toxic to humans.

3. Meet handling and marketing requirements in terms of weight, size, and shape.

4. Allow rapid cooling of contents and adequate ventilation to remove metabolic heat.

5. Be largely unaffected by moisture when wet or at high relative humidity.

6. Be cost-effective in relation to product value and required extent of protection.

The combined requirements of fresh and minimally processed produce and its transport environment often impose unusually severe conditions on the packaging used. As a result, higher package quality is usually needed for fresh fruits and vegetables than for manufactured goods of the same weight (International Trade Center UNCTAD/GATT 1988).

Packaging Protection Required for Fresh and Minimally Processed Produce

Four different types of mechanical injury to produce are: cuts, compressions, impacts, and vibrations. The susceptibilities of some fruits to mechanical injury are presented in Table 4-3 (Wills et al. 1989). Impact bruises result from dropping onto a hard surface and can be reduced by use of careful handling and use of in-package cushion pads or fillers. Compression damage results from incorrect packing, overfilling, and inadequate package performance. Vibration and abrasion damage is a result of product movement within the package during handling and shipping and can be minimized

Table 4-3
Susceptibility of Produce to Types of Mechanical Injury[a]

		Type of injury	
Produce	Compression	Impact	Vibration
Apple	S	S	I
Apricot	I	I	S
Banana, green	I	I	S
Banana, ripe	S	S	S
Cantaloupe	S	I	I
Grape	R	I	S
Nectarine	I	I	S
Peach	S	S	S
Pear	R	I	S
Plum	R	R	S
Strawberry	S	I	R
Summer squash	I	S	S
Tomato, green	S	I	I
Tomato, pink	S	S	I

S, susceptible; I, intermediate; R, resistant.
[a]From Guillou, R. Orderly development of produce containers. Proceedings, Fruit and Vegetable Perishables Handling Conference; University of California, Davis, CA, March 23–25, 1964; pp. 20–25.

through correct package sizing and fill density and use of internal packaging materials such as wraps, paddings, and trays. Ideally, the package must be able to perform under all temperature and humidity conditions that are likely to be encountered (International Trade Center UNCTAD/GATT 1988). Packaging is necessary for quality retention and shelf-life extension primarily as a means to reduce mechanical damage and retard microbial and physiological degradation.

Types of Packaging for Fresh and Minimally Processed Produce

The three categories of MPR produce packaging currently in use are: consumer or end-product user packaging (usually referred to as unit packaging), transport packaging, and unit load packaging.

Unit packaging includes (1) sealed polymeric film bags, (2) rigid or semirigid plastic trays sealed across the top with polymeric film, and (3) overwrapped trays (O'Beirne 1990) for sale to institutions (hotels, restaurants, and institutional feeding establishments [HRI]) and to consumer retail markets. As previously noted, the major requirement for unit packaging is the presence of gas and water vapor permeability characteristics compatible with the product. However, appearance (clarity and gloss), texture, condensation resistance, tensile strength, impact strength, heat sealability, and ease of formation/manufacturing/filling and utilization on production equipment are also important considerations (O'Beirne 1990).

Transport packages (also referred to as shipping containers or boxes) are used to facilitate manual handling and to collate and contain fixed quantities of unit packaged produce (International Trade Center UNCTAD/GATT 1988).

Unit load packaging is used to permit efficient mechanical handling of transport packages during distribution wherein shipping cases (boxes) are typically assembled into pallet loads for long-distance transport (International Trade Center UNCTAD/GATT 1988) via truck, train, ship, or airplane (Peleg 1985).

Unit Packaging

Many package types are used for unit packaging of fresh and minimally processed produce, as previously discussed, and include: wraps of PE or PVC often in the form of shrink-wrap, stretch film, or cling film; bags of perforated and unperforated PE and PP; and shallow trays of molded pulp, cardboard, thermoformed plastic, or expanded PS covered or sealed within polymeric film.

Transport Packaging

Transport packaging for produce is dominated by closed boxes made of corrugated fiberboard (Peleg 1985). Transport containers should be loaded onto carriers in a manner that takes maximum advantage of their inherent strength (Ashby et al. 1987). Any shipping container should be designed to meet the specific requirements of the particular produce commodity to be shipped (Hardenburg 1975). Wood and expanded PS boxes are also used but in a much more limited quantity due largely to economic considerations. The strength and versatility of the fiberboard box are largely determined by the materials used in its make-up, a proper manufacturer's joint, use of correct dimensions for proper fit of content, interior packing forms, and selection of a proper style of container (Fiber Box Association 1976). Corrugated fiberboard boxes are made from paperboard (>

0.2 mm thick) which is made from tree cellulose by either of two methods: (1) chemical and (2) semichemical. For boxes with net weights of 10 or more kg, the paperboard used is predominantly made by the Kraft process. Together with thickness (caliper) basis weight defines paperboard quality. Double-lined or double-faced corrugated (single board) is the major form of corrugated fiberboard used to manufacture containers (shipping or transport containers) for fresh produce. The corrugating medium is usually 0.2–0.3 mm thick and 122–137 g m^{-2} basis weight. Liners are 0.2–0.7 mm thick and 175–235 g m^{-2} basis weight. Both B and C flutes are commonly used for fabricating shipping or transport containers. Single- and double-wall corrugated are usually used for 10–25 kg capacity boxes. Many designs of corrugated box are used for fresh produce including regular slotted container (RSC), half telescopic container (HTC), and full telescopic container (FTC) with or without internal partitions or dividers. The RSC is the most popular transport container, but it has poor stacking strength. The HTC transport box is not significantly stronger than the RSC box. The FTC box can carry the highest stacking forces and is the most frequently used transport container for produce after the RSC. Other corrugated box designs for shipping fruits and vegetables include the one-piece box with a tuck-in cover and the self-locking tray (McGregor 1987). Regardless of fiberboard box style a minimum 19.3 kg cm^{-2} (275 psi) bursting test strength fiberboard is recommended for boxes intended for export (McGregor 1987). Various materials may be added to shipping containers to provide additional strength, for example, pads, wraps, and sleeves can reduce bruising and dividers or partitions provide additional product protection. Ventilation holes are usually used in these transport packages and the manufacturer's joint is made with tape, glue, or staples (Peleg 1985). Details of transport package descriptions, box styles, measurement methods, specifications, dimensions, and load capacity are found in Peleg (1985), Fiber Box Association (1976), the International Trade Center UNCTAD/GATT (1988), and Remes (1989, 1989a) and are available from various suppliers of transport packaging.

The United Nations Economic Commission for Europe (UN/ECE) Recommendation No. 222 contains a performance testing procedure for transport packaging of perishable goods including fresh fruits and vegetables. Transport packaging materials should be constantly monitored in order to maintain quality. Suppliers of transport packages should guarantee the performance qualities of their products as well as provide specifications of corrugated fiberboard transport packages including: flat crush test, short column compression test, puncture resistance test, Cobb test, and Mullen test (all at a specified relative humidity) (International Trade Centre UNCTAD/GATT 1988). The basic test methods (both American Society of Testing Materials and Technical Association of the Pulp and Paper Industry) used for corrugated and solid fiberboard boxes are listed by the Fiber Box Association (1976).

Unit Load Packaging

Unit load packaging usually involves the palletization of transport packages in order to reduce handling costs by facilitating mechanical handling, that is, loading and unloading by forklift trucks, and allowing for better utilization of storage space and a reduction of mechanical strains and damage (International Trade Center UNCTAD/GATT 1988, Peleg 1985). Most distribution centers are set up to store palletized loads in three-tier racks (McGregor 1987). According to McGregor (1987) advantages of using unit pallet loads include reduced handling of shipping containers and less product damage.

The two methods used in assembly of pallet loads are the modular and two-way systems. In the modular system of pallet loading, transport packages are oriented in the same direction, that is, when stacked on a pallet packages are placed directly on top of one another forming a series of separate columns. Because of their configuration, modular pallet loads have straight sides and vertical edges suitable for most pallet-load securing methods. In the two-way system of pallet loading, transport packages in each tier form a pattern such that some packages are oriented lengthwise and others crosswise on the pallet. Usually, the two-way system results in stacking one tier at a time with a different pattern among tiers so that the packages on successive tiers interlock with one another. Some two-way pallet loads have internal spaces on tiers and such loads may be difficult to secure on the pallet. However, some two-way configurations have horizontal cross-sections without spaces and can be secured in the same way as modular loads (International Trade Center UNCTAD/GATT 1988).

For best results with regard to shipping case stacking strength and pallet load stability, the shipping case stack on the pallet should be square with its edges, without horizontal spaces between containers. Most problems occur when a pallet load has horizontal spaces and the cases protrude outside the pallet, that is, when there is considerable "overhang" (Peleg 1985). Even when transport containers (cases) are properly aligned with pallet edges, strapping or over-wrapping pallet loads is highly recommended. Column stacks (modular pallet load) have no inherent stability and cannot be handled or transported without some external means of stabilization; however, column stacked palletloads provide maximal shipping container stacking strength since all container corners and sides are aligned (Peleg 1985).

Pallet Construction and Dimensions

Pallets for fresh fruit and vegetables are usually made of wood, and generally no pallet boards should be <12.5 mm thick. Pallets with boards covering their total surface, that is with spaces of no more than 70 mm between boards, are suitable for a range of package sizes. Pallets are made for two-way entry of truck forks or for four-way entry; four-way pallets should be used whenever possible and all four-way pallets have double-deck construction. Pallets made of materials other than wood such as chipboard, fiberboard, expanded polystyrene, and other plastics currently are not used much (in Europe) for fresh fruits and vegetables (Peleg 1985). Wood pallets must be strong enough to allow storage under load in three-tier racks and the design of the bottom of the pallet should not block air circulation (McGregor, 1987).

The International Organization for Standardization (ISO) in Geneva, Switzerland has agreed to standard pallet dimensions of 120 cm × 100 cm as the primary handling unit size for international trade. Most trucks and semitrailers will accommodate this pallet size with reasonably good surface utilization (Peleg 1985). In the United Kingdom some pallets of 121.9 cm × 101.4 cm remain in use, and in the United States this is the preferred pallet size (Ryall and Lipton 1979); for many purposes this modest deviation in size from the international standard pallet can be ignored. ISO has also agreed to standardize a 120 cm × 80 cm pallet. These two pallet sizes are used for distribution of fresh fruit and vegetables in Europe. However, in many cases these two pallet sizes are unsuitable as they are not adapted to the internal dimensions of refrigerated transport. In such cases, the internal dimensions of the transportation container should be used to derive a suitable pallet size—thus, the 104 cm × 100 cm pallet was derived from the normal internal dimensions of the 609.6 cm refrigerated intermodal container.

Table 4-4, taken from International Trade Center UNCTAD/GATT (1988), provides examples of transport container dimensions for

Table 4-4
Examples of Packs Suitable for Modular and Interlocking Stacking Patterns on the 1,200 × 1,000 mm and the 1,200 × 800 mm pallets

External Package Horizontal Dimensions (mm)	Suitability for 1,200 × 1,000 mm pallet indicated by "x"		Suitability for 1,200 × 800 mm pallet indicated by "x"	
	Modular	Interlocking	Modular	Interlocking
600 × 500	x			
600 × 400ᵃ		x	x	
600 × 333	x			
600 × 266			x	
600 × 250	x			
600 × 200	x	x	x	x
520 × 240		x		
500 × 400	x			
500 × 333		x		
500 × 300ᵃ	x			x
500 × 200	x			
433 × 333		x		
400 × 400			x	
400 × 333	x			
400 × 300ᵃ		x	x	
400 × 266			x	
400 × 250	x			
400 × 200	x		x	
380 × 240		x		
333 × 300	x			
333 × 200	x			
300 × 266			x	
300 × 250	x			
300 × 240				x
300 × 200	x	x	x	x
200 × 200	x	x		

ᵃRecommended by UN/ECE and OECD.
(From UNCTAD/GATT 1988.)

modular and interlocking stacking patterns on 120 cm × 100 cm and 120 cm × 80 cm pallets. Proliferation of shipping containers for produce results in different dimensions and many do not use space efficiently on the 120 cm × 100 cm pallet. The Organization for Economic Cooperation and Development (OECD) recommendations for four standard shipping containers are 60 cm × 40 cm, 50 cm × 40 cm, 50 cm × 30 cm, and 40 cm × 30 cm. The depth of each can vary depending on the commodity or product packed, and each size uses the standard 120 cm × 100 cm pallet well. These four sizes are promoted in the United States by the United Fresh Fruit and Vegetable Association through Project MUM (modularization, unitization, and metrication). Project MUM was developed by the United States fruit and vegetable industry and the USDA to encourage shipping container standardization and unit loads with the goal of utilizing 90–100% of the surface of the widely used 1,016 mm × 1219 mm (40 in. × 48 in.) standard pallet with no overhang and little underhang (McGregor 1987). Tables in McGregor (1987) show recommended MUM containers (shipping cases) arranged on a standard pallet and list current produce shipping containers and their proposed MUM replacements. Changing transport containers from the current many to these four standard metric sizes would result in better utilization of pallet space, and more efficient handling during distribution (Ryall and Pentzer 1982).

Securing Pallet Loads

One-side or two-way strapping by two or four bands will usually be adequate for stabilizing most unit loads. Angle bracing strips in places where strapping bands bear on the container edges should be used to spread the load over the container edge. Steel or plastic strapping bands can be used. Overwrapping by shrinkable and stretch plastic films or netting is also used to stabilize pallet loads. Heat shrink is being phased out in favor of stretch film overwrapping (Peleg 1985). Types of films used in stretch unit load overwrapping are extruded 0.0254 mm LDPE (stretched 15–25%) and 0.02 mm PVC film (stretched 30–40%).

According to the International Trade Center UNCTAD/GATT (1988) the best load stabilization is achieved by using full-length, corner post-style protectors and strapping. The corner posts are made of extruded plastic, metal, or multi-ply solid board and are "L"-shaped in cross-section. Strapping is usually made of PP. Three to four horizontal straps usually provide sufficient stability, but it is often also desirable to secure pallet loads vertically with two straps in the lengthwise direction (International Trade Center UNCTAD/GATT 1988).

Conclusions

MPR products, even as complex as, for example, a mixed salad of shredded lettuce, tomato wedges, shredded carrots, diced celery, and sliced mushrooms, require packaging that in general, has the functions and meets the requirements of some packaging materials currently utilized for fresh fruits and vegetables. But MPR products are normally subjected to greater postharvest processing stress and therefore increased efforts are necessary to ensure attainment of an adequate distribution, and storage shelf-life. Coincident with an intensive quality assurance/sanitation/GMP regimen, substantial attention to product temperature control and packaging parameters is virtually a mandatory requirement for achieving acceptable storage/ distribution life for MPR products. In the United States there is general agreement that for nationwide marketing from one or a few minimal processing sites a minimum 21-day processing-to-final purchase shelf-life is necessary. Minimal processing facilities utilized for only local or regional marketing require as few as 5 days of high-quality shelf-life.

Degradation of MPR product quality involves moisture loss, mechanical damage, microbial spoilage, and product tissue catabolic metabolism. Among those methods available to control or moderate these degradative processes packaging technology is vitally important. In particular, utilization of rigid, semirigid, and flexible polymeric materials to moderate moisture loss and retard the onset of product senescence by affecting the concentration of gases and water vapor within the package coupled with the use of acceptable transport packages are crucial to successful delivery of high-quality MPR products to consumers.

Modified atmosphere packaging of MPR products, using either passive or active methodology, requires careful selection of polymeric packaging material(s) especially with regard to their permeability to O_2, CO_2, and water vapor. It is necessary that the polymeric film selected be three to six or more times more permeable to CO_2 than to O_2. Polymeric films with potential to be used for MAP of MPR products include LDPE, LLDPE, MDPE, HDPE, PP, PVC, PS, EVA copolymers, ionomers, and polybutylene. Considerable research on the use of multi-ply thin films to provide optimum permeability characteristics as well as improved clarity, ink-printability, impact strength, and the like is being conducted by packaging material manufacturers. Using either existing or newly developed polymeric materials, selection of a MA package for MPR produce products must include empirical testing under conditions that simulate commercial operations including processing, MA packaging, transport packaging, and shipping.

Commercial plastic packaging materials usually include nonplastic components that have potential to migrate to contained foods. Thus, polymeric MA packaging materials must comply with all governmental regulations related to indirect food additives, and packaging suppliers must be able to certify such compliance.

Distribution of MPR produce products from the manufacturing site to the marketplace requires careful selection and utilization of transport and unit load packaging as well as unit packaging in order to provide reasonable assurance of protection from shipping abuse including mechanical damage such as bruising and compression. Thus, packaging considerations will continue to comprise a major aspect of production and delivery of high-quality MPR product to the marketplace.

References

Anon. 1979. Properties of packaging films. *Modern Packaging* **52**(12):36–38.

Anon. 1982. Standard tests for package materials. Package Engineering Including Modern Packaging Encyclopedia, pp. 32–34.

Anon. 1984. Films, properties chart. *The Packaging Encyclopedia—1984, Packaging* **29**(4):90–93.

Anon. 1991. U.S. resin sales to major markets. *Modern Plastics Int.* **21**(1):61–62.

Ashby, B.H., R.T. Hinsch, L.A. Risse, N.G. Kindya, W.L. Craig, Jr., and M.T. Turczyn 1987. Protecting Perishable Foods During Transportation by Truck. *Agricultural Handbook No. 669*. Washington, DC: USDA Office of Transportation.

ASTM. 1986. Standard test methods for determining gas permeability characteristics of plastic film and sheeting ASTM D 1434-82. In *Annual Book of ASTM Standards*, Section 8. Plastics Vol. 8.01. Plastics, pp. 613–628. Philadelphia: Business Copy Products.

ASTM. 1987. Standard test methods for water vapor transmissions of materials ASTM E 96-80. *Annual Book of ASTM Standards* Section 15. General Products, Chemical Specialties, and End Use Products, Vol. 15.09. Paper; Packaging; Flexible Barrier Materials, pp. 893–899. Philadelphia Business Copy Products.

Baijal, M.D. 1982. General considerations. In *Plastics, Polymer Science, and Technology*, D. Baijal (ed.), pp. 1–26. New York: John Wiley & Sons.

Ballantyne, A. 1986. MAP of selected prepared vegetables. *Technical Memorandum No. 436.* Chipping Campden, United Kingdom: Campden Food Res. Assoc.

Ballantyne, A., R. Stark, and J.D. Selman. 1988. Modified atmosphere packaging of shredded lettuce. *Int. J. Food Sci. Technol.* **23**:267–274.

Barmore, C.R. 1987. Packaging technology for fresh and minimally processed fruits and vegetables. *J. Food Quality* **10**:207–217.

Barmore, C.R. 1991. Personal Communication. Cryovac Div. of W.R. Grace Co., Inc. Duncan, SC.

Benning, C.J. 1983. *Plastic Films for Packaging Technology, Applications and Process Economics.* Lancaster, PA: Technomic Publishing Co.

Ben-Yehoshua, S. 1985. Individual seal-packing of fresh fruit and vegetables in plastic film—a new post harvest technique. *Hort Science* **20**:32–37.

Ben-Yehoshua, S., B. Shapiro, Z.E. Chen, and S. Lurie. 1983. Mode of action of plastic film in extending life of lemon and bell pepper fruits by alleviation of water stress. *Plant Physiol.* **73**(4):87–93.

Bhowmilk, S.R. and C.M. Sebris. 1988. Quality and shelf life of individually shrink-wrapped peaches. *J. Food Sci.* **53**:519–522.

Brecht, P.E. 1980. Use of controlled atmospheres to retard deterioration of produce. *Food Technol.* **34**(3):45–50.

Breder, C.V. 1988. Migration of packaging components into foods. Regulatory considerations. In *Food and Packaging Interactions,* J.H. Hotchkiss (ed.) pp. 159–169. Washington, DC: American Chemical Society.

Brody, A.L. 1970. *CRC Flexible Packaging of Foods.* London: Butterworths.

Brydson, J.A. 1982. *Plastics Materials,* 4th edit. London: Butterworths.

Crank, J. 1975. *The Mathematics of Diffusion,* 2nd edit. Oxford: Claredon Press.

Crompton, T.R. 1979. *Additive Migration From Plastics into Food.* London: William Clowes (Beccles).

Crosby, N.T. 1981. *Food Packaging Material—Aspects of Analysis and Migration of Contaminants.* Essex: Applied Science Publishers.

Datta, S.K. 1984. Polyvinylidene chloride. In *Plastics in Packaging,* S.A.P. Vaidya (ed.), pp. 142–148. Bombay: Indian Institute of Packaging.

Davies, J.K. 1987. Polypropylene random copolymers. In *Modern Plastics Encyclopedia,* Vol. 64, No. 10A, p. 75. New York: McGraw-Hill.

Deily, K.R. and S.S.H. Rizvi. 1981. Optimization of parameters for packaging of fresh peaches in polymeric films. *J. Food Process Engin.* **5**:23–41.

Demorest, R.L. 1989. Measuring oxygen permeability through today's packaging barriers. *J. Packaging Technol.* **3**(4):222–226.

Duncan, R.E. 1987. Ethylene-vinyl acetate. In *Modern Plastics Encyclopedia,* Vol. 64, No. 10A, p. 57. New York: McGraw-Hill.

El-Goorani, M.A. and N.F. Sommer. 1981. Effects of modified atmospheres on post-harvest pathogens of fruits and vegetables. In *Horticultural Reviews,* Vol. 3, Jules Janick (ed.), pp. 412–462. Westport, CT: AVI Publishing.

FDA. 1988a. *Code of Federal Regulations—Food and Drugs 21 Parts 170 and 199.* Washington, DC: U.S. Government Printing Office.

FDA. 1988b. *Code of Federal Regulations—Food and Drugs 21 Parts 100 to 169.* Washington, DC: U.S. Government Printing Office.

Frazier, W.C. and D.C. Westhoff. 1988. *Food Microbiology,* 4th edit. New York: McGraw-Hill.

Fiber Box Association. 1976. *The Fiber Box Handbook.* Chicago, IL.

Giacin, J.R. and J. Miltz. 1983. Characterizing polymeric materials. *Package Engin. Mod. Packag.* **28**(4):33–37.

Giacin, J.R., B. Harte, H.E. Lockhard, and M. Richmond. 1984. Package testing, present and future. *The Packaging Encyclopedia—1984, Packaging* **29**(4):35–44.

Gibbons, J.G. 1973. Barrier structures for packaging. *Packaging Technol.* **19**(130):15–19.

Gopal, N.G.S. 1984. Effect of ionizing radiation on packaging materials. In *Plastics in Packaging,* S.A.P. Vaidya (ed.), pp. 284–316. Bombay: Indian Instituté of Packaging.

Gosselin, B. and N.I. Mondy. 1989. Effect of packaging materials on the chemical composition of potatoes. *J. Food Sci.* **54**:629–631.

Griffin, Jr., R.C., S. Sacharow, and A.L. Brody. 1985. In *Principles of Package Development,* 2nd edit., p. 46. Westport, CT: AVI Publishing.

Hall, C.W., R.E. Hardenburg, and Er. B. Pantastico. 1975. Principals of packaging, part II-consumer packaging with plastics. In *Postharvest Physiology, Handling and Utilization of Tropical and Subtropical Fruits and Vegetables,* Er. B. Pantastico (ed.), pp. 303–313. Westport, CT: AVI Publishing.

Hardenburg, R.E. 1975. Principals of packaging, part I-general considerations. In *Postharvest Physiology, Handling and Utilization of Tropical and Subtropical Fruits and Vegetables,* Er. B. Pantastico (ed.), pp. 283–302. Westport, CT: AVI Publishing.

Hayakawa, K., Y.S. Henig, and S.G. Gilbert. 1975. Formulae for predicting gas exchange of fresh produce in polymeric film packages. *J. Food Sci.* **40**:186–191.

Henig, Y.S. and S.G. Gilbert. 1975. Computer analysis of the variables affecting respiration and quality of produce packaged in polymeric films. *J. Food Sci.* **40**:1033–1035.

Henkel, R.N. 1973. Introduction to plastics. *Mod. Packaging* **46**(12):128–131.

Hotchkiss, J.H. 1988. Experimental approaches to determining the safety of food packaged in modified atmospheres. *Food Technol.* **42**(9):55, 60–64.

Huxsoll, C.C. and H.R. Bolin. 1989. Processing and distribution alternatives for minimally processed fruits and vegetables. *Food Technol.* **43**(2):124–128.

Idol, R. 1991. Tyvec 1059B uncoated non-antistatic spunbonded olefin material specification. Buffalo, New York: Multiform Desiccants.

Institute of Food Technologists. 1990. Quality of fruits and vegetables—a scientific status summary by IFTs' expert panel on food safety and nutrition. *Food Technol.* **44**(6):99–106.

Institute of Food Technologists. 1991. *Food Packaging, Food Protection and the Environment: A Workshop Report.* Chicago, IL.

International Trade Center UNCTAD/GATT. 1988. *Manual on the Packaging of Fresh Fruits and Vegetables.* Geneva, Switzerland: International Trade Center UNCTAD/GATT.

James, D.G. 1984. Films, polyvinyl chloride. *The Packaging Encyclopedia—1984, Packaging* **29**(4):74–75.

Jenkins, W.A. and J.P. Harrington. 1991. *Packaging Foods with Plastics.* Lancaster, PA: Technomic Publishing.

Jurin, V. and M. Karel. 1963. Studies on control of respiration of McIntosh apples by packaging methods. *Food Technol.* **17**(6):104–108.

Kader, A.A. 1980. Prevention of ripening in fruits by use of controlled atmospheres. *Food Technol.* **34**(3):51–54.

Kader, A.A. 1986. Biochemical and physiological basis for effects of controlled and modified atmospheres on fruits and vegetables. *Food Technol.* **40**(5):99–104.

Kader, A.A., Zagory, D., and E.L. Kerbel. 1989. Modified atmosphere packaging of fruits and vegetables. *Crit. Rev. Food Sci. Nutr.* **28**:1–30.

Kanellis, A.K., T. Solomos, and K.A. Mattoo. 1989. Hydrolytic enzyme activities and protein pattern of avocado fruit ripened in air and in low oxygen, with and without ethylene. *Plant Physiol.* **90**:259–266.

Katsura, T. 1989. Present state and future trend of functional packaging materials attracting considerable attention. *Packaging Japan* **10**:21–26.

Kelsey, R.J. 1978. *Packaging in Today's Society.* New York: St. Regis Paper Co.

Kester, J.J. and O.R. Fennema. 1986. Edible films and coatings: a review. *Food Technol.* **40**(12):46–57.

King, Jr., A.D. and H.R. Bolin. 1989. Physiological and microbiological storage stability of minimally processed fruits and vegetables. *Food Technol.* **43**(2):132–135.

King, A.D., J.A. Magnuson, T. Torok, and N. Goodman. 1991. Microbial flora and storage quality of partially processed lettuce. *J. Food Sci.* **56**:459–461.

Kumar, K.R. and N. Balasubrahmanyam. 1984. Plastics in food packaging. In *Plastics in Packaging*, S.A.P. Vaidya (ed.), pp. 319–341. Bombay: Indian Institute of Packaging.

Labuza, T.P. and W.M. Breene. 1989. Applications of "Active Packaging" for improvement of shelf life and nutritional quality of fresh and extended shelf-life foods. *J. Food Processing Preser.* **13**:1–69.

Lakin, W.D. 1987. Computer-aided hermetic package design and shelf life prediction. *J. Packaging Technol.* **1**(3):82.

McGlasson, W.B. 1991. Personal Communication. Richmond NSW, Australia: University of Western Sydney, Hawkesbury.

McGregor, B.M. 1987. *Tropical Products Transport Handbook, Agricultural Handbook No. 668.* Washington, DC: USDA Office of Transportation.

Mannapperuma, J.D. and R.P. Singh. 1990. Modeling of gas exchange in polymeric packages of fresh fruits and vegetables. Abstract 646 (p. 227), 1990 IFT Annual Meeting. Anaheim, CA.

Mannapperuma, J., R.P. Singh, D. Zagory, and A.A. Kader. 1988. Unpublished results. University of California, Davis.

Marcellin, P. 1974. Conservation des fruits legumes en atmosphere controlee, a l'aide de membranes de polymeres. *Revue Gen. Froid* **3**:217.

Miles, D.C. and J.H. Briston. 1979. *Polymer Technology.* New York: Chemical Publishing.

Myers, R.A. 1989. Packaging considerations for minimally processed fruits and vegetables. *Food Technol.* **43**(2):129–131.

Nakhasi, S., D. Schlimme, and T. Solomos. 1991. Storage potential of tomatoes harvested at the breaker stage using modified atmosphere packaging. *J. Food Sci.* **56**:55–59.

O'Beirne, D. 1990. *Chilled Foods The State of the Art*, T. Gormley (ed.). Essex, United Kingdom: R.T. Elsevier Science Publishers.

Oswin, C.R. 1975. *Plastic Films and Packaging.* New York: Halsted Press, John Wiley & Sons.

Peleg, K. 1985. *Produce Handling, Packaging and Distribution.* Westport, CT: AVI Publishing.

Peters, D.W. 1987. Dispersion PVC. *Modern Plastics Encyclopedia,* Vol. 65, No. 10A, pp. 102–104. New York: McGraw-Hill.

Radian Corporation. 1986. *Polymer Manufacturing Technology and Health Effects.* Park Ridge, NJ: Noyes Data Corporation.

Remes, W.J. 1989. Part 1. An introduction to case packing. *J. Packaging Technol.* **3**(3):132–135.

Remes, W.J. 1989a. Part 2. An introduction to case packing. *J. Packaging Technol.* **3**(4):189–191.

Rice, J. 1989. Modified atmosphere packaging. *Food Processing* **50**(3):60–75.

Rolle, R.S. and W. Chism III. 1987. Physiological consequences of minimally processed fruits and vegetables. *J. Food Quality* **10**:157–177.

Ronk, R.J., K.L. Carson, and P. Thompson. 1989. Processing, packaging and regulations of minimally processed fruits and vegetables. *Food Technol.* **43**(2):136–139.

Rooney, M.L. 1989. Measuring packaging film attributes. *Food Australia* **41**:880–881.

Rosen, J.C. and A.A. Kader. 1989. Postharvest physiology and quality maintenance of sliced pear and strawberry fruits. *J. Food Sci.* **54**:656–659.

Russell, M.J. 1991. Packaging plastics: still exciting, still growing. *Chilton's Food Engin.* **63**(9):93–97.

Ryall, A.L. and W.J. Lipton. 1979. *Handling, Transportation and Storage of Fruits and Vegetables*, 2nd edit., Vol. 1, *Vegetables and Melons.* Westport, CT: AVI Publishing.

Ryall, A.L. and W.T. Pentzer. 1982. *Handling, Transportation and Storage of Fruits and Vegetables*, 2nd edit., Vol. 2, *Fruits and Tree Nuts.* Westport, CT: AVI Publishing.

Sacharow, S. 1976. *Handbook of Package Materials.* Westport, CT: AVI Publishing.

Sacharow, S. and R.C. Griffin, Jr. 1973. *Basic Guide to Plastics in Packaging.* Boston, MA: Cahners Publishing.

Saddik, M.F., M.R. El-Sherbeeny, and F.L. Bryan. 1985. Microbiological profiles of Egyptian raw vegetables and salads. *J. Food Protect.* **48**:883–886.

Schlimme, D.V. 1991. Unpublished data. College Park, MD. University of MD, Horticulture Department.

Shewfelt, R.L. 1986. Postharvest treatment for extending the shelf-life of fruits and vegetables. *Food Technol.* **40**(5):70–80.

Shewfelt, R.L. 1987. Quality of minimally processed fruits and vegetables. *J. Food Quality* **10**:143–156.

Smith, J.P., H.S. Ramaswamy, and B.K. Simpson. 1990. Developments in food packaging technology. Part II: storage aspects. *Trends Food Sci. Technol.* **1**(5):111–118.

Smith, S., J. Geeson, and J. Stow. 1987. Production of modified atmospheres in deciduous fruits by the use of films and coatings. *Hort Science* **22**:772–776.

Solomos, T. 1991. Personal Communication. College Park, MD: University of MD, Horticulture Department.

Swett, R.M. 1987. Introduction to polystyrene. In *Modern Plastics Encyclopedia*, Vol. 64, No. 10A, pp. 76–77. New York: McGraw-Hill.

Theis, E.N. 1987. Low density polyethylene. In *Modern Plastics Encyclopedia*, Vol. 64, No. 10A, p. 56. New York: McGraw-Hill.

Thompson, W.R. 1987. Introduction to polypropylene. In *Modern Plastics Encyclopedia*, Vol. 64, No. 10A, pp. 70–71. New York: McGraw-Hill.

Tolle, W.E. 1971. Variables affecting film permeability requirements for modified-atmosphere storage of apples. *USDA—ARS Technology Bull. 1422.* Washington, DC: U.S. Department of Agriculture.

Tomanek, C.J. and E.J. Meyer. 1987. Suspension PVC. In *Modern Plastics Encyclopedia*, Vol. 64, No. 10A, pp. 104–109: New York: McGraw-Hill.

Veeraju, P. and M. Karel. 1966. Controlling atmosphere in a fresh-fruit package. *Mod. Packaging* **40**(2):168–17, 254.

Wagner, M.K. and L.J. Moberg. 1989. Present and future use of traditional anti-microbials. *Food Technol.* **42**(1):143–147.

Watada, A.E. 1986. Effects of ethylene on the quality of fruits and vegetables. *Food Technol.* **40**(5):82–85.

Watada, A.E., K. Abe, and N. Yamauchi. 1990. Physiological activities of partially processed fruits and vegetables. *Food Technol.* **44**(5):116–122.

Wilbrandt, C.S. 1991. Gases and packaging materials utilized for chilled food in MAP. Unpublished report. Chicago, IL: Epstein Process Engineering, an A. Epstein Company.

Wills, R.B.H., W.B. McGlasson, D. Graham, T.H. Lee, and E.G. Hall. 1989. *Postharvest An Introduction to the Physiology and Handling of Fruit and Vegetables*, 3rd edit. New York: Van Nostrand Reinhold.

Zagory, D. and A.A. Kader. 1988. Modified atmosphere packaging of fresh produce. *Food Technol.* **42**(9):70–77.

5

Some Biological and Physical Principles Underlying Modified Atmosphere Packaging

Theophanes Solomos

Introduction

The practice of modified atmosphere packaging (MAP) for fresh and minimally processed refrigerated (MPR) fruits and vegetables is expanding rapidly, particularly for commodities with a relatively short storage life (Cameron 1989; Chinnan 1989; Hayakawa, Henig, and Gilbert 1975; Hobson and Burton 1989; Kader 1986; Mannapperuma and Singh 1990). The subject has been reviewed in the past from both a practical and a theoretical point of view (Chinnan 1989; Mannapperuma and Singh 1990). The beneficial effects of MAP are due in part to the decrease in O_2 and the increase in CO_2 levels, and in part to the decrease in water loss (Ben-Yehoshua et al. 1983; Biale 1946, 1960; Fidler et al. 1973; Isenberg 1979; Kader 1980, 1986; Kidd and West 1945; Lipton and Harris 1974; Smock 1979). In fact, in non-climacteric fruits such as citrus fruits, the prevention of water loss is the main factor contributing to the extension of their storage life (Ben-Yehoshua et al. 1983). (See Chapter 4 for packaging materials.)

In order to develop an appropriate modified atmosphere (MA) environment, the rates of O_2 uptake and CO_2 evolution, along with the permeability to O_2 and CO_2 of the film, must be known. In addition, the tolerance of the plant materials to the levels of CO_2 and O_2 engendered by MA must also be considered. The optimum levels of O_2 and CO_2 are known for a number of commodities (Fidler et al. 1973; Isenberg 1979; Kader 1985; Salveit 1989; Smock 1979). In the case of bulky plant organs such as fruits, it is advantageous to determine the diffusivity of their skin and flesh to O_2 and CO_2, in order to avoid the creation of partial anoxia at the center of the tissue, as this would be expected to contribute to spoilage and development of off-flavors during extended shelf-life periods (Kader 1986).

In this chapter we address both the biological and the physical aspects of MAP. We also attempt to address some problems encountered in the generation of non-steady-state predictive models.

Biological Responses of Plant Tissue to Low O_2 or High CO_2

Effects of Low O_2 on Senescence of Detached Plant Tissues

The effects of O_2 on fruit ripening include: (1) a diminution in the rate of respiration; (2) a delay in the climacteric onset of the rise in ethylene; and (3) a decrease in the rate of ripening (Blackman 1954; Burg and Burg 1967; Fidler et al. 1973; Kader 1986; Kannelis, Solomos, and Roubelakis-Angelakis 1991; Mapson and Robinson 1966; Smock 1979; Solomos 1982; Yang and Chinnan 1988a, b). It was observed by Blackman (1954) that the respiratory isotherms of O_2 uptake as a function of the external O_2 concentration are biphasic in nature in that they include an initial gradual decrease at relatively high O_2 levels, followed by a rapid decline as the levels of O_2 approach zero. The isotherm of CO_2 output follows that of O_2 up to the point where the rate of decline diminishes; in fact it may even increase as the O_2 level approaches zero (Biale 1960). The rise in CO_2 evolution at low levels of O_2 is obviously caused by the expected Pasteur effect which results in an increase in fermentation. As far as prolonging storage life is concerned, the range of O_2 levels that would be expected to be beneficial must be in the region between the point that induces the initial decline in respiration and that at which it generates partial anoxic environments. It should be under-

Table 5-1
Ethanol Content (mM)

Apple No.	Air	Apple No.	1.5% O_2
1	3.294	1	1.32
2	3.422	2	0.56
3	9.264	3	0.09
4	5.361	4	2.18
5	5.584	5	0.54
Avg	5.385	Avg	0.938

Gala apples were kept for 180 days in air and 1.5% O_2.

lined that in this region of O_2 levels, the tissue does not experience anoxia because (1) there is no accumulation of ethanol (Table 5-1), and (2) no symptoms of low O_2 injury develop even after a long time in storage (Fidler et al. 1973; Kader 1986; Lougheed 1987).

The biphasic nature of the O_2 isotherm as a function of external O_2 concentration has been attributed in turn to:

1. The existence of regulatory enzyme[s] that perceive[s] the level of O_2 and exert[s] a feedback inhibition on the initial steps of glucose oxidation, thus lowering respiration (Blackman 1954; Solomos 1982; Tucker and Laties 1985);

2. The effect of resistance to the diffusion of O_2 through the tissue (Chevillotte 1973; James 1953);

3. The presence of a terminal "oxidase" with an affinity for O_2 much smaller than that of cytochrome oxidase (Mapson and Burton 1962).

Work with apples and avocados (Solomos 1982, 1988; Tucker and Laties 1985) has shown that suggestion (2) is not a viable explanation of the biphasic nature of the O_2 isotherm. Suggestion (3), that the decrease in respiration at relatively high O_2 levels is due to the presence of an oxidase other than cytochrome oxidase, is rather difficult to assess. It is fair to say that neither cytochrome oxidase nor the alternative oxidase is expected to be curtailed by the levels of O_2 that initiate a diminution in the rate of respiration. Table 5-2 presents data that indicate that the apparent K_m for O_2 of the putative oxidase must be larger than 4 μM in order to produce an experimentally detectable decrease in CO_2 evolution. It is known that the

Table 5-2
Internal O_2 Concentration, Rate of Respiration, and Percentage of
V_{max} of Oxidases with Different $K_m^{O_2}$

Intercellular Partial Pressure of O_2 KP$_a$	CO_2 Output $(\mu l \cdot g^{-1} \cdot h^{-1})$	$K_m^{O_2}$ (μM)				
		0.05	2.2	2.5	3	4
		Percentage of V_{max}				
19.25	5.92	99.98	99.45	99.30	99.10	98.54
6.50	5.90	99.94	99.13	97.52	96.92	95.14
4.91	4.92	99.91	97.47	96.65	95.85	93.52
4.13	4.40	99.90	96.96	95.99	95.03	92.28
2.23	3.34	99.78	93.81	99.91	90.10	85.04
0.92	3.30	98.82	73.60	67.65	62.59	51.11
0.49	2.20	85.63	16.57	12.91	10.65	6.93

The data were calculated from the rate of respiration and diffusion coefficient of O_2 through the skin and flesh of "Gold" apples (Solomos 1987).

K_m for O_2 of the cytochrome oxidase is about 0.05 μM, whereas that of the alternative oxidase is 10- to 15-fold higher than that of cytochrome oxidase (Douce 1985; Siedow 1982; Solomos 1977; Tucker and Laties 1985). The data thus preclude the curtailment of either of the known mitochondrial terminal oxidases by relatively high O_2 concentrations. Plant tissues, however, contain terminal "oxidases" that are resistant to the combined inhibition of both cytochrome and alternative oxidase (Laties 1978; Theologis and Laties 1978). Neither the nature of the residual oxidases nor the degree of their participation in plant respiration is known with any degree of precision. Suffice it to say that they are predominantly cytosolic in origin, with a rather low affinity for O_2 (Solomos 1988). Because of this low O_2-affinity it could be argued that these "oxidases" may not be contributing to the decrease in respiration with decreasing external O_2 levels. It should be emphasized that in actively respiring plant tissues, such as avocados, the O_2 level is low enough to preclude any appreciable participation of the residual oxidases in the respiration of the fruit. Even in potato tubers, which have much lower rates of respiration than avocado fruits (Solomos and Laties 1976), the oxygen level at the center of the tuber drops to about 13% (Figure 5-1), a concentration that would be expected to severely curtail the

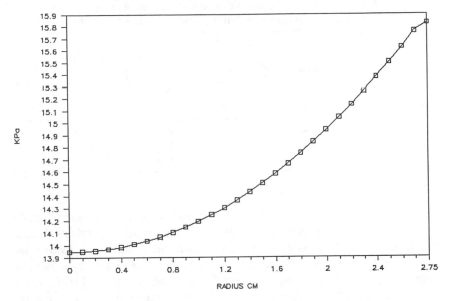

Figure 5-1   The oxygen distribution was calculated from the data concerning the diffusivity of CO_2 in the skin and flesh of potato tubers (Tables 5-11 and 5-12) and the assumption that the sum of the internal partial pressures of CO_2 and O_2 equals the partial pressure of the latter in the ambient atmosphere.

engagement of these "residual" oxidases (Solomos 1988). In addition, their curtailment must exert a feedback restraint on the initial steps of glucose oxidation and this is not compatible with the most likely known regulatory mechanisms of plant respiration (Davies 1980; Solomos 1988; Turner and Turner 1980; Wiskich 1980). In the case of climacteric fruits, it may be suggested that the effect of low O_2 on respiration is due to the diminution of ethylene action (Burg and Burg 1967). Therefore, on the basis of the above discussion, it appears that suggestion (1) is the most likely explanation of the effects of low O_2 on fruit respiration.

It was assumed in the past that the attendant decrease in respiration in response to a lowering of the external O_2 levels was an important facet of the mode of action of low O_2 in prolonging the storage life of fruits (Burton 1974). However, one may argue that the decrease in respiration reflects a metabolic depression engen-

Table 5-3
Effect of 1.5% O_2 on Sugar Accumulation and Activity of the Alternative Oxidase in Potato Tubers Stored at 1° C

| | Sugars (μmoles $\cdot$ g^{-1}) | | | Alternative oxidase nanomoles $O_2 \cdot$ min$^{-1} \cdot$ mg protein^{-1} | | |
| | 10° C | 1° C | 1° C | 10° C | 1° | 1° C |
Days	Air	Air	1.5% O_2	Air	Air	1.5% O_2
0	16.9	—	—	0.0	—	—
20	19.6	91.5	32.9	0.0	46.63	4.24
30	18.4	113.4	34.4	0.0	60.79	4.16

dered by hypoxia. In the first place, hypoxia affects metabolic events in tissues where ripening is not at issue and where ethylene is not involved. For instance, hypoxic conditions inhibited the accumulation of RNA, protein, and DNA synthesis associated with the wounding of potato tubers (Butler, Cook, and Vaya 1990). We have also observed that hypoxia (1.5% O_2) prevented the accumulation of simple sugars, and the induction of the alternative oxidase associated with storage of potato tubers at 1° C (Table 5-3). It should be pointed out that in potatoes chilling temperatures do not induce the biosynthesis of ethylene. Undoubtedly the delaying effects of low O_2 on the senescence of detached plant organs in general, and fruit ripening in particular, must involve a decrease in ethylene action. In a very perceptive paper, Burg and Burg (1967) suggested that the ethylene receptor contains a metal and when it is in its oxidized state, the binding of ethylene is enhanced. However the effect of hypoxia on ethylene biosynthesis and action may be indirect through the suppressive effects of hypoxia on the induction of 1-amino-cyclopropane-1-carboxylic acid (ACC) synthase and/or synthesis of transducer(s) of ethylene action. It has been reported previously that, in avocados, O_2 concentrations in the range of 2.5–5.5% suppressed the activity, appearance of isoenzymes, and accumulation of proteins of cellulase and polygalacturonase, associated with normal ripening (Kanellis, Solomos, and Roubelakis-Angelakis 1991). The suppressive effects on the cellulase protein were also reflected in the accumulation of its mRNA. Further, the intensity of inhibition of the synthesis of the above hydrolases was inversely related to the levels of O_2 under which the fruits were kept. In addition, the same range of O_2 concentrations that suppressed the synthesis of the above hydrolases induced the appearance of anaerobic isoenzymes of alcohol dehydrogenase (ADH). The rates of increase in the levels of cellulase, its mRNA and polygalacturonase, and the disappearance of the anoxic isoenzymes of ADH on reexposure of the fruits to air, were directly related to the previous levels of O_2 (Kanellis, Solomos, and Roubelakis-Angelakis 1990). The fact that similar ranges of O_2 concentrations on the one hand suppressed the rise in the enzymes associated with normal ripening, while at the same time inducing the synthesis of anoxic isoenzymes of ADH, indicates that the O_2-sensing mechanism is common for both processes. The induction of anoxic isoenzymes in response to hypoxia is easily understood because it is advantageous for the tissue to synthesize enzymes that increase the production of ATP in anoxia before oxygen is completely depleted. However, the extension of the storage life of fresh fruits and vegetables must be the consequence of metabolic depression which, unlike anoxia, is not deleterious to the long-term survival of the tissue. Metabolic depression is the most important adaptation for survival of intertidal organisms, which experience frequent transitions from normoxia to hypoxia (Storey and Storey 1990). Because the intensity of respiration could be considered to reflect the intensity of cellular metabolism, and because low oxygen invariably decreases the rate of respiration of such detached plant organs as fruits, flowers, and leaves, this indicates that hypoxia, by an as yet unknown mechanism, produces a decrease in metabolism, which in turn results in diminishing the rate of plant development and hence senescence. In short, the decrease in respiration may not be the cause of the decline in the rate of senescence, but rather a response to a metabolic depression, which diminishes the demand for biological energy.

It has been pointed out that low O_2 in preclimacteric tissues delays the onset of the climacteric rise in ethylene evolution (Mapson and Robinson 1966). Experimental results concerning the range of O_2 concentrations that delay the onset of ripening are limited. It appears that in the case of "Gala" apples the external O_2 concentration must fall below 8% in order to prolong the preclimacteric stage of the apples (Table 5-4). In short, the system that is involved in the induction of ACC synthase, a key regulatory enzyme in ethylene biosynthesis (Yang and Hoffman 1984), is saturated at O_2 levels above 7–8%. The data of Table 5-4 show, as expected, that the effect of low O_2 on the timing of the onset of ripening differs with the season.

Table 5-4
Days to Climacteric Under Different O_2 Concentrations

				Treatment			
Year	Harvest Date	Air	8% O_2	6% O_2	4% O_2	3% O_2	2% O_2
1987	8–24	19	24	40	66	109	>194
1988	8–26	22	—	—	89	>280	—
1989	8–22	21	—	45	76	103	—
1990	8–24	16	—	—	32	—	105
1991	8–27	9	—	—	—	—	45

Quantitative data concerning the effect of low O_2 on the rate of ripening are rather difficult to establish. At present it is not possible to state unequivocally the relationships between O_2 concentration and rate of ripening. Suffice it to say that low O_2 does indeed delay ripening, as has been amply demonstrated in a variety of fruits (Kader 1986; Knee 1980; Kanellis, Solomos, and Angelakis-Roubelakis 1991; Liu and Long-Jum 1986; Quazi and Freebairn 1970; Yang and Chinnan 1988a); Yang and Chinman (1988b) developed a mathematical expression for predicting the changes in the color of tomato fruits as a function of O_2 concentration.

A critical parameter that must be taken into consideration in designing proper MAP is the limit of O_2 below which the produce cannot be safely stored. This limit, as expected, varies with the produce, but it is important to realize that levels of O_2 that induce partial anaerobiosis will be detrimental to both longevity and quality of the produce. This limit can be assessed experimentally by measuring either the values of the respiratory quotient (RQ) or, preferably, the increase in ethanol content of the tissue. The latter may be a more reliable indicator than the RQ values, especially at levels of O_2 that initiate partial anaerobiosis, and that will be rather difficult to detect from the changes in the RQ. Because of its volatility, ethanol can be detected in the ambient atmosphere of MAP by removing a gas sample and determining the ethanol content by gas chromatography (Nakhasi, Schlimme, and Solomos 1991).

Effects of CO_2 on Senescence of Detached Plant Tissues

The mode of action of CO_2 on senescence is unclear. Burg and Burg (1967) suggested that CO_2 is a competitive inhibitor of ethylene. Recent experimental evidence indicates that CO_2 may indeed diminish the action of ethylene provided the concentration of the latter is less than 1 $\mu l \times L^{-1}$. In the case of apples, CO_2 enhances the inhibitory effects of low O_2 on respiration (Fidler et al. 1973), whereas CO_2 concentrations in the range of 1–27% do not affect the rate of respiration of peaches (Deily and Rivzi 1981). It should be pointed out that CO_2 is a metabolically active molecule participating in a number of carboxylating reactions. In addition, it is expected that high concentrations of CO_2 could alter the pH of the cytosol, which in turn may affect plant metabolism (Siriphanich and Kader 1986). Anoxic conditions generated by CO_2 induce changes in a number of intermediate metabolites that are different from those observed when the tissue is kept under nitrogen instead (Kader, personal communication). CO_2 is also required for the action of ACC oxidase (Kuai and Dilley 1992).

It is well known that tolerance to CO_2 differs greatly, not only between species but also between cultivars of the same species. For instance, Golden Delicious apples can tolerate high CO_2 concentrations, whereas McIntosh apples are damaged by even 3% CO_2 (Fidler et al. 1973). Strawberries can tolerate CO_2 levels as high as 20%, and storage of peaches in 10–15% CO_2 is beneficial (Deily and Rivzi 1981). In apples high CO_2 concentrations appear to inhibit succinic acid dehydrogenase (Hulme 1956). Storage of lemons under high concentrations of CO_2 leads to an accumulation of organic acids (Biale 1960). In lettuce, high CO_2 concentrations affect the metabolism of phenolic compounds (Siriphanich and Kader 1985a, b). Another beneficial effect of high CO_2 levels is their antimicrobial activity. At present it is impossible to predict the tolerance of a particular tissue to high levels of CO_2 (Kader 1986).

Effects of Slicing on Tissue Metabolism

The effects of wounding on plant metabolism have been studied extensively in tissues prepared from bulky plant organs such as tubers and roots. The vast literature on this subject has established that slicing induces profound quantitative and qualitative changes in tissue metabolism (Kahl 1974; Laties 1978). The observed changes include a rise in respiration, DNA and RNA synthesis, induction of new enzymes, membrane degradation, and the appearance of novel mRNA (apRees and Beevers 1960; Butler, Cooke, and Vaya 1990; Clicke and Hackett 1963; Kahl 1974; Laties 1978). The effect of slicing on respiration is probably the most extensively studied aspect of wounding in bulky plant organs (Laties 1978). These investigations have shown that slicing induces a three- to fivefold rise in respiration over that of the parent-plant organ. With aging there is a further two- to threefold increase in respiration (Laties 1978). This rise in respiration with aging of slices is critically dependent on protein and RNA synthesis, since the addition, within 8–10 h of slicing, of either protein or RNA synthesis inhibitors prevents the development of the respiratory rise with aging (Clicke and Hackett 1963; Kahl 1974). Neither the cause of this rise in respiration nor its metabolic significance is clear. However, the data indicate that inhibitors of respiratory development also inhibit a number of biochemical events, such as suberin formation and synthesis of phenolics, associated with aging of potato slices (Kahl 1974; Laties 1978).

A number of experiments show that the nature of both respiratory substrates and pathways changes with aging of slices. In particular, in fresh potato slices most of the respiratory CO_2 is derived from the α-oxidation of fatty acids arising out of the attendant breakdown of phospholipids in response to slicing, whereas carbohydrates are respiratory substrates of aged slices (Jacobson et al. 1970; Laties 1978). It has also been reported that in slices other than potatoes a large portion of CO_2 is produced by the pentose phosphate pathway (PPP) (apRees and Beevers 1960). In addition it should be mentioned that temperature and gas composition affect both respiratory substrates and pathways. Thus when potato slices are aged either in air, in the presence of 10% CO_2, or in a bicarbonate solution, suberin formation is prevented and the tissue develops callus (cf. Laties 1978). Moreover the respiration of aged slices is manolate-resistant and is presumed to comprise the PPP (Kahl 1974). This observation is important from the point of view of MAP because aging in high CO_2 levels may prevent the formation of color in potato slices.

The effects of hypoxia on minimally processed produce, in combination with high CO_2 concentrations, have not been studied in detail. However, based on the observations that hypoxia inhibits the synthesis of DNA, protein, and novel mRNA in potato slices (Butler, Cook, and Vaya 1990), it may be anticipated that the above conditions may repress the synthesis of those enzymes that are considered to exert adverse effects on the quality of tissue slices, for example, phenylalanine ammonia lyase (PAL), this being considered to increase the content of phenolics in the tissue, which in turn tend to increase in wounded plant tissues (Kahl 1974; Vritani and Asahi 1980). In addition MAP environments may suppress the rise in amylases,

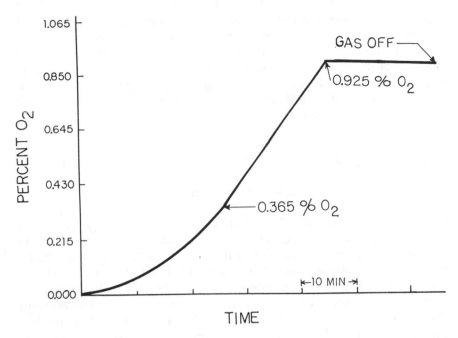

Figure 5-2   The rate of CO_2 uptake of slices suspended in air was followed polarographically. The slices were initially maintained under 0.925% O_2. At the indicated point the gas was turned off. The rate of O_2 uptake between 20.946% and 0.925% was of zero order.

thus diminishing the breakdown of starch prevalent in potato slices (Kahl 1974).

A number of experimental observations indicate that regardless of the origin of the respiratory reducing equivalents, the terminal electron acceptor is predominantly cytochrome oxidase, even in tissues that possess substantial cyanide-resistant respiration (Laties 1978; Solomos 1988). If this is the case in tissue slices, the oxygen concentration can be reduced to very low levels because of the high affinity for O_2 of the cytochrome oxidase, and because of the short diffusion path available to gases. For instance, in the case of sweet potato slices suspended in air at 25°C, the rate of O_2 uptake is of zero order with respect to its external concentration until the latter drops to about 0.4% (Figure 5-2). The ability to decrease the O_2 concentration to such low levels may be beneficial because it is expected to reduce the browning due to polyphenol oxidases (PPO), as the latter have a rather high K_m for O_2 (Beevers 1961).

At present there are no detailed studies concerning the effect of ranges of O_2 and/or CO_2 concentrations on either metabolism, longevity, or quality of cut tissue segments. It is to be expected, as in the case of intact tissues, that O_2 concentrations that engender partial anoxia will be detrimental to longevity and quality of the produce. This low limit of O_2 can be assessed in a manner identical to that described earlier for intact tissues.

Determination of Gas Diffusivities in Plant Tissues

General Considerations

In attempting to generate predictive MAP models, it is useful to know the permeability to gases of the tissue in order to calculate their concentration at the center of the organ, particularly when bulky fruits or vegetables are used. The diffusion barriers of a plant organ include the skin, the intercellular spaces, the cell walls, and plasmalemma. Previous work has established that the diffusion of gases through bulky plant organs such as fruits, roots, and tubers follows Fick's first law and the diffusion channels are predominantly gaseous in nature (Burg and Burg 1965; Burton 1974; Cameron and Yang 1980; Solomos 1987). Simple calculations with apples have shown that, assuming an aqueous diffusion barrier, the maximum radius that could maintain 1% O_2 at the center of the fruit would be about 0.7 cm (Solomos 1987). For fruits with rates of O_2 uptake much larger than apples, the radius would be even smaller. Similar observations have also been reported for potato tubers and apples by Burton (1974). The most convincing evidence for the gaseous nature of the diffusion paths is that provided by Burg and Burg (1965). These authors showed that the diffusivity of gases was inversely related to the external total pressure (Table 5-5), as would be expected from the ideal gas law. If the barrier was liquid in nature, the changes in external pressure would not be expected to affect the length of the mean free path because of the incompressibility of water.

Fick's first law states that the flux normal to the surface of a metabolically inert gas is given by (Crank 1970):

$$J = AD \frac{\partial c}{\partial x} \tag{5.1}$$

where J, in μmoles sec^{-1} per fruit, is the flux; A, in cm^2, is the surface available to diffusion; D, in cm^2 sec^{-1}, is the diffusion coeffi-

Table 5-5
Relationship Between External Pressure and Internal Concentration of C_2H_4[a]

External Pressure (kP$_a$)	Internal ethylene concentration (1)
101.3	472
76	319
37.3	190
25.3	88

[a]From Burg and Burg 1965.

cient; and $\partial c/\partial x$ is the concentration gradient with respect to distance. It is customary to replace $\partial c/\partial x$ with the difference in concentration, $\Delta c/\Delta x$. This is permissible only when the change in concentration with distance is linear (Jacobs 1967; Nobel 1983). In order to determine D, the concentration gradient must first be determined. In the case of non-steady-state conditions, the change in concentration with respect to time must also be known. In order to calculate the above gradients, the equation for Fick's second law must first be solved (Crank 1970; Jacobs 1967). The general equation for Fick's second law for a metabolically active gas in three dimensions is (Crank 1970):

$$\frac{\partial c}{\partial t} = D\left[\frac{\partial^2 c}{\partial x^2} + \frac{\partial^2 c}{\partial y^2} + \frac{\partial^2 c}{\partial z^2}\right] \pm v \qquad (5.2)$$

where v is the specific rate of evolution (+) or uptake (−) of the gas under consideration. The analytical solutions of Eq. (5.2) are numerous, depending on the boundary conditions and the initial distribution of the gas throughout the barrier. Eqs. (5.3) and (5.4) below represent the expression of Eq. (5.2) for a solid sphere and cylinder, respectively (Crank 1970; Jacobs 1967):

$$\frac{\partial c}{\partial t} = D\left[\frac{\partial^2 c}{\partial r^2} + \frac{2}{r}\frac{\partial c}{\partial r}\right] \pm v \qquad (5.3)$$

$$\frac{\partial c}{\partial r} = D\left[\frac{\partial^2 c}{\partial r^2} + \frac{1}{r}\frac{\partial c}{\partial r}\right] \pm v \qquad (5.4)$$

where r, in cm, is the radius of the sphere and cylinder. In cases

Table 5-6

Concentration of CO_2 with Distance and Time as Percent of Initial Amount Deposited at the Center of an Infinite Cylinder with a Diffusion Coefficient of 2.5×10^{-4} $cm^2 \cdot sec^{-1}$

Time (min)	Distance (cm)				
	1	1.5	2	2.5	3
10	12.688	1.370	0.061	0.001	0.000
11	14.223	1.880	0.111	0.003	0.000
15	18.755	4.253	0.533	0.037	0.001
20	21.854	7.182	1.512	0.204	0.018
30	24.009	11.433	4.046	1.064	0.208
40	24.119	13.826	6.344	2.330	0.685
50	23.581	15.109	8.102	3.636	1.365
60	22.843	15.763	9.378	4.809	2.126

where the peel of the tissue is considered, the above equations must be solved for hollow spherical and cylindrical shells. For nonmetabolic gases, there are analytical solutions for a hollow sphere and cylinder (Crank 1970).

Apart from the mathematical complexities, determining the diffusivity of gases under dynamical conditions introduces a number of uncertainties because of the nonhomogeneous nature of the diffusion barriers of a plant organ. For instance, the diffusion coefficients of CO_2 in the skin and flesh of potato tubers are about 6.90×10^{-7} and 2.50×10^{-4} cm^2 sec^{-1}, respectively. The existence of such a barrier in the flesh will generate appreciable concentration gradients within the flesh when the efflux of a gas is measured. To demonstrate this point, it is assumed that CO_2 is diffusing in an infinite cylinder of unit cross-section area, with a D_{CO_2} similar to that of potato tuber flesh. Table 5-6 describes the percentage distribution of a quantity M of CO_2 deposited at $x = 0$ and $t = 0$. The change in concentration with time and distance is given by (Crank 1970):

$$C(x, t) = \frac{M}{2\pi(Dt)^{1/2}} \times \exp - \left[\frac{x^2}{4Dt} \right] \qquad (5.5)$$

It may be seen from Table 5-6 that the concentration gradient is very substantial. Therefore the assumption that the concentration of a metabolically inert gas is uniform throughout the flesh is not valid (Cameron and Yang 1980).

Another uncertainty of the efflux method is the assumption that the equilibrium between the cellular solution and intercellular spaces is instantaneous. However, a number of observations indicate that this may not be the case. It was shown by Burton (1950) that the evacuation of O_2 from a small plug of potato tissue was rather lengthy. In addition, indirect experimental evidence indicates that the resistance to gas diffusion from the cell to the intercellular spaces may not be negligible (Chevillotte 1973). It is also expected that the solubility of the gas in aqueous solutions would affect the equilibrium distribution between the cell and the intercellular spaces, especially where short time intervals are concerned. A case in point is the changes in RQ in the course of the rapid climacteric rise in respiration. In preclimacteric avocados the RQ is close to unity, changes to less than one at the climacteric peak, and then returns toward unity at the postclimacteric stage (Solomos and Laties 1976). It was shown later that in bananas this pattern of changes was not metabolic in nature, but rather the result of the difference in the respective solubilities of CO_2 and O_2 in water (McMurchie et al. 1972). Because of this difference in solubilities, O_2, which has a smaller solubility in water than does CO_2, equilibrates with the intercellular spaces faster than does CO_2. Further, the efflux method requires a rather precise knowledge of the volume of the intercellular spaces and the solubility of the gas in the cellular liquid.

However, if appropriate experimental precautions are taken, it may be feasible to obtain reasonable approximations of gas diffusivities through the skin of a plant organ by following the efflux of metabolically inert gases. For instance, if the skin is thin, if the tissue is loaded with relatively high concentrations of the inert gas, if the volume of the vessel is small, and if the diffusion in the flesh is much larger than in the skin, then this method could give reasonable approximations of gas diffusivity through the skin. In order to avoid the generation of the concentration gradient along the flesh of potato tubers, the resistance to diffusion was calculated by considering only the initial linear part of the efflux isotherm of ethane (Banks 1985). This approach, however, introduces some uncertainties concerning the origin of the gas. It was assumed that the gas originated under the skin, which may not be correct because ethane, being nonpolar, is expected to dissolve in the waxy layers of the cuticle. In tissues with thick skin, the volume of the waxy layer can be appreciable. For instance, in a cylindrical tuber of radius 2.8 cm, length 12 cm and skin thickness 0.012 cm, the volume of the phellem is about 2.5 ml. It is also possible that some of the initial gas efflux may originate from the gas adsorbed on the tuber surface or present in gaseous cavities. This approach could be compared to the ion fluxes, where the initial flux contains a large component of the apparent free space and does not measure fluxes across the cellular membranes, these being the main barrier to ion fluxes between cells and ambient environment (Briggs, Hope, and Robertson 1961). It should be emphasized that any determination of gas diffusion is *meaningless* unless it is verified experimentally.

In view of both the mathematical complexities and uncertainties involved in the determination of the D of gases under non-steady-state conditions, I shall here consider only steady-state situations.

The steady-state solution of Eq. (5.2), $((\partial c)/\partial t) = 0)$, in one dimension, plane sheet, for a metabolically active gas is (Hill 1928)

$$C(x) = \frac{v}{2D} x^2 - \frac{\ell v}{D} x + C_0 \qquad (5.6)$$

where v, in μmoles cm^{-3} sec^{-1}, is the constant rate of output $(+)$ or uptake $(-)$ of the gas per unit tissue volume; ℓ, in cm, is half of the tissue thickness; and C_0, in μmoles cm^{-3}, is the concentration of the gas at $x = 0$, that is, the ambient atmosphere. Thus, the concentrations of CO_2 and O_2 at the center of the tissue C_i are:

$$C_i = C_0 \pm \frac{v}{2D} 1^2 \qquad (5.7)$$

The concentration of CO_2 and O_2 at the center of a sphere and cylinder are given by Eq. (5.8) and (5.9), respectively (Hill 1928):

$$C_i = C_0 \pm \frac{v}{6D} R^2 \qquad (5.8)$$

$$C_i = C_0 \pm \frac{v}{4D} R^2 \qquad (5.9)$$

where R, in cm, is the radius of either the sphere or cylinder. The other notations have been defined earlier.

In the case of metabolically inert hollow spherical and cylindrical shells, the flux of CO_2 per unit time at their surfaces is given by Eqs. (5.10) and (5.11), respectively (Crank 1970):

$$J_{r=R} = 4\pi D \frac{C_i - C_0}{R - R_i} R^2 \qquad (5.10)$$

$$J_{r=R} = 2\pi Dh \frac{C_i - C_0}{1n(R/R_i)} \qquad (5.11)$$

where R and R_i, in cm, are the outside and inside radii, respectively. In the case of a thin spherical wall, Eq. 5.10, it is assumed that $R \cdot R_i \approx R^2$. The other notations have been defined earlier. It should be pointed out that Eq. (5.11) may not be very accurate unless the surfaces of the cylindrical bases are small in comparison with the cylindrical surface, and the length is much larger than the radius. In the case of oxygen, the order of the concentration differences in Eqs. (5.10) and (5.11) is reversed, for example, $C_0 - C_i$. It is obvious from Eq. (5.11) that for an accurate determination of D, the values of R and R_i must be known with some degree of precision. It is customary to use Eq. (5.12), instead of Eq. (5.11):

$$J_{r=R} = 2\pi rh \frac{C_i - C_0}{\Delta r} D \qquad (5.12)$$

and to determine the apparent diffusion coefficient, $D' = (D/\Delta r)$. This could, depending on the dimensions, introduce appreciable error because $D' = R \times (D/\Delta r)$ (Abdul-Baki and Solomos 1993).

Finally the flux of oxygen through a metabolically inert plane sheet is given by Eq. (5.13) (Jacobs 1967):

$$J = AD (C_0 - C_1)/\Delta x \qquad (5.13)$$

It has been pointed out in the text that gases diffuse in and out of plant organs in gaseous channels. Thus the usually observed low diffusivities are due to the fact that only a small fraction of the tissue surface is available to gas diffusion. In Russet Burbank potato tubers the fraction of the surface permeable to gases varied with the tuber from 4.22×10^{-6} to 7.8×10^{-6}, the average being 6.22×10^{-6} (Abdul-Baki and Solomos 1993). It is thus apparent that Eq. (5.1) should be written as:

$$J = ADN \frac{dc}{dx}$$

where N is a number between 0 and unity representing the fraction of the surface that is permeable to gases (Burg and Burg 1965). On the basis of microscopic and gas diffusion measurements it was calculated that only 1/1,000 of the cross-section of the flesh of potato tubers was permeable to gases (Woolley 1962).

The diffusivity of gases through plant tissues could also be decreased by the degree of tortuosity of the path. However, in most plant tissues of interest for consumption, the thickness of the skin is rather small, hence the effect of a tortuous path will probably be insignificant.

It was mentioned earlier that for the determination of the diffusion coefficient of the gases for the cases considered above, one must measure the flux and the concentrations of the gases inside and outside the tissue.

Measurements of Intercellular Gases

Several methods have been used in the past to ascertain the internal concentration of gases in various fruits and vegetables. These methods include evacuation, manometric techniques, use of oxygen microelectrodes, and the removal of plugs of tissue which are then sealed in airtight vials (Solomos 1987).

The evacuation technique introduces the following uncertainties. In the first place, the values reflect the overall concentration of the gases in the tissue and not that at a particular point, for example, at the center, under the skin, etc. Further, the evacuated gases will contain not only those present in the intercellular spaces, which is required, but an unknown portion of the dissolved gases in the cellular sap. This in turn requires corrections that must include solubility of gases in the cell liquid but also, depending on time and intensity of respiration, the production or utilization of the gas within the time interval. The use of O_2 microelectrodes has produced measurements of some large O_2 gradients within the tissue (Brädle 1968). Readings of an oxygen microelectrode will vary greatly depending on whether the electrode is submerged in liquid or is in a gaseous phase. The use of manometric techniques, though reliable, requires the construction of special apparatus which makes it difficult to use for a large number of samples (Hulme 1951). Removal of plugs is a destructive method. In addition it introduces uncertainties in the subsequent analysis of the gases similar to those given above for the evacuation technique. Banks and Kays (1988) affixed small vials on the surface of potato lenticels and followed the changes in the concentration of CO_2 and O_2. It is expected that the concentrations of CO_2 and O_2 in the vials will reflect that under the skin. This method is better than any of the previous techniques but the uncertainty exists that the gases may diffuse laterally to adjacent lenticels if the pressure in the vial increases or the lenticel is partially blocked. Waldraw and Leonard (1939) removed small plugs of tissue to create cavities into which the inserted tubes were in turn sealed airtight. It is anticipated that, with time, the composition of the gas atmospheres of the tubes will equilibrate with the internal gas atmosphere of the tissue. Thus the composition of the fruit gases can be determined by analyzing the gas in the tubes. Trout et al. (1942) showed that the removal of up to 10 ml of gas from the internal cavity of apple fruit generated no appreciable drop in pressure, and the system returned to equilibrium rather rapidly. However, this may not be the case for plant organs with small intercellular spaces. With improvement in analytical techniques for measuring gases a small volume of samples—between 25 and 50 μl—can be used to accurately determine the concentrations of metabolically active gases, that is, O_2, CO_2, and C_2H_4. Several investigators have inserted hypodermic needles into the locule cavities of apple fruits to determine the internal concentration of C_2H_4 (Burg and Burg 1965). The hubs of the needles are sealed with a vaccine cap and samples are withdrawn from the needle with an airtight syringe. The concentration of C_2H_4 is then measured by gas chromatography (Burg and Burg 1965). This method can be improved upon further by gluing a chromatographic septum to the calix of the fruit and inserting the needle through the septum and into the locules (Solomos 1989). This technique facilitates sequential sampling and the needle can be replaced easily if it becomes blocked. The method has the additional advantage that it inflicts minimal injury and the needle can be kept in the fruit for long periods so that the effect of injury is dissipated. In the case of fruits, such as apples, with large locular cavities the injury effect may not be an issue. Further, because of the small volume of the needle, it is expected that its gas space will come into rapid equilibrium with the intercellular gases and, in addition, the removal of small volumes of sample gas is expected to represent that in the intercellular spaces adjacent to the needle tip. In this way gradients across the tissue can be ascertained.

Previous work has established, as expected, that the total internal gas pressure is equal to that of the ambient environment (Hulme 1951; Trout et al. 1942). That entails that the sum of the internal partial pressures of the gases should be equal to the surrounding atmosphere, approximately 1 atm. The data of Table 5-7 show that this is indeed the case for apple fruit. This in turn suggests that the sampling method does not introduce appreciable experimental error. The rate of gas exchange can be measured either by a static or a flow-through system (Henig and Gilbert 1975; Solomos 1987).

Experimental Determination of CO_2 Diffusivity in Apples and Potatoes

It has been pointed out earlier that the diffusion barriers from the cell to the ambient atmosphere include the skin, intercellular spaces,

Table 5-7
Internal Partial Pressure of Gases in Atmospheres in "Gala" Apples

	CO_2	O_2	N_2	Total $CO_2 + O_2 + N_2 + Argon$ + Water vapors
Experiment 1	0.022	0.181	0.772	1.002[a]
Experiment 2	0.026	0.183	0.777	1.012
Experiment 3	0.022	0.188	0.777	1.014

[a]Each reading represents the average of five apples.

cell walls, and plasmalemma. Most of the previous data were mainly concerned, apart from a couple of exceptions (Burton 1950; Solomos 1987; Woolley 1962), with measuring skin resistance (Banks 1985; Burg and Burg 1965; Cameron and Yang 1980). The main reason for this is that the experimental procedures that were used are not amenable to determining gas diffusion through the intercellular spaces of the flesh. Further, apart from a few exceptions, the calculated resistances have not been subjected to experimental verification. We shall here briefly describe methods for evaluating gas diffusion coefficients through both skin and flesh, as well as experimental procedures for ascertaining their validity. We shall confine ourselves to apples and potato tubers.

Apples

We have used varieties of apples whose geometry approaches that of a sphere (Solomos 1987). Within the cultivar we selected fruits whose equatorial and polar circumferences differed by < 5%. In order to subject the data to experimental verification, we altered the rate of CO_2 output by decreasing the external O_2 concentration and comparing the values of CO_2 diffusivities. The experimental arrangements were those described by Burg and Burg (1965), with minor modifications (Solomos 1987, 1989). The geometrical configuration of the skin of the apple was assumed to be a hollow spherical shell. It is apparent from Eq. (5.10) that the concentration of CO_2 under the skin, along with the respiration rates and fruit dimensions, must be known, so that D' can be calculated. The concentration of CO_2 under the skin can be measured by inserting a hypodermic needle just under the surface of the fruit, while the concentration at the center is obtained by inserting a hypodermic needle

Table 5-8
Diffusion Coefficient ($cm^2 \cdot sec^{-1} \times 10^{-4}$) of CO_2 in the Skin of "Gala"
Apples Under Different O_2 Levels at 15° C

	Apple No.					CO_2 output ($\mu l/G/H$)
	1	2	3	4	5	
Air	1.67	1.28	1.28	1.50	1.51	6.08
13.00	1.26	1.17	1.35	1.50	1.30	5.99
6.78	1.18	0.98	0.99	1.28	1.19	4.29
4.75	1.18	0.98	0.98	1.28	1.19	4.19
1.59	1.16	1.48	1.00	1.30	1.47	3.54
0.62	1.34	1.47	0.94	1.29	1.23	2.91
N_2	1.32	1.20	1.10	1.34	1.32	3.15
AVG	1.301	1.223	1.09	1.356	1.316	
STD	0.164	0.19	0.150	0.093	0.120	

through the calix into the locules. In most of the apple cultivars we used, the gradient between the center and the subcutin was rather small (0.2–0.6%) (Solomos 1987). In the case of "Gala," whose data are presented here, the gradient of CO_2 was between 0.1 and 0.2%, which falls within the experimental error for measuring CO_2. It has been demonstrated that in the case of ethylene, the use of the concentration at the center to represent that under the skin introduced an insignificant error in the values of D' (Solomos 1989). Thus the concentration of CO_2 under the skin is taken to be identical to that at the center. Table 5-8 shows the diffusion coefficient of CO_2 under different external O_2 concentrations. When the external O_2 concentration was decreased in steps from air to N_2 this of course affected the rate of CO_2 output. It may be seen from Table 5-8 that the diffusivities of CO_2 under different O_2 levels are in reasonable agreement.

The evaluation of the diffusivity of intercellular spaces poses some problems for apple fruit. Because of the small difference in CO_2 concentrations between the center and subcutin, Eq. (5.8) cannot be used to calculate D. We thus proceeded to peel the fruit, blot it dry with filter paper, and then measure the rate of respiration and internal CO_2 concentration. Within about 6–8 h the rate of CO_2 evolution was close to that of the intact fruit, probably because the dissolved CO_2 was dissipated. From the rate of CO_2 output and external and internal CO_2 concentrations, its diffusion coefficient in the intercellular spaces was calculated based on Eq. (5.8). The values ob-

Table 5-9
Diffusion Coefficient of CO_2 in the Flesh of Gala Apples

Experiment	$cm^2 \cdot sec^{-1} \cdot 10^{-3}$
1	1.46 (0.27)[a]
2	1.47 (1.27)
3	1.26 (0.27)
4	2.13 (0.95)

[a]Each value represents the average of five apples. The number in parentheses is the STD.

tained are presented in Table 5-9. Unfortunately the validity of these values cannot be tested experimentally because with time the outer layers of the fruit will form periderm, thus altering the internal concentration of CO_2.

Potato Tubers

We have used only Russet Burbank tubers because their geometry simulates a cylinder. (It should be stressed, however, that no tuber is exactly cylindrical.) The tubers were selected with the proviso that their length be greater than 11 cm, and that the circumference, measured at several points along the tuber, not vary by more than 10% (Abdul-Baki and Solomos 1993). The CO_2 concentrations under the skin and at the center were measured by gluing two chromatographic septa, 11 mm in diameter, on the surface in the middle of the tuber, each septum being 180° apart. Through the septa, two hypodermic needles were inserted, one at the center and the other under the skin. In addition the thickness of the lenticels was measured microscopically. From the rate of CO_2 output and the concentration of CO_2 under the skin, the diffusion coefficient of CO_2 in the skin was calculated using Eq. (5.11). In Table 5-10 the values of the D_{CO_2} are presented. It may be seen that there is appreciable variability between the tubers. These values are close to those reported previously for O_2 (Burton 1950). The validity of the data was tested by transferring the tubers from 10° to 27° C. From the observed values of CO_2 concentration under the skin, and the values of D_{CO_2} calculated from those obtained at 27° C (Jost 1960), we calculated the rate of CO_2 output at 10° C and compared it to that observed. The data of Table 5-11 indicate that the observed and calculated values of respiration are in good agreement.

Table 5-10
Diffusion Coefficient ($cm^2 \cdot sec^{-1} \cdot 10^{-7}$) of CO_2 in the Skin of Potato Tubers

Tuber No.	10° C	27° C
1	7.16	8.21
2	6.73	9.33
3	6.03	6.04
4	6.04	7.97
5	6.37	7.77
6	4.19	5.12
7	5.56	5.98
8	7.79	7.62
Avg	6.24	7.26

[a]The values of D_{CO_2} were calculated by inserting in Eq. (5.11) the observed fluxes and concentration of CO_2 under the skin and ambient atmosphere, along with dimensions of the tuber and skin thickness (0.012 cm).

Table 5-11
Comparison of Observed and Calculated Rates of CO_2 Evolution at 10° C.

27° C Tuber	($\mu moles \cdot sec^{-1} \times 10^{-2}$)	
	Observed	Calculated
1	2.97	2.92
2	2.37	1.83
3	2.63	2.96
4	2.34	1.69
5	2.34	1.65
6	2.39	2.20
7	2.56	2.68
8	2.70	2.86
Avg	2.54	2.35

The theoretical fluxes were obtained by inserting in Eq. (5.11) the calculated values of D_{CO_2} at 10° C from those observed at 27° C along with the theoretical CO_2 concentration under the skin, calculated as in Table 5-13, dimensions of the tuber, and the concentration of CO_2 in the ambient atmosphere.

Table 5-12
Diffusion Coefficient ($cm^2 \cdot sec^{-1} \times 10^{-4}$) of CO_2 in the Flesh of Potato Tubers

Tuber No.	10° C	27° C
1	1.67	1.90
2	2.17	2.23
3	2.63	3.10
4	2.68	2.90
5	2.90	2.46
6	2.30	2.67
7	3.65	3.81
8	1.96	2.10
Avg	2.50	2.65

[a]D_{CO_2} was calculated by inserting in Eq. (5.9) the experimental data of specific respiration, together with the CO_2 concentrations at the center and under the skin.

The diffusion coefficient of CO_2 in the flesh was calculated from the values of CO_2 concentrations at the center and under the skin, and rates of CO_2 output, based on Eq. (5.9) (Table 5-12). The accuracy of these values was tested by calculating the concentration of CO_2 under the skin from Eq. (5.9) along with the observed concentrations of CO_2 at the center, and the calculated values of D_{CO_2} at 10° C from the data at 27° C corrected for temperature (Jost 1960). It may seen from Table 5-13 that the observed and calculated values are in reasonable agreement.

Modeling for Appropriate Gas Environment in MAP

General Considerations

MAP is an inexpensive way to generate controlled atmosphere (CA) conditions within the package. The CA environment is generated through the interactions between produce respiration, film permeability to gases, and the ratio between total film area and produce weight. MAP is a dynamic system in that the internal concentration of gases changes continuously until it reaches a steady state, i.e. where the rate of O_2 and CO_2 fluxes equal their respective rates of utilization and production. Modeling thus includes a determination of the time it takes for the gases to reach their steady-state levels,

Table 5-13
Observed and Calculated Concentrations (μmoles $\cdot$ cm^{-3}) of CO_2 Under the Skin at 10° C

Tuber No.	Observed	Calculated
1	1.90	1.89
2	1.42	1.51
3	2.66	2.64
4	1.85	1.87
5	1.87	1.86
6	2.93	2.96
7	2.53	2.52
8	2.10	2.10
Avg	2.15	2.17

The theoretical values were obtained by inserting in Eq. (5.9) the calculated values of D_{CO_2} from their value at 27° C (Jost 1967), along with the observed CO_2 concentration at the center, and the specific respiration.

which must equal the desired concentrations for the produce under consideration. However, the non-steady-state part of the modeling is of limited practical value and may be ignored. Modeling can be carried out under steady-state conditions.

At any time the rate of changes in the concentrations of O_2 and CO_2 per unit volume of free gas space in the package can be expressed as:

$$\frac{d[O_2]}{dt} = \frac{P_{O_2}A\{[O_2]_{out} - [O_2]_{in}\}}{V} - \frac{R_{O_2}W}{V} \tag{5.14}$$

$$\frac{d[CO_2]}{dt} = \frac{P_{CO_2}A\{[CO_2]_{in} - [CO_2]_{out}\}}{V} + \frac{R_{CO_2}W}{V} \tag{5.15}$$

where $[O_2]$ and $[CO_2]$, in ml cm^{-3}, are the concentrations of O_2 and CO_2, respectively; P_{O_2} and P_{CO_2}, in ml/h cm^2 ml cm^{-3}, are the permeabilities of the film to O_2 and CO_2; A, in cm^2, is the area of the film; R_{O_2} and R_{CO_2}, in ml kg^{-1} h^{-1}, are the rates of O_2 uptake and CO_2 output, respectively; W, in kg, is the weight of the produce; and V, in cm^3, is the free gaseous volume of the package (void volume).

Obviously when the system reaches steady state, the changes in the package of CO_2 and O_2 concentrations with time are zero; hence

$$R_{O_2}W = P_{O_2}A\{[O_2]_{out} - [O_2]_{in}\} \tag{5.16}$$

$$R_{CO_2}W = P_{CO_2}A\{[CO_2]_{in} - [CO_2]_{out}\} \tag{5.17}$$

Rate of Respiration

The solutions of Eqs. (5.14) and (5.15) require a precise knowledge
of the rates of O_2 uptake and CO_2 evolution, which in turn vary
with the concentrations of O_2 and CO_2; that is, $R_{O_2} = f(O_2, CO_2)$ and
$R_{CO_2} = g(O_2, CO_2)$. Further, the effect of O_2 or CO_2 on the rate of
respiration is also dependent on the stage of maturity. For instance,
in preclimacteric "Gala" apples the rate of CO_2 output decreases
when the external O_2 concentration drops below 8.10 kPa (8%),
whereas in the climacteric kind the rate of CO_2 output is of zero
order with respect to the external O_2 concentration up to 2.53 kPa
(2.5%) (unpublished observations). The rates of O_2 uptake and CO_2
output can be determined using a flow-through system. Here a stream
of gas is passed through the tissue which is enclosed in a jar. The
levels of O_2 and CO_2 in the outlet stream are monitored. This method
is probably the most accurate. However, it is not practicable to measure the rate of respiration under a number of combinations of O_2
and CO_2. Alternatively, the tissue may be enclosed in a vessel and
the changes in O_2 and CO_2 in the head space can be measured. At
any instant the change in the concentrations of O_2 and CO_2 will be
dependent on the rate of respiration, the volume of the gas space
in the vessel, and the weight of the tissue. Therefore

$$R_{O_2} = \frac{V_0}{W} \frac{d[O_2]}{dt} \qquad (5.18)$$

This method has the advantage that the rate of respiration can be
determined under a variety of O_2 and CO_2 concentrations. However, if rapid changes in the rate of respiration are involved, they
could introduce some uncertainty, especially with bulky plant organs, because of the large differences between the solubilities of O_2
and CO_2 in water. It is thus expected that the external O_2 levels will
reach equilibrium between the concentrations in the intercellular gas
spaces and the ambient atmosphere faster than will CO_2. It has been
noted earlier in the text that this can introduce appreciable experimental error in the values of RQ. Nevertheless if appropriate ratios
of the volume of the respiratory vessel to weight of tissue are chosen, it is possible that the concentration of gases in the ambient and
fruit atmospheres will be close to equilibrium because the changes
occur gradually. A number of authors have determined the rate of
O_2 uptake by scrubbing the CO_2 in the vessel (Cameron 1989; Henig
and Gilbert 1975). Because of the absorption of CO_2, the pressure
in the jar will decrease with time. This may introduce some ex-

perimental errors because of possible contamination from air during the withdrawal and subsequent injection of the gas into the gas chromatogram. Cameron (1989) has measured the rate of O_2 depletion by enclosing an O_2 electrode in the jar, thus avoiding the above source of experimental error. Once the relationship between rates of O_2 uptake and CO_2 output as a function of both O_2 and CO_2 levels is determined, an expression is generated by various interpolation techniques. A number of interpolation methods have been used in the past to express the rates of O_2 uptake and CO_2 output as a function of O_2 and CO_2 concentrations. Henig and Gilbert (1975) divided the isotherms showing the percentage of gas versus time into linear and curvilinear segments. The latter part was plotted on semilogarithmic paper and both segments were subjected to regression analysis for the determination of the coefficients and intercepts. Hayakawa, Henig, and Gilbert (1975) expressed the rate of respiration in stepwise linear segments which were subsequently used to develop a predictive MAP model. Cameron (1989) fitted the O_2 depletion data to an exponential function, whereas Yang and Chinnan (1987, 1988a) used polynomial interpolations.

Unfortunately previously published modeling work was mainly concerned with intact tissue. There is a scarcity of experimental data regarding the optimal MAP conditions as well as the effects of O_2 and CO_2 on the rate of respiration of tissue segments.

It was mentioned above that previous work with tissue slices cut from such plant organs as tubers and roots has established that slicing invokes an immediate two- to fourfold increase in respiration over the parent organs (Laties 1978). In addition, there is a further two- to threefold increase with aging. The latter increment depends on temperature and on whether the aging takes place with slices that are submerged in aerated liquid or in moist air (cf. Laties, 1978). The facts that (1) slice respiration is mediated mainly by cytochrome oxidase with a K_m for O_2 of 0.05 μM (Solomos 1988; Theologis and Laties 1978), and (2) the resistance to diffusion through the flesh is lower than that through the skin indicate that tissue slices at relatively low temperatures can be maintained at rather low O_2 concentrations. For instance, the diffusion of O_2 in potato flesh is about 2.9×10^{-4} cm^2 sec^{-1} (Table 5-11). If it is assumed that at 10° C the rate of O_2 uptake is 9 μl kg^{-1} h^{-1}, and the ambient O_2 concentration is 2%, then the O_2 level at the center of a slice 2 cm thick will be about 0.4%, which will result in a 6.7 μM O_2 solution in the adjacent cells, a concentration that is unlikely to limit cytochrome oxidase. We have observed that the rate of O_2 uptake of sweet potato slices

2 mm thick at 25° C is of zero order with respect to its external level until the latter decreases below 0.5% (Figure 5-2).

The effect of temperature on MAP modeling must also be considered because it affects both the rate of respiration and film permeability to gases. The effects of temperature on plant respiration can be expressed as Arrhenius-type equations (James 1953). In chilling-sensitive tissues there is an increase in the energy of activation at low temperatures (Lyons 1973). Further, in a number of tissues, low temperatures may induce a rise in respiration. A classic example is potato tubers, where storage at 1° C evokes a rise in respiration above that observed at 10° C (Isherwood 1973).

Changes in the permeability of gases through the film with temperature can also be expressed by an Arrhenius-type equation (Mannapperuma and Singh 1990). The authors have determined the energy of activation in a number of commercially available films.

Steady-State Modeling

The most important aspect of MAP modeling is the design of the proper packaging for generating the appropriate gas environment for long-term storage of the commodity. Usually, the establishment of the steady-state CA environment takes about 24 h, which is adequate for most commodities. In cases where the creation of the desired gas composition has to be accelerated, the package can be flushed with the appropriate gas mixture before sealing. It should be underlined that the time for the system to reach its final steady-state is determined by the parameters that are used for the creation of the long-term desired gas composition. A detailed knowledge of the transient changes in the gas composition is of limited practical value, though very interesting from a theoretical point of view.

It has been noted above that under steady-state conditions the concentrations of O_2 and CO_2 inside the package can be considered constant, although small changes occur gradually due to changes in the respiratory activity of the tissue under the new gas environment. Thus $(d[O_2]_{in}/dt)$ and $(d[CO_2]_{in}/dt)$ are zero. And the equilibrium fluxes can be determined from Eqs. (5.16) and (5.17). It is apparent from these equations that the internal concentrations of O_2 and CO_2 will be determined from the rates of O_2 uptake and CO_2

evolution, weight of the tissue, and area and permeability properties of the film. Combining Eqs. (5.16) and (5.17) we obtain:

$$\frac{R_{O_2}}{R_{CO_2}} = \frac{P_{O_2}}{P_{CO_2}} \frac{[O_2]_{out} - [O_2]_{in}}{[CO_2]_{in} - [CO_2]_{out}} \tag{5.19}$$

It is evident that both the RQ and the ratio of permeabilities of O_2 over CO_2 will be critical in establishing a particular CA environment. For most tissues, RQ is close to one, in particular for tissue slices of bulky plant organs such as tubers and roots (Laties 1978). Assuming a value for RQ of 1, Eq. (5.18) can be rearranged to become:

$$[CO_2]_{in} = \frac{P_{O_2}}{P_{CO_2}} [O_2]_{out} + [CO_2]_{out} - \frac{P_{O_2}}{P_{CO_2}} [O_2]_{in} \tag{5.20}$$

A plot of $[O_2]_{in}$ against $[CO_2]_{in}$ will result in a straight line with a slope equal to the permeability ratio, as $[CO_2]_{out}$ can be neglected, and the $P_{O_2}/P_{CO_2} \cdot [O_2]_{out}$ is constant. Figure 5-3 illustrates the relationship between $[O_2]_{in}$ and $[CO_2]_{in}$ for 1/2, 1/4, 1/5, and 1/6 permeability ratios of O_2 over CO_2. These ratios were chosen because they are the most common in the commercially available films. For a successful MAP package the combination of internal concentrations of O_2 and CO_2 will fall close to the line for a given permeability ratio.

Eqs. (5.16) and (5.17) show that the area of the film, along with the weight of the tissue, will be critical in establishing a desired MA environment. If W/A is denoted by ρ, then

$$[O_2]_{in} = [O_2]_{out} - \frac{R_{O_2}}{P_{O_2}} \rho \tag{5.21}$$

$$[CO_2]_{in} = [CO_2]_{out} + \frac{R_{CO_2}}{P_{CO_2}} \rho \tag{5.22}$$

In this way an appropriate W/A ratio can be selected to move the internal CO_2 and O_2 concentrations toward the point where the lines of Figure 5-3 intersect the right-hand y-axis.

Jurin and Karel (1963) determined the steady-state internal oxygen concentration from the intercept of the plot of the experimental rates of respiration and flux across the film as a function of O_2 concentration. Cameron (1989) fitted the curve showing oxygen depletion versus time to an exponential equation

$$[O_2] = a\{1 - e^{-(btc)^d}\} \tag{5.23}$$

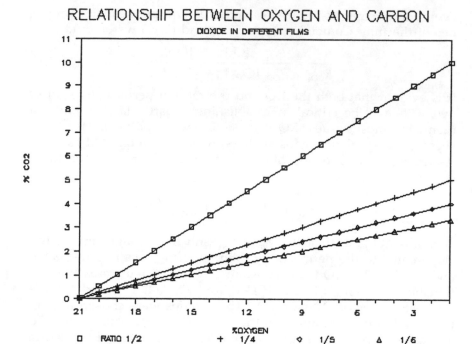

Figure 5-3   Steady-state relationship between the internal concentrations of CO_2 and O_2.

where a, b, and c are constants. The rate of respiration at steady state was calculated by multiplying the time derivative of Eq. (5.23) by the V/W ratio, where V, in lit, and W, in kg, are the void volume of the vessel and weight of tomato fruits, respectively. The transient changes were ignored; only steady-state modeling was considered. It should be noted that Eq. (5.23) may not always be appropriate to use with plastic bags because of the changes in the void volume due to film shrinkage. Changes in V are produced by the decrease in the internal pressure due to differences in the permeabilities of O_2 and CO_2. This necessitates a decrease in volume so that the internal total gas pressure equals the ambient pressure (see later). Eqs. (5.16) and (5.17) are more appropriate because the volume is not a variable.

In summary, for modeling an appropriate MA package, first the desired concentration of gases for a particular commodity can be selected from the compilation of previous data (Isenberg 1979; Kader

1985; Salveit 1989). Then from the values of respiration under the chosen MA environment the appropriate film and W/A (ρ) ratio can be determined.

Dynamic Modeling

Non-steady-state modeling can predict both the time from the start until the virtual steady-state is established, and the steady-state concentrations of O_2 and CO_2 in the package. In order to generate the appropriate expressions, the equations expressing the rate of respiration as $f(O_2, CO_2)$ must be inserted into Eqs. (5.14) and (5.15). The results in the literature differ somewhat (Chinnan 1989; Hayakawa, Henig, and Gilbert 1975; Mannapperuma and Singh 1991). These differences could be partly biological in nature because of the inherent variability in biological material, and because of the limited number of determinations that are usually used. The differences could also be due to physical considerations in assessing the rate of respiration and changes in internal package gas concentrations during the transient stage.

In order to illustrate the latter point, we assume a solid sphere with a diffusion coefficient similar to that for O_2 in the Russet "Burbank" potato tuber (2.94×10^{-4} cm^2 sec^{-1}). Further, at zero time the sphere contains no O_2 and is transferred to a vessel where the O_2 concentration is maintained constant at 9.1 μmoles cm^{-3} O_2 (air concentration at 10° C). It is also assumed that oxygen is not utilized by the tissue. It can be shown that for boundary conditions $C(R,t)$ = C_0, $t > 0$ and $C(0,t) = 0$ for $0 < t < t_2$, and initial conditions $C(r,0)$ = 0, the solution of Eq. (5.2) is:

$$C(r,t) = C_0 + \frac{2RC_0}{\pi r} \sum_{n=1}^{\infty} \frac{(-1)^n}{n} \sin \frac{n\pi r}{R} \cdot \exp\left(-\frac{n^2\pi^2}{R^2} \cdot Dt\right) \quad (5.24)$$

where C_0, in μmoles $\cdot$ cm^{-3}, is the concentration of O_2 in the ambient atmosphere; R, in cm, is the radius of the sphere; t, in sec, is the time; and D, in cm^2 sec^{-1}, is the diffusion coefficient. It may be seen from Figure 5-4a and b that even after 10 min the concentration of O_2 at $r = 1$ cm is almost zero. Figure 5-4b demonstrates the distribution of O_2 along the radius after 1 h. It should be noted that the gradient would have been steeper if the utilization of O_2 had been incorporated into the solution of Eq. (5.2) and if the resistance to O_2 diffusion of the skin had also been included. Even if the initial

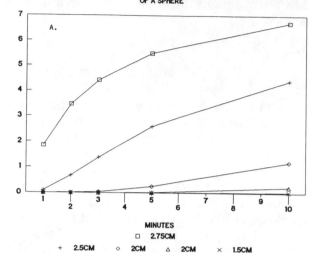

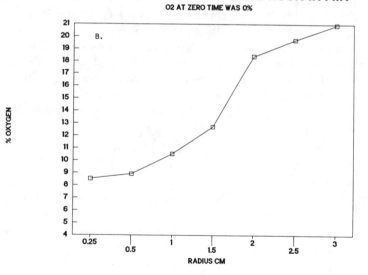

Figure 5-4   The distribution of oxygen along the radius of a sphere with a diffusion coefficient similar to that in potato flesh. (A) Changes with time in O_2 concentration at a number of points along the radius. (B) Distribution of oxygen across the sphere after 1 h.

O_2 distribution is not zero, the concentration gradient could be appreciable (Crank 1970).

It is likely that under rapid changes in the external O_2 concentration in a closed system, an appreciable concentration gradient of oxygen along the organ will be developed. Under these conditions the rate of respiration of the cells on the periphery will differ from those at the center of the organ because of the substantial differences in O_2 concentration. Further, the changes in respiration calculated from the gas isotherms may represent part of the respiration of the organ, because the contribution of the cells at the center may not be perceived.

It has been noted above that because of the differences in O_2 and CO_2 permeabilities through the film a partial vacuum is generated inside the package which in turn produces a decrease in void volume in order that the internal pressure may equal the ambient pressure. In short, the void volume is also a function of time, and Eq. (5.14) should be written as follows:

$$\frac{d[O_2]}{dt} = \frac{P_{O_2}A\{[O_2]_{out} - [O_2]_{in}\}}{V(t)} - \frac{R_{O_2}W}{V(t)} \tag{5.25}$$

A note of caution is also appropriate regarding the global validity of the rates of respiration calculated from the gas isotherms. In general, a number of interpolations produce a unique function. This, however, may not be the case for all methods of interpolation (Lancaster and Salkauskas 1986). Although the uniqueness of the local expression may be assured this may not necessarily reflect the biochemical behavior of the system. For instance, the rate of respiration of a number of plant tissues is of zero order at concentrations of O_2 from 15% to 100% (Burton 1974; James 1953; Tucker and Laties 1985). If the local expressions reflected the biochemical events that underly plant respiration, then extension of the interpolation to concentrations of O_2 larger than those in air will result in respiration being independent of O_2.

It should also be noted that the relationship between O_2 and respiration is enzymatic in nature and may involve more than one terminal oxidase whose affinities for oxygen may differ. Furthermore, the suppression of respiration may be the result of a metabolic depression involving alterations in the kinetic properties and/or amount of key regulatory respiratory enzymes (Storey and Storey 1990). It may thus be more appropriate to develop mathematical expressions reflecting the kinetics of multienzyme sequences (Goldbeter 1991) rather than the usual interpolating techniques that are frequently used in the literature.

Experimental Dynamic MAP Modeling

The literature on dynamic MAP modeling has been reviewed previously (Chinnan 1989; Mannapperuma and Singh 1991). Here, a limited amount of previous research, representing different approaches to deriving predictive mathematical expressions, will be considered.

Deily and Rivzi (1981) produced analytical formulae for predicting the gas concentration and the time necessary to reach the final dynamic equilibrium for peach fruits. The authors observed that the O_2 depletion isotherm consisted of linear and exponential segments with an inflection point at about 5% O_2 and 20% CO_2. Further, the rate of respiration was unaffected by CO_2 concentrations in the range of 1–27%. Since the optimal MAP environment for peach storage was found to be 10–15% O_2 and 15–25% CO_2, and since the rate of respiration is constant under these conditions, the authors solved Eqs. (5.14) and (5.15) for constant R_{O_2} and R_{CO_2}. The analytical formulae derived for calculating O_2 and CO_2 are:

$$y(t) = \bar{y} + (y_a - \bar{y}) \cdot \exp(-AP_{O_2}t/V) \qquad (5.26)$$
$$z(t) = \bar{z} + (z_a - z) \cdot \exp(-AP_{CO_2}t/v) \qquad (5.27)$$

where $\bar{y}$ and $\bar{z}$ are the steady-state levels of O_2 and CO_2, calculated from the steady-state solution of Eqs. (5.14) and (5.15) and from limit $(y(t)/t\rightarrow\infty)$. y_a and z_a are the internal concentrations of O_2 and CO_2 at $t = 0$. The analytical formulae were tested by comparing the experimental and predicted gas concentrations using different films. Table 5-14 shows a good agreement between observed and calculated values.

Henig and Gilbert (1975) solved Eqs. (5.14) and (5.15) numerically using the experimental results of the respiration rate as a function of external O_2 and CO_2 concentrations. The authors validated the computer modeling with the experimental data. The experimental results with a VF-71 film package were in good agreement with the computer-predicted results (Figure 5-5) (Henig and Gilbert 1975). The authors also tested the validity of the computer model by altering the variables of the inputs, for example, permeability, weight/void volume ratio, and film area. Their results showed that the predicted steady-state values of CO_2 and O_2 concentrations were similar to those expected.

Table 5-14
Parameters and Results of Analytical and Experimental Determination
of Model Packages of Peach Fruits

Parameters	Package Types		Film Overlaps on Foam Trays		
	Bags	Super-L.-Bags[a]	Super Firm	Barrier Bag	Poly-olefin
W	0.21	212.30	0.32	0.23	0.31
R_y	7.84	7.84	7.84	7.84	7.84
R_z	7.55	7.55	7.55	7.55	7.55
S	0.12	1.11	0.04	0.04	0.03
V	2.34	2.32	533.90	439.60	614.00
K_y	166.67	166.67	166.67	0.10	0.06
K_z	200.00	200.00	200.00	5.54	0.29
$\hat{y}(\%)$	12.48	11.92	—	—	—
$\hat{z}(\%)$	6.62	7.05	—	—	—
t	96.00	108.00	20.00	10.00	10.00
Analyt.					
$O_2\%$	15.99	15.55			
$CO_2\%$	4.12	4.61			

W, S, and V are the weight, surface, and void volume of the package, respectively. R_y and R_z are the rates of O_2 uptake and CO_2 output respectively and K_y, K_z the permeabilities to O_2 and CO_2 respectively of the films. $\hat{y}$ and $\hat{z}$ are the steady-state levels of O_2 and CO_2, respectively.
From Deily and Rivzi 1975.

Hayakawa, Henig, and Gilbert (1975) derived an analytical solution of Eqs. (5.14) and (5.15) using Laplace transforms. The rate of respiration was expressed as linear segments:

$$R_{O_2} = a_i[O_2] + p_i[CO_2] + q_i \qquad (5.28)$$
$$R_{CO_2} = d_i[O_2] + e_i[CO_2] + f_i \qquad (5.29)$$

where a_i, p_i, q_i, d_i, e_i, and f_i are constants, and $[O_2]$ and $[CO_2]$ are the analytical expressions determining the O_2 and CO_2 levels. Because of computational complications the authors assumed that the rate of O_2 uptake of tomato fruits was not critically affected by CO_2, hence $p_i = 0$. Similarly it was assumed that the rate of CO_2 output was not significantly affected by the external O_2 levels. There is some uncertainty concerning the latter assumption because usually the rate of CO_2 evolution parallels that of O_2 uptake as a function of external O_2 concentrations up to the inflection point. Nevertheless, the pre-

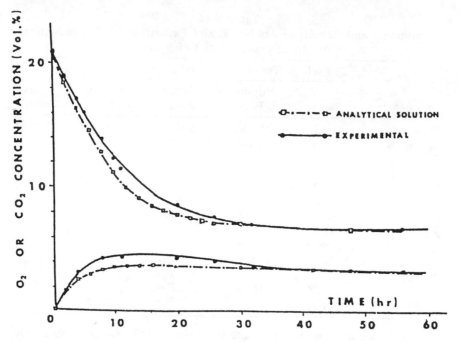

Figure 5-5 Changes with time in O_2 and CO_2 concentrations in a RMF-61 film package of tomato fruits. (From Henig and Gilbert 1975.)

dicted transient changes in O_2 and CO_2 concentrations were similar to those observed experimentally (Figure 5-6).

Yang and Chinnan (1987) measured the rates of O_2 uptake and CO_2 output under 20 combinations of external O_2 and CO_2 concentrations. These data were subsequently used to develop a computer-predictive model by expressing the rates of O_2 uptake and CO_2 output as a second-degree polynomial of O_2, CO_2, and time (Yang and Chinnan 1988a):

$$R_{O_2} = a_0 + a_1 C_0 + a_2 C_c + a_3 t + a_4 C_o^2$$
$$+ a_5 C_c^2 + a_6 t^2 + a_7 C_0 C_c + a_8 C_o t + a_9 C_c t \tag{5.30}$$

where C_o and C_c are the concentrations of O_2 and CO_2, respectively, and $a_0 \ldots a_9$ are constants. The calculated values were tested by comparing them with the experimental observations at two arbitrary combinations of O_2 and CO_2 levels (Figure 5-7). The prediction of the steady-state concentrations of O_2 and CO_2 was achieved by iterative techniques which minimize the sum of the squares of the O_2

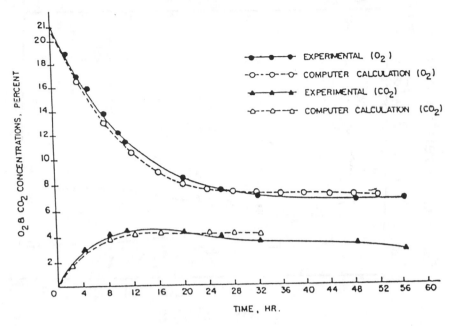

Figure 5-6   A comparison between experimental and computed O_2 and CO_2 concentrations in RMF-61 film package of tomato fruits. (From Hayakawa, Henig, and Gilbert 1975.)

and CO_2 fluxes at small time-intervals as the system approaches steady state (Yang and Chinnan 1988b). An innovative aspect of the above work is the development of expressions to predict quality attributes, such as color, as a function of O_2 and CO_2. This is very useful because it may eventually lead to the determination of the apparent K_m for O_2 of the enzyme(s) whose activity is restricted by O_2, producing a slowing of metabolic reactions involved in plant senescence in general and fruit ripening in particular.

Concluding Remarks

The biological aspects underlying the beneficial effects of low O_2 or high CO_2 on the shelf-life of plant tissues are not as yet understood. Recent results using molecular biological techniques, however, have begun to shed some light on the mechanism of low O_2 action. It appears that hypoxia induces the expression of anoxic genes, while

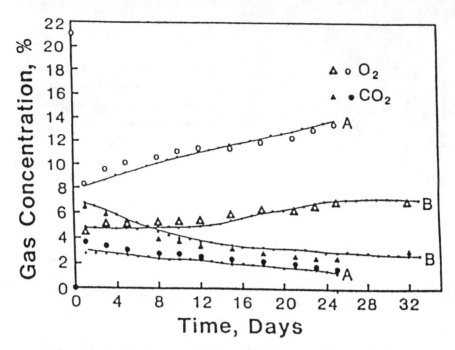

Figure 5-7   A comparison between experimental (○ ▲ · ▲) and computed (−) results of the atmosphere in two packages (A and B) made from cryo-pack E-type film. Both packages had the same surface area (1,392 cm^2). Packages A and B contained two and four tomatoes, respectively. (From Yang and Chinnan 1988.)

suppressing those genes that are involved in plant development and that eventually lead to plant senescence. In short, hypoxia produces a metabolic depression that arrests the rate of senescence. Future research should be directed towards the identification of genes involved in the induction of metabolic depression so that the molecular aspects of MAP on plant tissues will be better understood.

MAP environments have a great potential for extending the shelf-life of semiprocessed plant tissues because a number of tissue slices can be stored in relatively low O_2 or high CO_2 environments. In addition, MAP modeling for segments is less complex than with intact tissues because the relationship between respiration and, at least, O_2 correlation is easier to assess in slices than in intact bulky plant organs.

The development of transient predictive MAP models is limited by the availability of respiratory data in response to changes in the external concentrations of O_2 or CO_2 in forms that can be used to develop predictive MAP modeling. It should be noted that the development of steady-state MAP models is feasible if the optimal gas composition for the storage of a commodity, the rate of respiration, and film permeabilities are known. One aspect that has been given very scant attention is the development of models predicting the effect of low O_2 and/or high CO_2 on quality attributes. Such studies would be very useful in identifying the affinity for O_2 of the enzymes whose activity is restricted at relatively high O_2 concentrations and that may be involved in the perception of O_2 and/or CO_2 levels.

References

Abdul-Baki, A.A. and T. Solomos. 1993. The diffusivity of CO_2 in the skin and the flesh of potato tubers (*Solanum tuberosum* cv Russet Burbank) *J. Am. Hort. Sci.*, (in press.)

apRees, T. and H. Beevers. 1960. Pentose phosphate pathway as a major component of induced respiration of carrot and potato slices. *Plant Physiol.* **35**:839–847.

Banks, N.H. 1985. Estimating skin resistance to gas diffusion in apples and potatoes. *J. Exp. Bot.* **36**:1842–50.

Banks, N.H. and S.J. Kays. 1988. Measuring internal gases and lenticel resistance to gas diffusion in potato tubers. *J. Am. Hort. Sci.* **113**:577–580.

Beevers, H. 1961. *Plant Respiration*. New York: Row, Paterson and Co.

Ben-Yehoshua, S., B. Shapiro, Z. Even-Chen, and S. Lurie. 1983. Mode of action of plastic film in extending life of lemon and bell pepper fruits by alleviation of water stress. *Plant Physiol.* **73**:87–93.

Biale, J.B. 1946. Effect of oxygen concentration on respiration of avocado fruit. *Am. J. Bot.* **33**:363–373.

Biale, J.B. 1960. Respiration of fruits. In *Hanbuch Der Plantephysiologie. Encyclopedia of Plant Physiology*, Vol. XII/2, J. Wolf (ed.), pp. 536–592. Berlin: Springer-Verlag.

Blackman, F.F. 1954. *Analytical Studies in Plant Respiration*. London: Cambridge University Press.

Brädle, R. 1968. Die Verteilung der Sauerstoffkonzentration in fleischigen Spercherorganen (Apfel, Bannanen, and Kartollknollen) Ber. Schwiez. Bot. Ges. **78**:330–64.

Briggs, G.E., A.B. Hope, and R.N. Robertson. 1961. *Electrolytes and Plant Cells*. Oxford: Blackwell Scientific Publications.

Burg, S.P. and E.A. Burg. 1965. Gas exchange in fruits. *Physiol. Plant.* **18**:870–886.

Burg, S.P. and E.A. Burg. 1967. Molecular requirements for the biological activity of ethylene. *Plant Physiol.* **42**:144–151.

Burton, W.G. 1950. Studies on the dormancy and sprouting of potatoes. I. The oxygen content of potato tuber. *New Phytol.* **49**:121–34.

Burton, W.G. 1974. Some biophysical principles underlying the controlled atmosphere storage of plant material. *Ann. Appl. Biol.* **78**:149–168.

Butler, W., C. Cook, and M.E. Vaya. 1990. Hypoxic stress inhibits multiple aspects of potato tuber wound process. *Plant Physiol.* **93**:264–270.

Cameron, A.A. 1989. Modified atmosphere packaging: a novel approach for optimizing package oxygen and carbon dioxide. In Controlled Atmosphere Research Conference, Wanatchee, WA.

Cameron, A.C. and S.F. Yang. 1980. A simple method for the determination of resistance to gas diffusion in plant organs. *Plant Physiol.* **70**:21–23.

Cameron, A.A., W.E. Boylan-Pett, and J. Lee. 1989. Design of modified atmosphere systems. Modeling oxygen concentrations within sealed packages of tomato fruits. *J. Food Sci.* **54**:1413–1416, 1421.

Chevillotte, P. 1973. Relation between the reaction of cytochrome oxidase–oxygen uptake in cells *in vivo*. The role of diffusion. *J. Theor. Biol.* **39**:277–295.

Chinnan, M.S. 1989. Modeling gaseous environment and physio-chemical changes of fresh fruits and vegetables in modified atmospheric storage. American Chemical Society Symposium 189–202.

Clicke, R.E. and D.P. Hackett. 1963. The role of protein and nucleic acid synthesis in the development of respiration in potato tuber slices. *Proc. Natl. Acad. Sci. USA* **50**:243–250.

Crank, J. 1970. *The Mathematics of Diffusion.* Oxford: Clarendon Oxford Press.

Davies, D.D. 1980. Anaerobic production of organic acids. In *The Biochemistry of Plants. A Comprehensive Treatise*, Vol. 2, D.D. Davies (ed.), pp. 581–611. New York: Academic Press.

Deily, K.R. and S.S.H. Rizvi. 1981. Optimization of parameters for packaging of fresh peaches in polymeric films. *J. Food Proc. Engin.* **5**:23–41.

Douce, R. 1985. *Plant Mitochondria.* New York: Academic Press.

Fidler, J.C., B.G. Wilkinson, K.L. Edney, and R.O. Sharples. 1973. The biology of apple and pear storage. Research Review. No. 3. *Commonwealth Bureau of Horticulture and Plant Crops.* East Malling, Maidstone Kent, U.K.

Geankoplis, C.J. 1983. *Transport Processes and Unit Operations.* Boston: Allyn and Bacon.

Goldberter, A. 1991. Models for oscillation and excitability in biochemical systems. In *Biological Kinetics*, pp. 107–154. Cambridge University Press.

Goodenough, P.W. and T.H. Thomas. 1981. Biochemical changes in tomatoes stored in modified gas atmospheres. I. Sugars and acids. *Ann. Appl. Biol.* **98**:507–.

Hayakawa, K.I., Y.S. Henig, and S.G. Gilbert. 1975. Formulae for predicting gas exchange of fresh produce in polymer film package. *J. Food Sci.* **40**:186–191.

Henig, Y.S. and S.G. Gilbert, 1975. Computer analysis of the variables affecting respiration and quality in produce packaged in polymeric films. *J. Food Sci.* **40**:1033–1035.

Hill, A.V. 1928. Diffusion of oxygen and lactic acid through tissues. *Proc. R. Soc. Biol. Ser. B.* **104**:39–96.

Hobson, G. and K.S. Burton. 1989. The application of plastic film technology to the preservation of fresh horticultural produce. *Prof. Horticult.* **3**:20–23.

Hulme, A.C. 1951. Apparatus for the measurement of gaseous conditions inside apple fruits. *Exp. Bot.* **2**:65–85.

Hulme, A.C. 1956. Carbon dioxide injury and the presence of succinic acid in apples. *Nature* **178**:218.

Isenberg, M.F.R. 1979. Controlled atmosphere storage of vegetables. *Hort. Rev.* **1**:337–394.

Isherwood, A.C. 1973. Starch–sugar interconversion in *Solanum tuberosum*. *Phytochemistry* **12**:2579–2591.

Jacobs, M.H. 1967. *Diffusion Processes*. New York: Springer-Verlag.

Jacobson, B.S., B. Smith, S. Epstein, and G.G. Laties. 1970. The prevalence of carbon-13 in respiratory carbon dioxide as an indicator of the type of endogenous substrate. *J. Gen. Physiol.* **25**:1–17.

James, W.O. 1953. *Plant Respiration*. Oxford: Oxford Press.

Jost, W. 1960. *Diffusion in Solids, Liquids and Gases*. New York: Academic Press.

Jurin V. and M. Karel. 1963. Studies on control of respiration of McIntosh apples by packaging methods. *Food Technol.* **17**:104–108.

Kader, A.A. 1980. Prevention of ripening in fruits by use of controlled atmospheres. *Food Technol.* **34**:51–54.

Kader, A.A. 1985. Modified atmospheres: an index reference list with emphasis on horticultural commodities. Supplement No. 4. *Post Harvest Hort Series 3*, University of California, Davis.

Kader, A.A. 1986. Biochemical and physiological basis for effects of controlled and modified atmospheres on fruits and vegetables. *Food Technol.* **40**:94–104.

Kahl, G. 1974. Metabolism in plant storage tissue slices. *Bot. Rev.* **40**:263–314.

Kannelis, A.K., T. Solomos, and K.A. Roubelakis-Angelakis. 1990. Suppression of cellulase and polygalacturonase and induction of alcohol dehydrogenase isoenzymes in avocado fruit mesocarp subjected to low oxygen stress. *Plant Physiol.* **96**:269–274.

Kidd, F. and C. West. 1945. Respiratory activity and duration of life of apples. *Plant Physiol.* **20**:467–504.

Knee, M. 1980. Physiological responses of apple fruits to oxygen concentrations. *Ann. Appl. Biol.* **96**:243–253.

Kuai, J. and D.R. Dilley. 1992. Extraction, partial purification and characterization of 1-aminocyclopropane-1-carboxylic acid oxidase from apple fruit. *Postharvest Biol. Techn.* **1**:203–211.

Lancaster, P. and K. Salkauskas. 1986. *Curve and Surface Fitting*. New York: Academic Press.

Laties, G.G. 1978. The development and control of respiratory pathways in slices of plant storage organs. 1978. In *Biochemistry of Wounded Plant Tissues*, Ed. G. Kahl (ed.), pp. 421–466. Berlin: Walter de Gruyter.

Lau, O.L. and N.E. Looney. 1978. Effects of pre-storage high carbon dioxide treatment on British Columbia and Washington State Golden Delicious apples. *J. Am. Soc. Horticult. Sci.* **103**:341–344.

Lipton, W.J. and C.M. Harris. 1974. Controlled atmosphere effects for fresh vegetables and fruits, why and when. In *Postharvest Biology and Handling of Fruits and*

Vegetables, Vol. 2. N.F. Haard and D.K. Salunkhe (ed.), pp. 340 Westport, CT: AVI Publishing.

Liu, F.W. and C. Long-Jum. 1986. Responses of daminozide-sprayed McIntosh apples to various concentrations of oxygen and ethylene simulated CA storage. *J. Am. Soc. Horticult. Sci.* **111**:400–403.

Lougheed, E.C. 1987. Interactions of oxygen, carbon dioxide, temperature and ethylene that may induce injuries in vegetables. *HortScience* **22**:791–794.

Lyons, S.M. Chilling injury in plants. 1973. *Annu. Rev. Plant Physiol.* **24**:445–446.

Mannapperuma, J.D. and R.P. Singh. 199. Modeling of gas exchange in polymeric packages of fresh fruits and vegetables. Abstract 646. Inst. Food Technol. Annual Meeting, Dallas, TX.

Mapson, L.W. and Burton, W.G. 1962. The terminal oxidases of potato tuber. *Biochem. J.* **82**:19–25.

Mapson, L.W. and J.E. Robinson. 1966. Relation between oxygen tension, biosynthesis of ethylene, respiration and ripening changes in banana fruit. *J. Food Technol.* **1**:215–225.

McMurchie, E.J., B.W. McGlason, and J.L. Eaks. 1972. Treatment of fruit with propylene gives information about the biogenesis of ethylene. *Nature* **237**:235–236.

Nakhasi, S., D. Schlimme, and T. Solomos. 1991. Storage potential of tomatoes harvested at the breaker stage using modified atmosphere packaging. *J. Food. Sci.* **55**:55–59.

Nobel, P.S. 1983. *Biophysical Plant Physiology*. San Francisco: Freeman and Company.

Quazi, M.H. and H.T. Freebairn. 1970. The influence of ethylene, oxygen and carbon dioxide on ripening of bananas. *Bot. Gaz.* **131**:5–14.

Salveit, M.E. 1989. A summary of requirements and recommendations for the controlled and modified atmosphere storage of harvested vegetables. In: Controlled Atmosphere Research Conference, Wenatchee, WA.

Siau, J.F. 1984. *Transport Processes in Wood*. Berlin: Springer-Verlag.

Siedow, J.N. 1982. The nature of cyanide-resistant pathway in plant mitochondria. *Rec. Adv. Phytochem.* **16**:47–84.

Siriphanich, J. and A.A. Kader. 1985a. Effects of CO_2 on total phenolics, phenylalanine amonia lyase, and polyphenol oxidase in lettuce tissue. *J. Am. Soc. Hort. Sci.* **110**:249–253.

Siriphanich, J. and A.A. Kader. 1985b. Effects of CO_2 on cinnamic acid 4-hydroxylase in relation to phenolic metabolism in lettuce tissue. *J. Am. Soc. Horticult. Sci.* **110**:333–335.

Siriphanich, J. and A.A. Kader. 1986. Changes in cytoplasmic and vacuolar pH in harvested lettuce tissue as influenced by CO_2. *J. Am. Soc. Horticult. Sci.* **111**:73–77.

Smock, R.M. 1979. Controlled atmosphere storage of fruits. *Horticult. Rev.* **1**:301–336.

Solomos, T. 1977. Cyanide-resistant respiration in higher plants. *Annu. Rev. Plant. Physiol.* **28**:279–97.

Solomos, T. 1982. Effect of oxygen concentration on fruit respiration: nature of respiratory diminution. In *Controlled Atmospheres for Storage Transport of Perishable Ag-*

ricultural Commodities, D.G. Richardson and M. Meheriuk (eds.), pp. 161–170. Beaverton, OR: Timber Press.

Solomos, T. 1987. Principles of gas exchange in bulky plant tissues. *HortScience* 22:766–771.

Solomos, T. 1988. Respiration in senescing plant organs: its nature, regulation, and significance. In *Senescence and Aging in Plants*, L.D. Nooden and A.C. Leopold (eds.), New York: Academic Press.

Solomos, T. 1989. A simple method for determining the diffusivity of ethylene in 'McIntosh apples'. *Scientia Horticult.* 39:311–318.

Solomos, T. and G.G. Laties. 1976. Effects of cyanide and ethylene on respiration of cyanide-sensitive and cyanide-resistant plant tissues. *Plant Physiol.* 58:47–50.

Storey, K.D. and J.M. Storey. 1990. Metabolic rate depression and biochemical adaptation in anaerobiosis, hibernation and estimation. *Q. Rev. Biol.* 65:145–174.

Theologis, A. and G.G. Laties, 1978. Relative contribution of cytochrome-mediated and cyanide-resistant electron transport in fresh and aged potato slices. *Plant Physiol.* 2:232–237.

Trout, S.A., E.G. Hall, R.N. Robertson, F.M.V. Hackney, and S.M. Sykes. 1942. Studies in the metabolism of apples: preliminary investigations on internal gas composition and its relation to changes in stored Granny Smith apples. *Aust. J. Exp. Biol. Med. Sci.* 20:219–231.

Tucker, M. and G.G. Laties. 1985. The dual role of oxygen in avocado fruit respirations: kinetic analysis and computer modeling of diffusion-affected respiratory oxygen isotherms. *Plant Cell Environ.* 8:117–127.

Turner, J.S. and D.H. Turner. 1980. The regulation of glycolysis and pentose pathway. In *The Biochemistry of Plants: A Comprehensive Treatise*, Vol. 2, D.D. Davies (ed.), pp. 279–316. New York: Academic Press.

Uritani, I. and T. Asahi. 1980. Respiration and related metabolic activity in wounded and infected plant tissues. In *The Biochemistry of Plants A Comprehensive Treatise*, Vol. 2, D.D. Davies (ed.), pp. 463–485. New York: Academic Press.

Waldraw, C.W. and E.R. Leonard. 1939. Studies on tropical fruits: IV. Methods in the investigation of respiration with special reference to banana. *Ann. Bot.* 3:27–42.

Wiskish, J.T. 1980. Control of the Krebs Cycle. In *The Biochemistry of Plants. A Comprehensive Treatise*, Vol. 2, D.D. Davies (ed.), pp. 243–278. New York: Academic Press.

Woolley, 1962. Potato tuber tissue respiration and ventilation. *Plant Physiol.* 37:793–798.

Yang, C.C. and M.S. Chinnan. 1987. Modeling of color development of tomatoes in modified atmosphere storage, *A.S.A.E.* 30:548–553.

Yang, C.C. and M.S. Chinnan. 1988a. Modeling the effect of CO_2 on respiration and quality of stored tomatoes. *A.S.A.E.* 31:920–925.

Yang, C.C. and M.S. Chinnan. 1988b. Computer modeling and color development of tomatoes stored in polymeric film. *J. Food Sci.* 55:869–872.

Yang, S.F. and N.E. Hoffman. 1984. Ethylene biosynthesis and its regulation. *Annu. Rev. Plant Physiol.* 35:155–189.

6

Biological and Biochemical Changes in Minimally Processed Refrigerated Fruits and Vegetables

Patrick Varoquaux and Robert C. Wiley

Introduction

In recent years there has been a rapid expansion in the sale of pre-packed/precut fresh fruits and vegetables in North America and in Europe. Because the tissue integrity of these products has been altered during processing, they are more perishable than the original raw materials (Rolle and Chism 1987; Shewfelt 1986). Like whole fruits and vegetables, minimally processed refrigerated (MPR) produce deteriorates after harvesting due to physiological aging and microbial spoilage. Injury stresses (Figures 6-1 and 6-2) caused by processing also result in cellular decompartmentalization or delocalization of enzymes and substrates which leads to various biochemical deteriorations such as browning, off-flavors, and texture breakdown (Varoquaux 1987). Moreover, peeling and cutting facilitate primary infection of the plant tissues by epiphytic and phytopathogenic microorganisms.

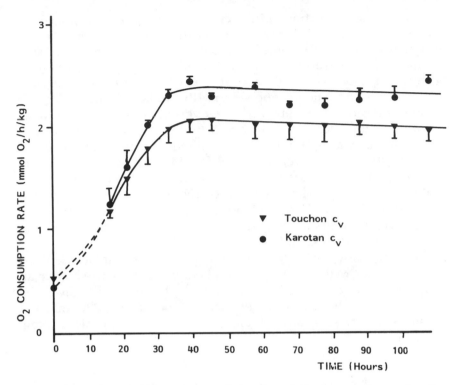

Figure 6-1 Change in respiratory intensity of fresh grated carrots after standard processing (2 cultivars). Grated carrots were stored in air at 10° C. (From Carlin 1989.)

Ready-to-use fruits and vegetables were developed about 30 years ago in the United States (Garrott and Mercker 1954). Recent investigations in the United States, Japan, and Europe have sought to improve the like-fresh characteristics of these products and to extend their shelf-life, thus allowing distribution within an adequate area (Huxsoll and Bolin 1989). Achievement of this aim is possible through optimization of all unit operations during processing, preservation, and marketing.

The first part of this chapter is devoted to a review of the physiological, biochemical, and microbial degradation mechanisms of MPR fruits and vegetables. The second part deals with the effects of processing and distribution techniques on the mechanisms of quality deterioration.

Some minimal treatments use chemical compounds applied by spraying or dipping. Chemical preservative treatments may result in a change in taste or smell. Unfortunately, some very efficient chemicals such as sorbic and benzoic acids or sulfiting agents have been found to be potentially harmful to some segments of the population. These treatments, applied to MPR fruits and vegetables, are being more carefully scrutinized by government regulators in most countries. Moreover, all additives, whether natural or useful nutrients, are increasingly rejected by individual consumers of ready-to-use fresh fruits and vegetables. Safe additives, such as critic and ascorbic acids or their combinations, are not effective enough in controlling browning of shredded lettuce (Bolin et al. 1977), and their beneficial effects are short term for pear (Rosen and Kader 1989) and apple slices (Varoquaux and Varoquaux 1990). Chemical preservatives are covered in Chapter 3.

There are many postharvest physiology reviews of intact plant tissues, including Wills et al. (1989) and Kays (1991). This chapter attempts to cover additional information that relates primarily to biological and biochemical changes that may occur in MPR fruits and vegetables. These are physiological, biochemical, and microbiological in nature.

Mechanisms of Quality Deterioration

Physiological Disorders (Primarily Injury Stress)

The effects of processing, packaging, and storage on the maintenance of the quality of minimally processed fruits and vegetables is analyzed in a later section.

Desiccation, chilling injury, and CO_2 injury, which are widely known disorders in stored intact fruits and vegetables, are well covered in Wills et al. (1989) and Kays (1991). Wounding stress results in metabolic activation. The main physiological manifestations of this phenomenon include increased respiration rate (Figure 6-1) and, in some cases, ethylene production (Rosen and Kader 1989). The response depends on the magnitude of the stress.

The O_2 consumption rate of shredded endive is only 1.2 times that of intact endive (Chambroy 1989). This ratio increases to 1.4 for broccoli (Ballantyne 1987) and to 2 for shredded lettuce (Ballantyne 1986). For more damaged plant tissue, respiration averages three to seven times that of the intact tissue, for example, four to seven for grated carrots (Carlin 1989; MacLachlan and Stark 1985). This increase in the metabolism of minimally processed fruits and vegetables results in rapid consumption of oxygen in the packaging. Bolin and Huxsoll (1991) found about four times the oxygen concentration in an intact head of lettuce compared with shredded lettuce after about 16 days of modified atmosphere packaging (MAP) storage at 2° C.

Many examples of wound-induced ethylene production in fruit and vegetable tissues have been extensively reviewed. Because ethylene contributes to the neosynthesis of enzymes involved in fruit maturation (Yang and Hoffman 1984), it may play a part in physiological disorders of sliced fruits.

The stimulation of ethylene production by stress typically occurs after a time lag of 10–30 min and subsides later after reaching a peak within several hours (Yang and Pratt 1978). When tomato is cut into small disks, ethylene production increases to about 20-fold that of whole fruit (Watada, Abe, and Yamauchi 1990).

Immediately after slicing, and for 2 h at 20° C, the ethylene production rate of kiwifruit decreases. Then, 2–4 h later, it increases sharply, peaks at seven times that of intact fruit, and decreases slightly or remains constant after about 10 h (Varoquaux et al. 1990). This confirms the results of Watada, Abe, and Yamauchi (1990), who found ethylene production rates 16-fold higher in sliced kiwifruit than in intact fruits. These authors suggested that the continual increase in rate was probably due to stimulation of ethylene production by endogenous ethylene as well as slicing. The ethylene production rate was found to be proportional to the injured surface area, and hence to the intensity of the stress. Ethylene production by sound, unstressed kiwifruit tissues is negligible, compared to uninjured tissue, whatever the maturity of the fruit (Vial 1991).

Rosen and Kader (1989) found an increase in ethylene production in sliced strawberry but not in sliced pear.

Injury stress may also enhance the susceptibility of plant tissue to ethylene (Lafuente et al. 1989).

Biochemical Reactions

Enzymes and substrates are normally located in different cellular compartments and their transfer is actively regulated. Processing results in destruction of surface cells and injury stress of underlying tissues. Enzymatic reactions cause sensory deteriorations such as off-flavor, discoloration, and loss of firmness.

Off-flavor

Enzymatic peroxidation of unsaturated fatty acids is the most dramatic example of the biochemical modifications of natural aromas of vegetables that have been minimally processed. This peroxidation is catalyzed by lipoxidase and leads to the formation of numerous aldehydes and ketones (Hildebrand 1989).

It has been shown that the concentration of n-hexanal, a by-product of hydroperoxide degradation, is well correlated with postharvest development of off-flavor in peas (Bengtsson et al. 1967). Gowen (1928) reports that vine-shelled peas develop a strong off-flavor within 4–6 h at room temperature. Bruising of peas has been shown to be an important factor in the development of delayed off-flavor. Hand-shelled peas do not deteriorate in flavor as rapidly as vine-shelled peas. This oxidative reaction also occurs, to a lesser extent, in French beans and potatoes, both of which are currently minimally processed. The hydroperoxides are unstable, may be cytotoxic, and particularly affect proteins and membranes (Watada, Abe, and Yamauchi 1990). Damage to the membrane can result in disruption of the diffusion barrier and thus generation of physiological disorders.

Discoloration

The main color deterioration that occurs in bruised plant tissues is enzymatic browning (Mayer 1987). The enzymatic reactions involved in the brown discoloration are still under investigation (Figure 6-2). The enzymatic activities markedly depend on pH; a 0.5 reduction in the natural pH of apple results in a 50% decrease in chloroplast polyphenoloxidase (PPO) activity (Harel et al. 1964).

Ortho-benzoquinones are very reactive and unstable in aqueous solutions. They are converted into phenolics by a reducing agent such as ascorbic acid and also undergo polymerization into melanins (Bu'Loch 1960; Whitaker 1972).

Other reactions can alter the natural color of fresh fruits and vegetables but color changes are not specifically caused by minimal processing. Conversion of chlorophylls into pheophytins, for example, may be caused by acidification of cellular cytoplasm, a reaction that is responsible for the degreening of broccoli (Ballantyne et al. 1988b).

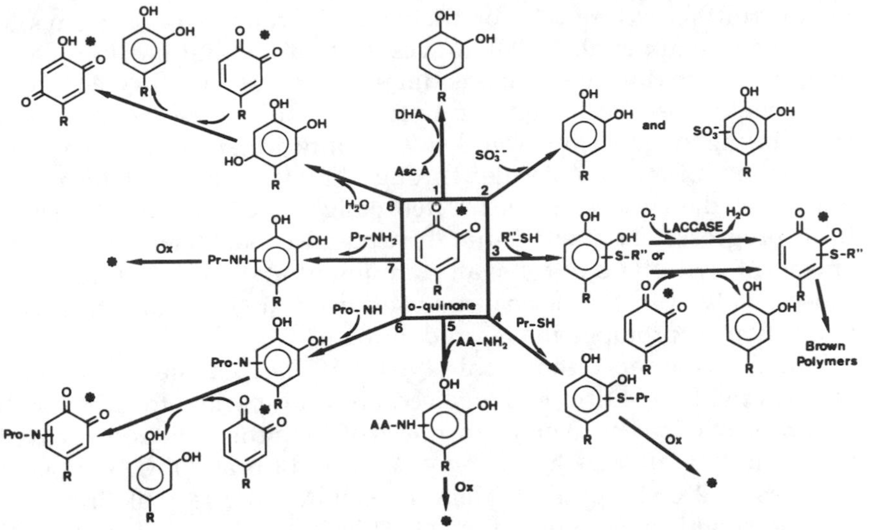

Figure 6-2   Enzymatic browning: the role of inhibitors on the formation of brown polymers from *o*-quinone. (From Rouet-Mayer et al. 1992.)

Destruction of chlorophyll by ethylene has been reported to be due to increased chlorophyllase activity (Amir-Shapira et al. 1987). The chlorophyll change may also result from the loss of membrane integrity that occurs with senescence hastened by ethylene (Rolle and Chism 1987). Other degradative enzymes have been reported, such as chlorophyll oxidase, chlorophyllase, lipolytic acid hydrolase, and peroxidase–hydrogen peroxide systems. The results reported by Watada, Abe, and Yamauchi (1990) indicate that the chlorophyll degradation pathway probably differs among plant species and it is unknown if ethylene activates other pathways. It seems that chlorophyll degradation constitutes a good marker of the physiological condition of green plant tissues (Yamauchi and Watada 1991). Coupled oxidation of carotenoids with lipoxidase-catalyzed hydroperoxides may result in discoloration of grated carrots.

Loss of Firmness

Slicing plant tissue generally results in loss of firmness, as observed with apple slices by Ponting, Jackson, and Watters (1972). There have been many reviews on loss of firmness in intact plant tissues (Doesburg 1965; Kertesz 1951).

Kiwifruit slices lose 50% of their initial firmness in < 2 days at 2° C. Varoquaux et al. (1990) suggested that textural breakdown of kiwifruit slices during storage is due to enzymatic hydrolysis of cell wall components. Pectinolytic and proteolytic enzymes liberated from cells damaged by slicing could diffuse into inner tissues. The migration rate of macromolecules through kiwifruit tissue, determined with labeled enzymes, is unexpectedly high, because the radioactive front progresses at about 1 mm/h (Cuq and Vial 1989). The mechanisms of hydrolysis of cell wall component after slicing differ from those involved in the normal maturation of kiwifruit in which solubilization of protopectins is predominant.

Watada, Abe, and Yamauchi (1990) emphasized the role of ethylene in the loss of firmness of sliced kiwifruit packed together with banana sections. The average firmness of 1 cm thick slices decreased by about 25% after 24 h and by 40% after 48 h at 20° C. Exposure of slices to 2 or 20 ppm ethylene accelerated the loss of firmness. But, as stated by Varoquaux et al. (1990), the loss of firmness of sliced kiwi begins immediately after cutting at the same softening rate as that after 6 or 12 h. Therefore, the texture breakdown is not primarily provoked by the neosynthesis of enzymes initiated by ethylene. Nevertheless, Watada, Abe, and Yamauchi (1990) suggested that "wound ethylene" can increase the permeability of membranes and perhaps reduce phospholipid biosynthesis, which can upset the dynamic processes of cellular structure and membrane integrity.

Microbial Spoilage

Microflora responsible for spoilage of MPR fruits and vegetables include a large number of fungi and bacterial species. These are reviewed in Chapter 7. Among gram-negative bacteria, pseudomonadacea and enterobacteriacea prevail. Gram-positive microorganisms, mainly represented by lactic acid bacteria and numerous yeast species, have so far been detected in mixed salads and grated carrots (Denis and Picoche 1986). Only phytopathogenic or epiphytic bacteria able to induce sensory deteriorations affected by processing and packaging conditions are considered in this chapter.

Pectinolytic bacteria such as *Erwinia carotovora* (Brocklehust et al. 1987), *Pseudomonas marginalis* (Nguyen-The and Prunier 1989), and *Pseudomonas viridiflava* (Carlin et al. 1989) were identified in minimally processed and fresh vegetables (Manvell and Ackland 1986) and in vacuum-packed sliced carrots (Buick and Damoglou 1987).

These microorganisms were identified in both raw and processed vegetables (Lund 1988; Mundt and Hammer 1968).

All spoilage mechanisms are interdependent and contribute to disorders in MPR fruits and vegetables. The plant response to these stresses is cellular delocalization, which results in biochemical reactions alone or may be superimposed on other spoilage manifestations (namely alcoholic or lactic acid fermentations).

Effects of Processing and Marketing Techniques on Quality

Processing

The successive operations in the processing of MPR vegetables are summarized in Figure 6-3 (Anon. 1989). (Also see Figure 1–1.) Each step may play a role in the spoilage mechanisms. Bruises in minimally processed fruit and vegetables lead to further deterioration, with loss of quality and shelf-life. Damage that occurs to cells next to the cut surfaces will also be very detrimental (Bolin and Huxsoll 1991; Huxsoll and Bolin 1989). The most damaging unit operations are those that alter tissue integrity.

Bolin et al. (1977) showed that compared to chopping, slicing improved the shelf-life of shredded iceberg lettuces and that the cutting blades should be as sharp as possible (Figure 6-4). Later work has shown that tearing by hand was more beneficial to lettuce than shredding by machine (Bolin and Huxsoll 1991). In general, shelf-life for most commodities is enhanced by reducing machine-to-product and product-to-product impacts.

Bolin et al. (1977) also claimed that total microbiological pollution of shredded lettuces was closely correlated to quality deterioration (Figure 6-5). To reduce microbial pollution, it is necessary to remove all the heavily contaminated external parts of the raw material, especially those in contact with soil. For example, roots and tubers should be carefully peeled and green salads severely trimmed. After cutting, the plant fragments should be thoroughly washed, although this operation may be very detrimental to the taste and flavor of grated roots or tubers and, to a lesser extent, shredded foodstuffs, because of the possibility of leaching flavor compounds. Disinfection can be performed using chlorinated water (Adams et al. 1989). Chlorine in the disinfection bath reduces the count of mesophilic aerobic bacteria according to an apparent first-order reaction (Figure 6-6).

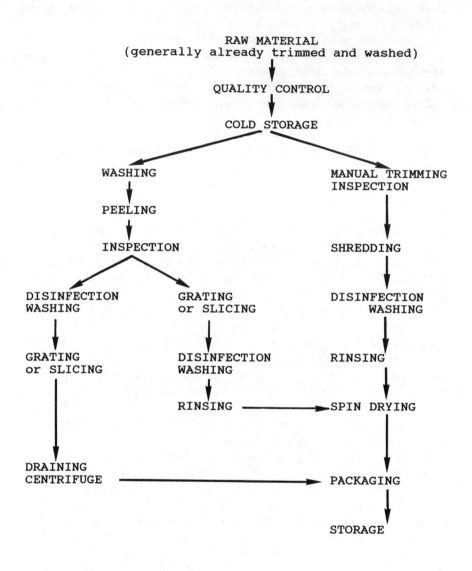

roots and tubers   **leaf vegetables**

Figure 6-3 Minimally processed vegetables. Flow diagram of processing lines.

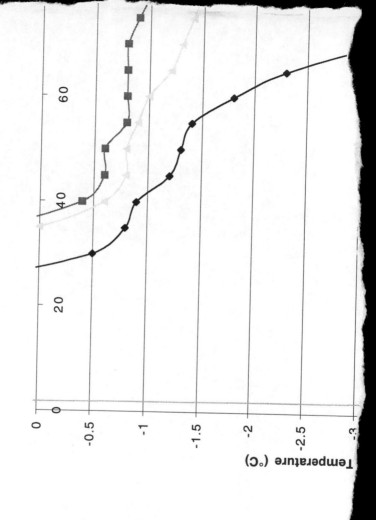

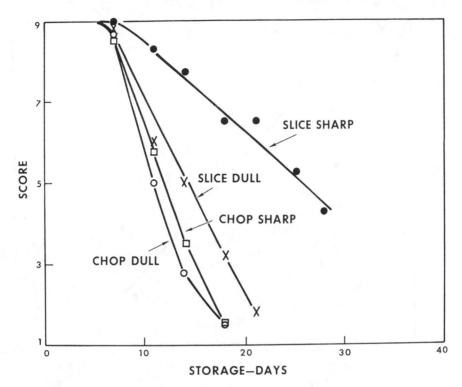

Figure 6-4 Effect of cutting method on storage life of shredded lettuce. (From Bolin et al. 1977.)

An optimal concentration of 120 ppm active chlorine on shredded salads was suggested by Mazollier (1988). It is noteworthy that chlorine only delays microbial spoilage and does not show any beneficial effects on biochemical or physiological disorders (Bolin et al. 1977). Washing with clean water removes the free cellular contents that are released by cutting. Cellular fluids contain active PPO and phenolic compounds responsible for rapid brown discoloration (Bolin et al. 1977).

Draining should be efficient because water droplets on the product surface result in microbial proliferation. Herner and Krahn (1973) indicated the importance of keeping cut lettuce dry, even advocating not rinsing at all before storage.

Conversely, excessively efficient draining, using a centrifuge, bruises plant tissue and is responsible for rapid biochemical deteriorations, although the shelf-life of lettuce was extended by cen-

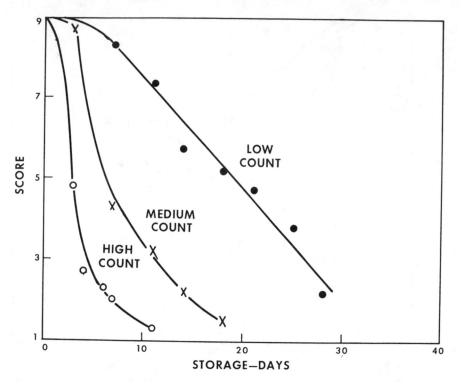

Figure 6-5   Effect of initial microbial count on storage stability of shredded lettuce. (From Bolin et al. 1977.)

trifugation (Bolin and Huxsoll 1991). According to Ryall and Lipton (1972), a detectable texture breakdown is noted if moisture loss exceeds 5%.

After draining, the minimally processed product must be packed for retail sale. Proper packaging should protect the fresh product from physical damage and surface abrasion caused by handling. It should also prevent microbial cross-contamination during distribution.

Polymeric membranes generally exhibit a high resistance to the diffusion of water vapor (see Chapter 4). Maintenance of high relative humidity is essential to the development of defense mechanisms. Below 75% relative humidity (RH), cells surrounding an injury are damaged by desiccation and are incapable of lignin synthesis (Ben-Yehoshua 1987).

High RH maintains the turgor of fruit and vegetable tissues but it may cause condensation on the commodity, creating conditions

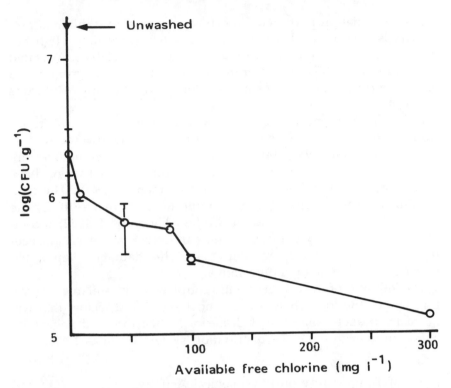

Figure 6-6   Effect of chlorine concentration on the count of mesophilic aerobic bacteria on washed lettuce leaves. pH increased from 7.3 for unchlorinated water to 9.4 for 300 mg L^{-1} of free chlorine. I indicates ranges in replicate experiments. (From Adams et al. 1989.)

favorable growth for phytopathogenic and epiphytic flora (Zagory and Kader 1988). Excessive RH may also result in the exudation of cellular sap which causes proliferation of saprophytes (Tomkins 1962).

Among other possible functions of packaging reviewed by Smith et al. (1989), pouches or overwrapping films should create an optimal modified atmosphere to keep the product under optimal physiological conditions.

The effects of MAP on MPR fruits and vegetables are reviewed later in this chapter and in Chapter 5.

Temperature

The chill chain used with MPR fruits and vegetables should begin as soon as possible after harvesting. Early precooling of raw material dramatically extends the shelf-life of minimally processed products.

A substantial proportion of French salads grown for minimal processing is vacuum-cooled less than 4 h after harvesting. High humidity air precooling is also workable for leafy vegetables. As stated by Bolin et al. (1977), temperature has one of the most pronounced effects on the storage life of shredded lettuce (and of any MPR fruits or vegetables).

French regulations imposed 8° C as a maximum temperature for MPR fruits and vegetables in 1987. This limit was lowered to 4° C in 1988 (Scandella 1988), but minimally processed commodities are often stored or distributed at higher temperatures (Anon. 1988; Scandella 1989; Scandella, Derens, and Benhamias 1990). The temperature chosen for investigations should range from 8 to 10° C. The English Guidelines for Handling Chilled Food (IFST 1982) recommend a storage temperature range of 0° C to 8° C for salad vegetables, noting that some vegetables may suffer damage if kept at the lower end of this temperature range.

The quality of raw ingredients coupled with suitable control throughout the food chain are the most significant factors that will normally predetermine the shelf-life of MPR fruits and vegetables before they even enter the distribution system (Lioutas 1988).

Effect of Temperature on Physiological Activity

Lowering temperature reduces respiration and delays senescence. There is a linear relation between the logarithm of the O_2 consumption rate and temperature. The respiration rate of shredded endive as a function of temperature is shown in Figure 6-7; also included is the equation for endive. The effect of a 10° C increase in temperature on the respiration rate, Q_{10}, averages 2 for most fruits and vegetables, but may range from 1 to 5.

Maintenance of a stable, low temperature is the key to success for packed MPR fruits and vegetables. When the storage temperature is increased to 10° C, the steady state is reached sooner (Ryall and Lipton 1972) and the gas composition within the pouches during shelf-life will be quite different (Figure 6-8).

At temperatures higher than 10° C, CO_2 concentration increases sharply due to enhanced metabolism and microbial proliferation. The chill chain temperature must therefore be taken into account for modified atmosphere packaging developments (Chapter 4).

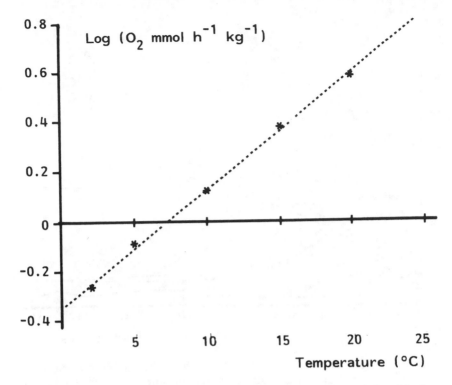

Figure 6-7   Effect of temperature on O_2 consumption rate of shredded endives in air. (From Chambroy 1990.)

Effect of Temperature on Biochemical Reactions

Because biochemical reactions are catalyzed by enzymes, biochemical change in MPR fruits and vegetables is, in part, the consequence of the effect of temperature on enzyme activities (Arrhenius' law).

The kinetics of loss of firmness of kiwifruit slices, as a function of temperature, are shown in Figure 6-9. All other enzymatic reactions are temperature dependent. For example, difference in flavor is not readily apparent in peas held at 4° C for up to 4 h. At 25° C, flavor differences are noticeable within 2 h, and at 37° C, off-flavor is inhibitory after only 1 h (Weckel et al. 1964).

Decreasing temperature also alleviates degradative change in color of injured plant tissues, thereby reducing tyrosinase and o-diphenoloxidase activities. As shredded lettuces darken during storage, discoloration is accompanied by a loss in visual green pigmentation

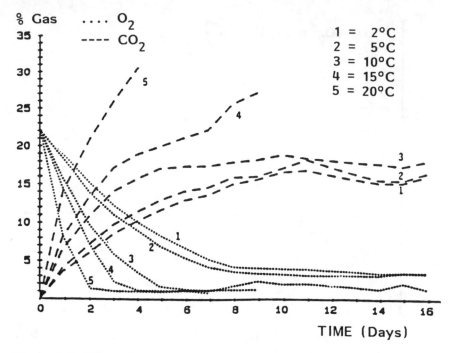

Figure 6-8   Effect of temperature on atmosphere change within propylene
packs of shredded endives versus duration of storage. (From Chambroy
1989.)

(Bolin et al. 1977; Bolin and Huxsoll 1991), likely due to coupled
oxidations. Loss in green color, measured as reflectance (*a*) versus
storage duration at several temperatures, is shown in Figure 6-10.

In bruised fruits and vegetables, the effect of temperature on enzymatic activities responsible for biochemical damage is indissocia-
ble from its effect on normal postharvest changes. Thus when plant
tissues are stored at temperatures inducing chill injuries (Marcellin
1982), the inner structures of cells disintegrate and biochemical change
occurs more intensively than in controls kept at higher temperatures. Hence, the optimal temperature minimizes tissue senescence
and thus delays cell delocalization.

Effect of Temperature on Microorganism Growth

Lowering temperature also reduces microbial proliferation on MPR
fruits and vegetables. In the properly controlled chill chain, cold-

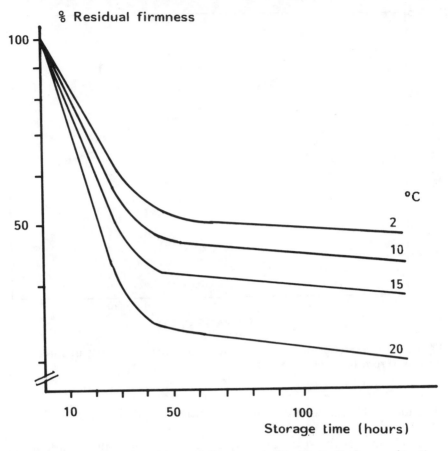

Figure 6-9   Logarithm of loss of firmness in kiwifruit slices as a function of storage time in sealed "clarylene" pouches. (From Varoquaux et al. 1990.)

tolerant microorganisms would grow slowly and eventually cause spoilage with consequent reduction in the shelf-life of the commodity (Manvell and Ackland 1986).

Lactic acid bacteria grow above 2° C in shredded endive packed in polypropylene (40 m), and at 6 and 10° C they develop faster than total flora, as shown in Figure 6-11.

In salad trays overwrapped with a cling film held at 7° C, lactic acid bacteria formed a low proportion of the total population, whereas at 30° C lactic acid bacteria formed a dominant population. These differences between population types led to the development of tests indicating shelf-life expiration or temperature abuse (Manvell and

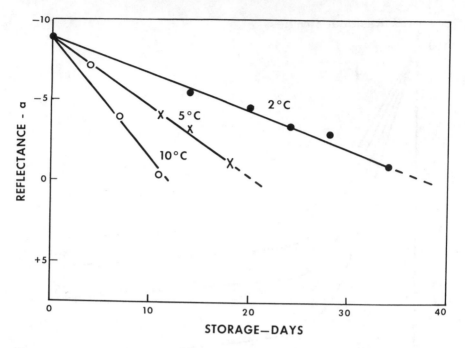

Figure 6-10   Effect of storage temperature on green color loss in shredded lettuce. (From Bolin et al. 1977.)

Ackland 1986) (see temperature–time indicator [TTI], Chapters 3 and 4).

Enrichment of the storage atmosphere with CO_2 results in a slower development of mesophilic flora compared to the air control and in more rapid growth of lactic acid bacteria at 6 and 10° C (Nguyen-The and Carlin 1988).

Modified Atmosphere Packaging

Retail sale demands that ready-to-use commodities be packaged, and as a consequence the atmosphere composition within the pack changes due to the respiration of living tissues. This change can be detrimental or beneficial to the overall quality of the commodity; it can also produce contradictory effects on the different spoilage mechanisms. Controlled atmosphere (CA) and MAP have become the subject of a tremendous number of research projects over the

TOTAL MESOPHILIC ON L.P.G.A.

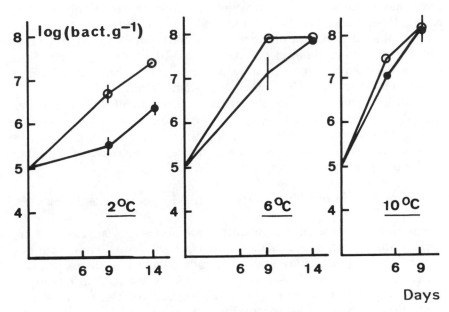

LACTIC ACID BACTERIA ON M.R.S.

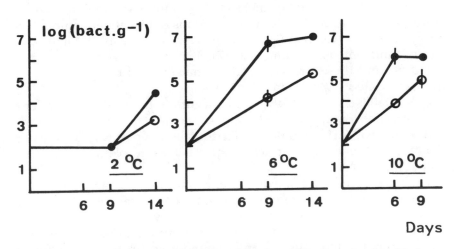

Figure 6-11 Changes in total flora and lactic acid bacteria in shredded endive packed in polypropylene pouches under air (O—O) or air +20% CO_2 (●—●) as a function of storage duration at 2, 6, and 10° C. (From NGuyen The and Carlin 1989.)

last decade. This research has provided a good, basic understanding of CA/MAP which is useful in developing MAP applications for minimally processed fruits and vegetables (Brecht 1980; Isenberg 1979; Kader 1986; Marcellin 1977; Smock 1979; Wolfe 1980).

Several studies have examined the potential for the use of sealed polymeric films to generate a favorable modified atmosphere within the package environment (Cameron et al. 1989; Daun and Gilbert 1974; Geeson et al. 1985; Zagory and Kader 1988).

Modified atmosphere (MA) can reduce the incidence of physiological disorder, microbiological spoilage, and biochemical deterioration, each of which alone or in conjunction results in changes in color, texture, flavor, and, as a consequence, in the commercial value of the commodity (see also Chapter 5).

Effects of MA on the Physiology of MPR Fruits and Vegetables

Respiration in plants is the oxidative metabolism of sugars and organic acids to end products CO_2 and H_2O with concurrent production of energy. MAP may lower the metabolism and decrease both O_2 consumption and CO_2 production (Laties 1978). The effects of low O_2 and high CO_2 on respiration are additive. The optimal concentrations of both gases in combination are difficult to predict without actual measurements in a variety of atmospheres. However, the potential respiration rate of most roots or bulbs is stimulated when stored under elevated CO_2 concentrations. This phenomenon has been shown for celeriac (Weichmann 1977a), carrots (Weichmann 1977b), and onions (Adamicki 1977). If O_2 is reduced or CO_2 elevated beyond the tolerance levels of the commodity, respiration is then associated with anaerobic metabolism.

It is established that high CO_2 concentrations inhibit several enzymes of the Krebs cycle including succinate dehydrogenase (Ranson et al. 1957). This would inhibit the aerobic pathway and result in accumulation of succinic acid, which is toxic to plant tissue (Bendall et al. 1960).

The difference between external and internal O_2 concentrations is determined by the resistance of the plant tissue to gas diffusion which depends on the species and stage of maturity.

Water condensation on the commodity reduces diffusion whereas temperature has little effect (Cameron and Reid 1982). The anaerobic metabolism pathway is responsible for the production of CO_2, ethanol, aldehydes, and other chemical compounds that produce off-flavors, off-odors, and discoloration. In theory, the O_2 level within the cell which induces anaerobic metabolism is as low as 0.2%, and that outside the product 1%–3% (Burton 1974).

The ratio of CO_2 production to O_2 consumption, known as the respiratory quotient (RQ), is, theoretically, 1 in true aerobic metabolism. In actual measurements it ranges from 0.7 to 1.3 (Forcier et al. 1987). CO_2 levels as low as 5% may induce physiological disorders in common mushroom (Lopez-Briones 1991) and asparagus exhibits surface pitting when stored in >10% CO_2 (Lipton 1977). The average CO_2 toxicity threshold ranges from 10 to 30% depending on plant and storage factors. Crisp head lettuce in storage with elevated CO_2 is strongly affected by O_2 concentration (Steward and Uota 1972); however, this is not the case for Romaine lettuce (Lipton 1987). Cultivation conditions such as irrigation, climate, and fertilization can modify plant tissue susceptibility to CO_2 injury. Krahn (1977) found that the outer leaves of crisp head lettuce are not injured by 2% CO_2 but the inner leaves and midribs show damage. Also, shredded head lettuce seems to tolerate higher levels of CO_2.

The effect of CO_2 on cell ultrastructures (Frenkel and Patterson 1974) and membranes (Sears and Eisenberg 1961) could account for its toxicity. It can be postulated that CO_2 dissolution, which enhances acidity in the cell medium, may participate in the physiological disorder. Optimum concentrations of O_2 and CO_2 should minimize the respiration rate without danger of anaerobic metabolism.

Commodities vary widely in their tolerance of different atmospheres (Lougheed 1977). A classification of fresh fruits and vegetables according to their tolerance to reduced O_2 and elevated CO_2 has been presented by Kader et al. (1989). Yet little is known about the atmosphere requirements of minimally processed commodities.

Although many polymeric films are available for packaging purposes, relatively few have been used to wrap or pack fresh fruits and vegetables. Until recently none exhibited suitable permeabilities for commodities with high O_2 requirements. Proper permeabilities to both O_2 and CO_2 should range for the most susceptible plant tissues from 6,000 to 150,000 $ml \cdot m^{-2} \cdot atm^{-1} \cdot day^{-1}$ and up.

The extent to which the MA differs from the external atmosphere is determined primarily by the permeability of the polymeric film, the ratio of its area of gas diffusion to the mass of the plant tissue, the respiration rate of the enclosed product, and the package headspace. The gas diffusion rate through the polymeric film is proportional to the difference in partial pressures between the internal and external media. This gas flow tends to compensate respiratory ex-

Table 6-1
Effect of Film Permeability on Fresh Minimally Processed Grated Carrots Stored for 2 Days at 10° C

Films	D950	A	B	C	D
Thickness (μm)	40	30	30	30	30
Permeability[a] to O_2	6,060	6,000	9,000	11,000	22,000
Permeability[a] to CO_2	18,000	6,000	9,000	11,000	22,000
Gaseous composition at steady state (n = 5)					
CO_2 (%)	19.6	21.6	19.7	27.0	16.5
O_2 (%)	1.5	1.6	2.2	1.6	5.1
Respiration rate in air (mol/kg·h)	2.2	2.3	2.1	2.6	1.8
Confidence interval at 5% level (n = 5)	±0.04	±0.10	±0.11	±0.19	±0.11
(RRp/RRa) × 100	3	11	33	27	61
Respiratory quotient inside the pack	17	6.2	1.5	2.2	1.2

RRp, respiration rate pouch; RRa, respiration rate air.
Supplier D950: Grace-Cryovac, Epernon—France.
Supplier A, B, C and D: Courtaulds Packaging, Avignon—France.
[a]Permeability to gas in ml/m^{-2}·day·atm, at 25° C.
(From Carlin et al. 1990.)

changes. Mathematically, the two phenomena should generate within the package a steady-state MA. As shown in Table 6-1, the respiration rates of grated carrots after 2 days at 10° C in pouches in the least permeable films, D 950 and A, are the most reduced respectively to 3 and 11% of that of the control that is placed in air. The respiratory quotient with these films reached a value above 6, indicating a shift to anaerobic metabolism. In B, C, and D films the RQ was similar to the RQ of control in air, that is about 1.5.

Gas exchanges might also be affected by the metabolism of microorganisms present on grated carrots. Because the respiration of grated carrots does not markedly increase during 2-day storage at 10° C and the number of mesophilic aerobic bacteria increases from 105 to 109 per gram, the contribution of microorganisms to gas exchange is small in pouches stored for only 2 days (Carlin 1989).

The relationship between MA composition and respiration rate is unclear. For example, the CO_2–O_2 concentrations were similar in A and D 950 films (Table 6-1), whereas the respiration rate (RR) was 10 times higher in film A. The O_2 and CO_2 concentrations within packs cannot fully account for the actual turnover of these gases. Conversely, there is a good relation between the respiratory quotient of the commodity and the gas turnover within the package.

This is in accordance with the results of Tomkins (1967), who assumed that MA conditions can alter the RQ which in turn affects the atmosphere created by the respiration of the commodity within the package (Carlin et al. 1990c).

Passively modified atmospheres develop very slowly in pouches of vegetables whose O_2 consumption rate is low, such as lettuce or endive. Biochemical reactions may cause deterioration long before an efficient equilibrated MA can be established and shelf-life is only slightly extended.

The atmosphere may be modified initially just before sealing. This can be done by pulling a slight vacuum and injecting a controlled gas mixture or by flushing with the same gas mixture. Flushing is less efficient than compensated vacuum but it is compatible with high-speed filling machines and for fragile plant organs it is less detrimental to tissue integrity.

Figure 6-12 shows the gas composition changes in shredded endives packed in polypropylene (40 μm) at 10° C as a function of time and percentage of CO_2 in the mixture injected at sealing. In this example, O_2 consumption rates are not markedly affected by additional CO_2, but for elevated CO_2 concentrations diffusion rates exceed CO_2 production through respiration and therefore the CO_2 concentration decreases. In endives, anaerobic metabolism seems difficult to trigger because injection of pure N_2 in the bags results in a decrease in CO_2 production rate compared to other samples (Chambroy 1989).

Several workers have attempted to model the interaction between foodstuff respiration and package atmosphere in an effort to provide an analytical basis for MAP design (Kader et al. 1989). As stated by Zagory and Kader (1988), prediction of the equilibrium gas composition and the time taken to reach equilibrium should take into account at least:

1. The effect of changing O_2 and CO_2 concentrations on respiration rate
2. The effect of switching, even partially, to anaerobic metabolism

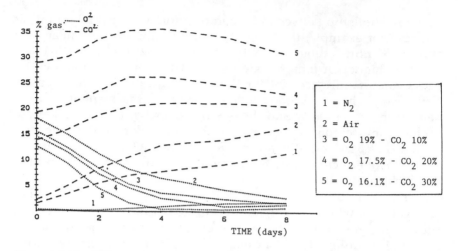

Figure 6-12   Effect of initial atmosphere composition on gas concentration changes within polypropylene packs of shredded endives versus duration of storage at 10° C. (From Chambroy 1989.)

3. The permeability of the film to O_2 and CO_2 (and the effect of moisture on the gas diffusion coefficients)
4. The effect of temperature on film permeability to both O_2 and CO_2, and on the respiration rate
5. The surface area and head space of the package
6. The resistance of the commodity to gas diffusion through its tissue
7. The optimal atmosphere for the commodity of interest, including biochemical reaction and microorganism growth

No model to date has integrated all of these variables.

Mathematical equations that fit gas composition changes in packaged plant organs have been developed recently (Cameron et al. 1989; Yang and Chinnan 1988). All models are based on two ordinary first-order differential equations representing first the gas exchange through polymeric films and second the plant tissue respiration. The gas exchange through the film or through perforations placed between two volumes obeys Fick's law (Emond et al. 1991). The respiration rate of living tissues is affected by the atmospheric composition. But Henig and Gilbert (1975) found with packaged tomatoes that the O_2 consumption rate with complete absorption of CO_2 was constant in the range of 11–21% O_2; below this value O_2

consumption rate decreased linearly with O_2 concentration. Henig and Gilbert (1975) also claimed that when CO_2 accumulation occurred concomitantly with O_2 reduction, there was a significant but surprisingly low reduction in the O_2 consumption rate. They therefore suggested that two straight lines could be used to approximate the relation between O_2 consumption rate and O_2 concentration. (Also see Chapter 5.)

This model was dismissed by Cameron, Boylan-Petit, and Lee (1989) as approximate and not based directly on O_2 measurement. Nevertheless, their own model is valid for scientific purposes but is of little use for optimizing parameters for MAP.

By using the Henig and Gilbert (1975) approach it becomes possible to solve the two differential equations:

$$X(O_2\%) = \frac{KS\,x_0}{KS \div \alpha m} \div \frac{\alpha m\,x_0}{KS \div \alpha m}\,e - \left[\frac{KS \div \alpha m}{V}\right]t \qquad (6.1)$$

$$\frac{1}{O_2(EMA)} - \frac{\alpha m}{KS\,x_0} + \frac{1}{x_0} \qquad (6.2)$$

where

   X = concentration O_2 (%) at time t
   X_0 = initial concentration of O_2
   K = O_2 diffusivity through the film
   S = surface area of the film
   V = headspace
   m = weight of plant tissue
   t = storage time
   α = proportionality between respiration intensity and O_2 concentration

The approximate equation (6.1) is not useful in practice, but as time passes the O_2 concentration tends toward the steady-state concentration (equilibrated modified atmosphere, EMA)

Equation (6.2) shows that the reciprocal of O_2 at steady state is directly proportional to the reciprocal of the film permeability. This model was validated with experimental data concerning apricots stored under MA (Chambroy et al. 1990) and common mushroom (Lopez-Briones 1991). Figure 6-13 shows that experimental data on MAP mushrooms fit the model reasonably well over a very large range of film permeability. However, there are great differences between mathematical and experimental data for CO_2 content within the pouches as already stated by Hayakawa, Henig-and-Gilbert (1975).

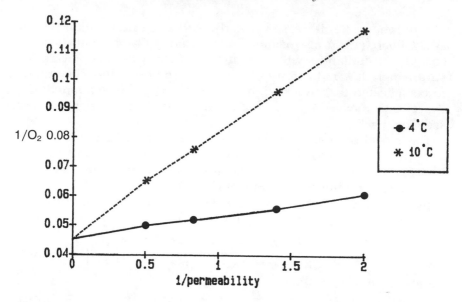

Figure 6-13   Double-reciprocal plot of O_2 concentration (%) within pouches at steady state (EMA) and film permeabilities (ml $O_2/m^{-2} \cdot atm^{-1} \cdot day^{-1}$). Packaged whole mushroom stored at 4 and 10° C. (From Lopez-Briones 1991.)

It has been recently demonstrated that the approximate model is not valid for MA containing less than 3% O_2 or over 15% CO_2. The proportionality between respiration rate and O_2 concentration cannot be extrapolated to anoxic conditions.

It may be assumed that apricot and mushroom metabolisms rapidly switch to partial anaerobic metabolism under MA storage. The metabolism switch has little effect on O_2 concentration but markedly affects CO_2 production. These models permit good predictive estimations of generated MA as a function of simple physical parameters such as surface area, thickness of the film, and weight of tissue. This approach may prove useful once the optimal film permeability has been determined by CA and experimental testing.

As described above in the review of physiological disorders, slicing plant tissue may increase ethylene production, especially in pre-climacteric fruit. High CO_2 levels inhibit the action of ethylene so that plant tissues do not respond to the presence of this compound (Burg and Burg 1969) and reduce ethylene synthesis (Buescher 1979).

Conversion of 1-aminocyclopropane-carboxylic acid to ethylene catalyzed by ethylene-forming enzyme is an oxidative reaction and is therefore reduced at low oxygen partial pressure (Kader 1980) and inhibited under anaerobic conditions (Yang 1985). Curiously, CO_2 inhibits ethylene production during tomato ripening but has little or no effect on wound-induced ethylene production by tomato (Buescher 1979). A similar result was found by Rosen and Kader (1989) with sliced pear.

The effects of ethylene neoformation on physiological and biochemical changes in MPR fruits have yet to be investigated.

Effects of MA on Biochemical Reactions in MPR Fruits and Vegetables

MAs may inhibit enzymatic systems responsible for deterioration in quality during storage but may also reduce tissue senescence and microbial spoilage, both of which result in cellular delocalization.

Effect of MA on Enzyme Activities

Lowering O_2 in a storage atmosphere reduces the reaction rate of enzyme-catalyzed oxidations because O_2 is a substrate (Murr and Morris 1974). Polyphenoloxidase and tyrosinase, the enzymes responsible for brown discoloration of plant tissue, have a low affinity for O_2 compared with cytochrome oxidase. Hence, the packaging of plant tissues with high browning potentiality under vacuum or nitrogen in high-barrier film prevents any discoloration even after 10 days at $10°$ C, but the process may trigger anaerobic metabolism and growth of lactic acid bacteria (Varoquaux and Varoquaux 1990).

Mazollier et al. (1990) claim that nitrogen flushing shredded lettuce before sealing reduces browning of the sliced surfaces but enhances the risk of lactic fermentation. This confirms the results of Ballantyne et al. (1988a), who optimized color stability of shredded lettuce with MA stabilized at 1–3% O_2 and 5–6% CO_2.

Color change in broccoli florets is minimal in a 2–3% O_2, 2–3% CO_2 equilibrium MA, but lower concentrations result in off-odors that markedly shorten shelf-life (Ballantyne et al. 1988b). Because of the experimental design of the reported research, the effect of low O_2 cannot be separated from the effect of increased CO_2.

CO_2 may inhibit polyphenoloxidase activity (Murr and Morris 1974), but the direct inhibition of this enzyme was not fully demonstrated. Another important effect of CO_2 is increased acidity in plant tissues. Because intracellular pH values are normally regulated within narrow limits, only elevated CO_2 concentrations (as high as 5%) will lower intracellular pH. Bown (1985) proposed that the accumulation of respiratory CO_2 is responsible for the reduction in pH, as dissolved CO_2 diffuses slowly compared to gaseous CO_2. Bertola, Chaves and Zaritzky (1990) determined that the specific resistance to CO_2 diffusion of tomato peel was about 200 times as great as that of the stem scar. Dissociation of carbonic acid into bicarbonate and hydrogen ions could affect the activity of enzymes. Tolerance of plant tissues to CO_2 can be determined by their buffering capacity.

Using nuclear magnetic resonance, Siriphanich and Kader (1986) estimated cytoplasmic and vacuolar pH in lettuce tissue as affected by elevated CO_2 concentrations. Lettuce exposed to air at 20° C and then stored for 6 days at 0° C with 16% CO_2 in air showed pH decreases of about 0.4 and 0.1 units in the cytoplasm and vacuole, respectively.

Since MRP fruits and vegetables are stored at low positive temperatures and peripheral tissues are bruised, dissolution of CO_2 should be much greater than in intact organs kept at ambient temperature. This acidification could explain either the marked reduction in activity of enzymes under MA or the phytotoxicity of CO_2. High CO_2 concentrations reduce texture loss of strawberries even after transfer of the berries to air (Kader 1986).

Maintenance of firmness of strawberry in MAP is the result of the improvement of the physiological conditions compared to normal air storage. CAs retard senescence and delay softening of fruit (Knee 1980). MAP does not alter the softening rate of kiwi slices, demonstrating that atmosphere composition has no effect on pectinolytic or proteolytic enzymes (Lecendre 1988).

Effect of MA on the Microbiological Spoilage of MPR Fruits and Vegetables

Published reviews have mentioned the effects of MAP and CA on the postharvest diseases microorganisms can cause (Eckert and Sommer 1967; El-Goorani and Sommer 1981; Harvey 1978; Lougheed et al. 1978; Smith 1963).

Microbial deterioration of minimally processed fruits and vegetables is covered in Chapter 7. Here we review the interdependence of the physiological, biochemical, and microbial spoilage mechanisms as affected by processing and packaging technics. Interaction among these mechanisms will be analyzed for two models: grated carrots and shredded endives. These commodities account for about 85% of ready-to-use fruits and vegetables sold in France (overall production: 30,000 metric tons in 1989).

Spoilage of Grated Carrots

Loss of firmness and off-flavor occurring in spoiled grated carrots are associated with the following characteristics: MA with excessively high CO_2 levels (over 30%) and low O_2 levels (below 1.5%); high number of lactic acid bacteria and yeasts; and production of ethanol, acetic, and lactic acids. Therefore, the deterioration of fresh grated carrots is typically a lactic acid fermentation, which can spontaneously occur in preparations of fermented sliced carrots (Andersson 1984; Niketic-Aleksic et al. 1973).

All isolated lactic acid bacteria were identified as *Leuconostoc mesenteroïdes*, commonly present on plants (Mundt and Hammer 1968) and on minimally processed vegetables (Denis and Picoche 1986). However, initial contaminations by *L. mesenteroïdes* do not markedly differ from one pack to another, so the count of this bacterium at packaging is not sufficient to determine the storability of the commodity (Carlin et al. 1989).

The next step in the attempt to improve grated carrot shelf-life is to study spoilage mechanisms under CAs. Carlin et al. (1990b) demonstrated that the growth of both lactic acid bacteria and yeasts on grated carrots was faster when CO_2 content increased from 10 to 40%, regardless of O_2 concentration (Figure 6-14).

Lactic acid bacteria were not found to be the primary cause of spoilage since the growth of *L. mesenteroïdes* on a sterile medium is unaffected by low O_2 content (Lucey and Condon 1986) or by high CO_2 concentrations (Figure 6-15).

Storing grated carrots in a CO_2-enriched CA produces high K^+ leakage. Other electrolytes and nutrients, especially sugars, are exuded.

Leakage of alpha-amino compounds was measured by Romo-Parada et al. (1989) to determine the increase in membrane permeability of cauliflower during storage under various CAs. They found that O_2 in the CA did not affect leakage, but CO_2 over 10% significantly enhanced it. This exudate provides a substrate for microbial growth (Tomkins 1962). Moreover, Atkinson and Baker (1987) have shown that the activation of K^+/H^+ exchange in beans by *Pseudomonas syringae pv syringae* induces host plasmalemma transport of sucrose, and allows the proliferation of the pathogen in intercellular spaces.

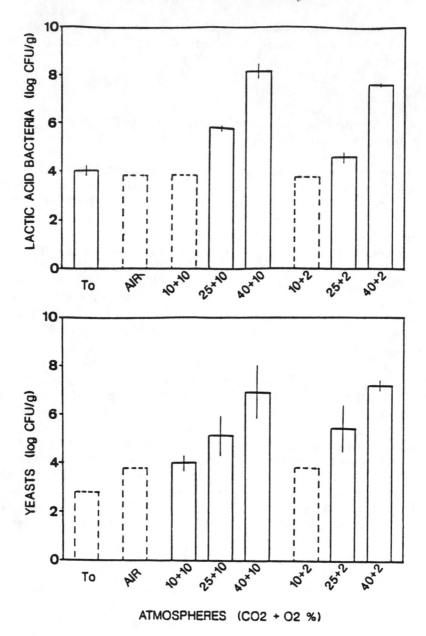

Figure 6-14   Counts of lactic acid bacteria and yeasts on grated carrots under controlled atmospheres after 10 days of storage at 10° C. Counts in dashed lines were below the detection level. To, initial count. Bars represent standard deviation. (From Carlin et al. 1990.)

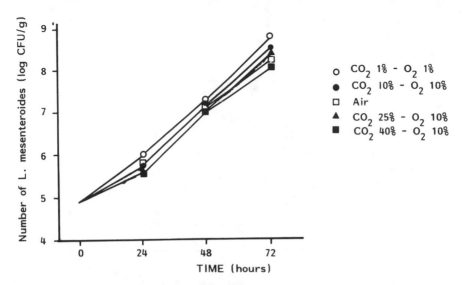

Figure 6-15   Growth at 10° C of *Leuconostoc mesenteroïdes* on a sterile carrot medium under controlled atmospheres. (From Carlin et al. 1990.)

Potassium leakage is lower in CA containing both 10% CO_2 and 10% O_2 than in air. In the same way, the catabolism of sucrose, whose concentration is the main factor in the taste quality of carrot (Rumpf and Hansen 1973), is lower in 10, 25, and 40% CO_2, 2% O_2, and in 25% CO_2 and 10% O_2 than in air or in other CAs.

Thus, MAs containing 15–20% CO_2, 5% O_2 would retard the senescence and microbial spoilage of grated carrots by reducing their physiological activity (Carlin et al. 1990c). These results confirm that the film currently used in France for packaging grated carrots, namely polypropylene, 40 μm in thickness, is not permeable enough to both O_2 and CO_2 to ensure good preservation of the commodity.

Ethanol production in the head space of grated carrot markedly decreases when the film permeability to gases increases. Ethanol is a good marker of spoilage though it may be either a by-product of anaerobic fermentation or an end-metabolite of several microorganisms, or both. As expected, grated carrots packaged with the least permeable film (permeability to $O_2 < 6000$ ml·m^{-2}·atm.$^{-1}$·day^{-1}) switched to anaerobic metabolism, with K^+ leakage as a consequence (Figure 6-16). Use of highly permeable films (20,000 ml·m^{-2}·atm^{-1}·day^{-1} and over) results in a better physiological con-

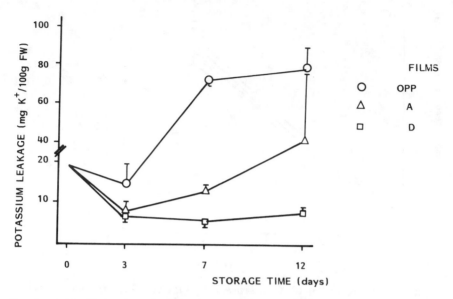

Figure 6-16   Potassium leakage from carrots in pouches as a function of storage time at 10° C for different film permeabilities. (From Carlin 1989.)

dition of the commodity and, therefore, prevents any microbial spoilage.

Conversely, these highly permeable films favor a high respiration rate (about 1 mmol O_2 kg^{-1} h^{-1}) and induce a faster consumption of carbohydrates which causes a noticeable loss in palatability of the carrots. It must be noted that the MA generated in packs depends on the storage temperature. At low temperature (about 2° C) physiological activity and microbial growth are reduced sufficiently to delay the development of spoilage, even with the least permeable film. But at storage temperatures at 10° C, the use of highly permeable films such as P-Plus D is justified to reduce spoilage (Table 6-2).

Spoilage of Shredded Endives

Phytopathogens such as *Erwinia carotovora* have been found on prepacked fresh vegetables but are not markedly pathogenic in minimally processed commodities (Lewis and Garrod 1983). Pectinolytic *Pseudomonas fluorescens* and *Pseudomonas viridiflava* are well known as soft rot bacteria on stored vegetables (Lund 1983). They may also

Table 6-2
Effect of Film Permeability on the Quality of Minimally Processed
Grated Carrots Stored at 10° C

	Films		
	Polypropylene	P-Plus A	P-Plus D
Permeability to O_2			
ml/m^2·day·atm	1,000	6,000	22,000
% of spoiled packs after			
7 days	100	0	0
14 days	100	75	8

(From Carlin et al. 1990.)

induce spoilage of shredded endives (Nguyen-The and Prunier 1989). Strains of pectinolytic *Pseudomonas marginalis* isolated from minimally processed shredded endives show a strong spoilage capacity on the commodity though these bacteria are present in both spoiled and apparently sound packs (Nguyen-The and Carlin 1988).

CA enriched in CO_2 up to 50%, reduces the *in vitro* growth of pseudomonads and *Erwinia* spp. (Figure 6-17). Surprisingly, the same CA does not modify epiphytic proliferation of *Pseudomonas marginalis* on salad leaves, but CA or MA containing over 15% CO_2 reduces or eliminates soft rot on endive leaves that were previously inoculated with a heavily concentrated *Pseudomonas marginalis* suspension (Table 6-3). The same phenomenon is observed when leaves are inoculated with a sterile growth medium of *P. marginalis*. The presence, in the ultrafiltrate, of active pectinolytic enzymes, can account for the considerable soft rot also shown in Table 6-3. Increasing CO_2 to 20% reduces the necrosis, and at 40% it prevents any damage.

It is remarkable that MA, with high CO_2 concentrations up to 40%, have no effect on soft rot induced by *Aspergillus niger* growth medium (Nguyen-The and Carlin 1988). Since *P. marginalis* produces pectate lyases (Lund 1983) with an optimum pH of 6–8, and *Aspergillus niger* a polygalacturonase active at pH 4–5, it is postulated that the beneficial effects of CO_2 on soft rot induced by *P. marginalis* are due to the acidification of cell medium provoked by dissolved CO_2 (Table 6-3).

Deterioration of shredded endives by both pectinolytic and lactic acid bacteria can be prevented by storing and marketing the commodity under a MA containing 20–30% of CO_2 and 1–3% of O_2 de-

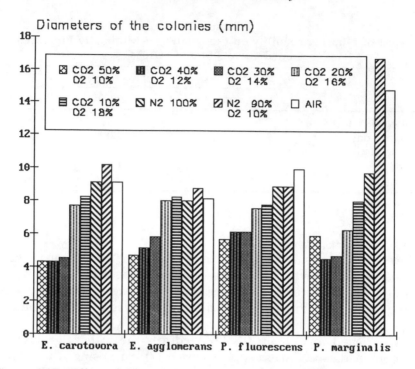

Figure 6-17   Effect of CO_2 on the in vitro growth of bacteria isolated from minimally processed endive. The percentage of CO_2 varies from 10 to 50% (Colony diameter in mm on LPGA after a 9-day incubation at 10° C). (From NGuyen-The 1989.)

pending on the maturity stage and cultivation conditions of the raw endive. A MA suitable for shredded endives can be created by use of a polypropylene film (35–40 μm thick), provided that the storage and distribution temperature never exceeds 10° C with a sell-by date of 1 week, which may be too short for North American markets.

Conclusions and Future Directions

The mechanisms of MPR fruit and vegetable deterioration are similar to those of intact plant organs, observed differences being quantitative and not qualitative.

Development of these new commodities for the retail market is strongly dependent on their microbiological safety and on freshness.

Table 6-3
Effect of CA on the Development of Soft Rot on Inoculated Endive Leaves

CA		Inoculum			
% CO$_2$	% O$_2$	H$_2$O (control)	Ps m (heavy)	Filtrate Ps. m	Filtrate A. niger
40	10	0	0	0	+++
20	10	0	0	(+)	+++
0	22	0	++	++	++

Ps. m, Pseudomonas marginalis; A. niger, Aspergillus niger. 0, no spoilage; (+), no browning, slight soft rot; ++, browning soft rot; +++, general browning and soft rot. (From Nguyen-The and Carlin 1989.)

Freshness may be improved by two nonexclusive means: (1) adaption of processing technology to the raw material, and (2) matching of the raw material to the processing and preservation methods. Both approaches rely on multidisciplinary research that simultaneously uses the basic principles of plant physiology, biochemistry, microbiology, and engineering. Examples include attempt to minimize browning of endives by selection of cultivars and determination of the optimal harvest time.

The suitability of carrot cultivars for "ready-to-use" processing has also been investigated (Hilbert 1990), and the susceptibility of carrot tissue to both increasing CO$_2$ and decreasing O$_2$ was found to be the primary spoilage factor. Current investigations are focused on the mechanisms of cell delocalization in ready-to-use commodities.

Optimization of Processing of MPR Fruits and Vegetables

Optimization of ready-to-use processing method requires:

- Limitation of initial bruising of plant tissues
- Minimization of wound injury during peeling and cutting and other size reduction operations
- Determination of optimal draining conditions to remove moisture
- Identification of an optimal MA which slows senescence, enzyme activity, and microbial growth but that does not trigger

anaerobic metabolism (this must be studied for each commodity)

• Ensuring refrigerated temperatures by using temperature–time indicators (TTI) placed on packaging.

Recent investigations have pointed out the importance of MA composition on the spoilage mechanisms of plant tissues. For some commodities the permeability of commercially available film is not high enough for both O_2 and CO_2 to match their respiratory requirements. New films have recently been developed in the United States, and England and tested in France. Curiously, intact plant organs with high respiration rates such as asparagus, spinach, mushroom, and to a lesser extent cauliflower and broccoli, are the first to benefit from these new films.

Matching of Raw Material and Processing Requirements

Minimal processing is too young an industry for the plant geneticists to have selected or created cultivars and hybrids adapted to its specific requirements. The first step is to define selection criteria in terms of objective chemical or physical determinations as established for fruits and vegetables for freezing or canning. This may prove a difficult task. For example, the browning potential of blended tissues is proportional to their phenolic compound content (Carlin et al. 1990a). Phenolics in plants such as peaches (Lee et al. 1990) and endives (Varoquaux et al. 1991) generally decrease during maturation, theoretically leading to reduced sensitivity of overmature fruits and vegetables to enzymatic browning. However, it is well established that overripe produce scores poorly in MPR processing. Biochemical parameters are not the limiting factors of the brown discoloration of MPR commodities.

Cellular delocalization seems to be the key mechanism that induces enzymatic browning of sliced plant tissues (Watada, Abe, and Yamauchi 1990). The most promising measurement would be rapid testing of susceptibility to cell delocalization. This requires more basic research into the cell response to various stresses.

Further Research Options

Injection of Various Gases at Packaging

Carbon monoxide is utilized in the United States for long-distance bulk transportation of some fruits and vegetables. The toxicity of this gas is not compatible with its use in retail packaging for distribution in Europe.

The effects of nitrogen protoxide on MPR fruits and vegetables are still unclear, but a beneficial effect on the browning of sliced apples and peeled potatoes has been reported (Varoquaux 1991). Further investigation of the effect of this gas on bacterial growth and enzyme activities is needed.

Ionization

Ionization with gamma radiation or accelerated electron beams allows disinfection of prepacked minimally processed commodities. However, even at very low doses (0.5–1 kGy), irradiation induces dramatic softening and off-odors. The effect of irradiation on prepacked salads is still controversial.

CA Atmosphere Packaging

Gas composition in CA packaging can be actively regulated by means of O_2 and CO_2 generators or scavengers (Lioutas 1988; Myers 1989). This technique is well adapted to nonrespiring produce. The feasibility of CA packaging for fresh plant tissues seems very remote.

Research carried out in Europe on highly perishable products aims to achieve a shelf-life of 1 week or 10 days at most. As pointed out by Lioutas (1988), the same operation will require a shelf-life of 21 days to have a chance in the United States market. Such a goal, if realistic, would be a tremendous challenge for fundamental and technical researchers.

References

Adamicki, F. 1977. Respiration rate of onion bulbs depending on the temperature, O_2 and CO_2 concentrations of atmosphere. *Acta Horticult.* **62**:15–22.

Adams, M.R., A.D. Hartley, and L.J. Cox. 1989. Factors affecting the efficacity of washing procedures used in the production of prepared salads. *Food Microbiol.* **6**:69–77.

Amir-Shapira, D., E.E. Goldschmidt, and A. Altman. 1987. Chlorophyll catabolism in senescing plant tissues *in vivo* breakdown intermediates suggest different degradative pathways for citrus fruit and parsley leaves. *Proc. Natl. Acad. Sci. USA* **84**:1901–1905.

Andersson, R. 1984. Characteristics of the bacterial flora isolated during spontaneous lactic acid fermentation of carrots and red beets. *Lebensm. Wiss. Technol.* **17**:282–286.

Anon. 1988. IVème gamme. Qualité-hygiène à l'ordre du jour. *Agro-industries.* **42**:107–108.

Anon. 1989. 4ème gamme. CTIFL ed. Paris, 86 pp.

Atkinson, M.M. and C.J. Baker. 1987. Alteration of plasmalemma sucrose in phaseolus vulgaris by *Pseudomonas syringae pv. syringae* and its association with K^+/H^+ exchange. *Phytopathology* **77**:1573–1578.

Ballantyne, A. 1986. Modified atmosphere packaging of selected prepared vegetables. Technical memorandum n°436, Chipping Campden, UK: Campden Food Res. Assoc.

Ballantyne, A. 1987. Modified atmosphere packaging of selected prepared vegetables. Technical memorandum n°464, Chipping Campden, U.K.: Campden Food Res. Assoc. 68p.

Ballantyne, A., R. Stark, and J.D. Selman. 1988a. Modified atmosphere packaging of shredded lettuces. *Int. J. Food Sci. Technol.* **23**:267–274.

Ballantyne, A., R. Stark, and J.D. Selman. 1988b. Modified atmosphere packaging of broccoli florets. *Int. J. Food Sci. Technol.* **23**:353–360.

Bendall, D.S., S.L. Ranson, and D.A. Walker. 1960. Effect of CO_2 on the oxidation of succinate and reduced diphosphopyridine nucleotide by *Ricinus* mitochondria. *Biochem. J.* **76**:221–225.

Bengtsson, B.L., I. Bosund, and I. Rasmussen. 1967. Hexanal and ethanol formation in peas in relation to off-flavor development. *Food Technol.* **21**:478–482.

Ben-Yehoshua, S. 1987. Transpiration, water stress, and gas exchange. In *Postharvest Physiology of Vegetables*, J. Weichmann (ed.), p. 113. New York: Marcel Dekker.

Bertola, N., A. Chaves, and N.E. Zaritzky. 1990. Diffusion of carbon dioxide in tomato fruits during cold storage in modified atmosphere. *Int. J. Food Sci. Technol.* **25**:318–327.

Bolin, H.R. and C.C. Huxsoll. 1991. Effect of preparation procedures and storage parameters on quality retention of salad-cut lettuce. *J. Food Sci.* **56**:60–62, 67.

Bolin, H.R., A.E. Stafford, A.D. Jr. King, and C.C. Huxsoll. 1977. Factors affecting the storage stability of shredded lettuce. *J. Food Sci.* **42**:1319–1321.

Bown, A.W. 1985. CO_2 and intracellular pH. *Plant Cell Environ.* **8**:459–465.

Brecht, P.E. 1980. Use of controlled atmospheres to retard deterioration of produce. *Food Technol.* **34**(3):45–63.

Brocklehurst, T.F., C.M. Zaman-Wong, and B.M. Lund. 1987. A note on the microbiology of retail packs of prepared salad vegetables. *J. Appl. Bacteriol.* **63**:409–415.

Buescher, R.W. 1979. Influence of carbon dioxide on postharvest ripening and deterioration of tomatoes. *J. Am. Soc. Horticult. Sci.* **104**:545–547.

Buick, R.K. and P.A. Damoglou. 1987. The effect of vacuum-packaging on the microbial spoilage and shelf-life of "ready-to-use", sliced carrots. *J. Sci. Food Agric.* **38**:167–175.

Bu'Loch, J.D. 1960. Intermediates in mechanism formation. *Arch. Biochem. Biophyis.* **91**:189–193.

Burg, S.P. and E.A. Burg. 1969. Interaction of ethylene, oxygen and carbon dioxide in the control of fruit ripening. *Qual. Plant Matter. Veg.* **19**:185–200.

Burton, W.G. 1974. Some biophysical principles underlying the controlled atmosphere storage of plant material. *Ann. Appl. Biol.* **78**:149–168.

Cameron, A.C. and M.S. Reid. 1982. Diffusive resistance: importance and measurement in controlled atmosphere storage. Symposium Series. Oregon State University, School of Agriculture. **1**:171–180.

Cameron, A.C., W. Boylan-Petit, and J. Lee. 1989. Design of modified atmosphere packaging systems: modeling oxygen concentrations within sealed packages of tomato fruits. *J. Food Sci.* **54**:1413–1416.

Carlin, F. 1989. Altérations microbiologiques et désordres physiologiques de carottes râpées prêtes à l'emploi. Thèse de Docteur-Ingénieur de l'Institut National Agronomique Paris-Grignon. 8 juin 1989.

Carlin, F., C. Nguyen-The, P. Cudennec, and M. Reich. 1989. Microbiological spoilage of fresh "ready-to-use" grated carrots. *Sci. Alim.* **9**:371–386.

Carlin, F., C. Nguyen-The, and P. Varoquaux. 1990a. La conservation des produits de la 4ème gamme. *Ind. Agric. Alim.* **10**:931–944.

Carlin, F., C. Nguyen-The, Y. Chambroy, and M. Reich. 1990b. Effects of controlled atmospheres on microbial spoilage, electrolyte leakage and sugar content on fresh, "ready-to-use" grated carrots. *Int. J. Food Sci. Technol.* **25**:110–119.

Carlin, F., C. Nguyen-The, G. Hilbert, and Y. Chambroy. 1990c. Modified atmosphere packaging of fresh "ready-to-use" grated carrots. Use of varied polymeric films. *J. Food Sci.* **55**:1033–1038.

Chambroy, Y. 1989. Physiologie et température des produits frais découpés. Colloque AFF, Avignon, 8–10 novembre 1988. *Rev. Gen. Froid.* **3**:78–92.

Chambroy, Y., M. Souty, G. Jacquemin, and J.M. Audergon. 1990. Maintien de la qualité des abricots après récolte. 9ème Colloque sur les Recherches Fruitières. Avignon. 341–350.

Cuq, J.L. and C. Vial. 1989. Personal communication. USTL—Place Eugène Bataillon—F-34000 Montpellier.

Daun, H. and S.G. Gilbert. 1974. Film permeation: the key to extending fresh product shelf-life. *Pack. Eng.* **19**:50–53.

Denis, C. and B. Picoche. 1986. Microbiologie des légumes frais prédécoupés. *Ind. Agric. Alim.* **103**:547–553.

Doesburg, J.J. 1965. Pectic Substances in fresh and preserved fruits and vegetables. I.V.V.T. Communication NR. 25. The Netherlands: Institute for Research on Storage and Processing of Horticultural Produce Wageningen.

Eckert, J.W. and N.F. Sommer. 1967. Control of diseases of fruits and vegetables by postharvest treatment. *Ann. Rev. Phytopathol.* **5**:391–431.

El-Goorani, M.A. and N.F. Sommer. 1981. Effects of modified atmosphere on postharvest pathogens of fruits and vegetables. *Horticult. Rev.* **3**:412–461.

Emond, J.P., F. Castaigne, C. Toupin, and D. Desilets. 1991. Mathematical modeling of gas exchange in modified atmosphere packaging. *Trans. ASAE* **34**:239–245.

Forcier, F., G.S.V. Raghavan, and Y. Gariepy. 1987. Electronic sensor for the determination of fruit and vegetable respiration. *Rev. Int. Froid.* **10**:353–356.

Frenkel, Ch. and M.E. Patterson. 1974. Effect of carbon dioxide on ultra-structures of bartlett pears. *Hort. Science* 9:338–340.

Garrott, W.N. and A.E. Mercker. 1954. The commercial potato peeling industry. In Proc. 6th Annual Potato Utilization Conf., p. 22, U.S. Dept. of Agriculture and Cornell University, Ithaca, N.Y.

Geeson, J.D., K.M. Browne, K. Maddison, J. Sheppard, and F. Guaraldi. 1985. Modified atmosphere packaging to extend the shelf-life of tomatoes. *J. Food Technol.* 20:339–349.

Gowen, P.L. 1928. Effect on quality of holding shelled peas. *Canner* 66:112–115.

Harel, E., A.M. Mayer, and Y. Shain. 1964. Catechol oxidases from apples, their properties, subcellular location and inhibition. *Physiol. Plant.* 17:921–930.

Harvey, J.M. 1978. Reduction of losses in fresh market fruits and vegetables. *Ann. Rev. Phytopathol.* 16:321–341.

Hayakawa, K., Y.S. Henig, and S.G. Gilbert. 1975. Formulae for predicting gas exchange of fresh produce in polymeric film package. *J. Food Sci.* 40:186–191.

Henig, Y.S. and S.G. Gilbert. 1975. Computer analysis of variables affecting respiration and quality of produce packaged in polymeric films. *J. Food Sci.* 40:1033–1035.

Herner, R.H. and T.R. Krahn. 1973. Chopped lettuce should be kept dry and cold. Yearbook Prod. Mark. Assoc., p. 130 in Bolin et al. (1977).

Hilbert, G. 1990. Influence du procédé de fabrication des carottes râpées de 4ème gamme: pouvoir d'altéteration des levures sur ces carottes. *Maîtrise Biochimie— Toulouse*, 28 pp.

Hildebrand, D.F. 1989. Lipoxygenases. *Physiol. Plant.* 76:249–253.

Huxsoll, C.C. and H.R. Bolin. 1989. Processing and distribution alternatives for minimally processed fruits and vegetables. *Food Technol.* 43:124–128.

IFST, 1982. Guidelines for the handling of chilled food.

Isenberg, F.M.R. 1979. Controlled atmosphere storage of vegetables. *Horticult. Rev.* 1:337–394.

Kader, A.A. 1980. Prevention of ripening in fruits by use of controlled atmosphere. *Food Technol.* 32(3):51–54.

Kader, A.A. 1986. Biochemical and physiological basis for effects of controlled and modified atmospheres on fruits and vegetables. *Food Technol.* 40(5):99–104.

Kader, A.A., D. Zagory, and E.L. Kerbel. 1989. Modified atmosphere packaging of fruits and vegetables. *Crit. Rev. Food Sci. Nutr.* 28:1–30.

Kays, S.J. 1991. *Postharvest Physiology of Perishable Plant Products*. New York: Van Nostrand Reinhold.

Kertesz, Z.I. 1951. *The Pectic Substances*. New York-London: Interscience.

Knee, M. 1980. Physiological responses of apple fruits to oxygen concentrations. *Ann. Appl. Biol.* 96:243–253.

Krahn, T.R. 1977. Improving to keeping quality of cut head lettuce. *Acta. Horticult.* 62:79–92.

Lafuente, M.T., M. Cantwell, S.F. Yang, and V. Rubatsky. 1989. Isocoumarin content of carrots as influenced by ethylene concentration, storage temperature and stress conditions. *Acta. Horticult.* 258:523–534.

Laties, G. 1978. The development of control of respiratory pathways in slices of plant storaged organs. In *Biochemistry of Wounded Plant Tissues*, Kahl G. (ed.), p. 421. Berlin: Walter de Gruyter.

Lecendre, I. 1988. Le kiwi de 4ème gamme. Etude de la fermeté des tranches après découpe. Mémoire de Fin d'Etudes ENSBANA. Dijon, 25p.

Lee, C.Y., V. Vogan, A.W. Jaworski, and S.K. Brown. 1990. Enzymatic browning in relation to phenolic compounds and polyphenoloxidase activity among various peach cultivars. *J. Agric. Food Chem.* **38**:99–101.

Lewis, B.G. and B. Garrod. 1983. Carrots. In *Post-Harvest Pathology of Fruits and Vegetables*, C. Dennis (ed.), pp. 103–124. London: Academic Press.

Lioutas, T.S. 1988. Challenges of controlled and modified atmosphere packaging: A food company's perspective. *Food Technol.* **42**(9):78–86.

Lipton, W.J. 1977. Recommendations for CA storage of broccoli, Brussels sprouts, cabbage, cauliflower, asparagus and potatoes. *Mich. State Univ. Hort. Rept.* **28**:277–281.

Lipton, W.J. 1987. Carbon dioxide induced injury of Romaine lettuce stored in controlled atmospheres. *HortScience* **22**:461–463.

Lopez-Briones, G. 1991. Augmentation de la durée de vie du produit frais: application au Champignon *Agaricus bisporus*. Thèse, Université de Reims. 17 décembre 1991.

Lougheed, E.C. 1987. Interactions of oxygen, carbon dioxide, temperature and ethylene that may induce injuries in vegetables. *HortScience* **22**:791–794.

Lougheed, E.C., D.P. Murr, and L. Berard. 1978. Low pressure storage for horticultural crops. *HortScience* **13**, 21–27.

Lucey, C.A. and S. Condon. 1986. Active role of oxygen on NADH oxidase on growth and energy metabolism of Leuconostoc. *J. Gen. Microbiol.* **132**:1789–1796.

Lund, B.M. 1983. Bacteria spoilage. In *Post-Harvest Pathology of Fruits and Vegetables*, C. Dennis (ed.), pp. 218–257. London: Academic Press.

Lund, B.M. 1988. Bacterial contamination of food crops. *Asp. Appl. Biol.* **17**:71–82.

MacLachlan, A. and R. Stark. 1985. Modified atmosphere packaging of selected prepared vegetables. Technical memorandum n°412, Chipping Campden, UK: Campden Food Res. Assoc., 78 pp.

Manvell, P.M. and M.R. Ackland. 1986. Rapid detection of microbial growth in vegetable salads at chill and abuse temperatures. *Food Microbiol.* **3**:59–65.

Marcellin, P. 1977. Use and potential development of controlled atmosphere in the storage of fruits and vegetables. *Int. Inst. Refrig. Bull.* **59**:1151–1158.

Marcellin, P. 1982. Nouvelles tendances de la conservation des fruits et légumes par réfrigération. *Rev. Gén. du Froid.* **3**:143–151.

Mayer, J. 1987. Polyphenol oxidases in plants. Recent progress 1987. *Phytochemistry* **26**:11–20.

Mazollier, J. 1988. IVe gamme. Lavage désinfection des salades. Infos-CTIFL. **41**:20–23.

Mazollier, J., M.C. Bardet, and F. Bonnafoux. 1990. La laitue en IVe gamme. Info-CTIFL. **59**:23–26.

Mundt, J.O. and J.L. Hammer. 1968. *Lactobacilli* on plants. *Appl. Microbiol.* **16**:1326–1330.

Murr, D.P. and L.L. Morris. 1974. Influence of O₂ and CO₂ on *o*-diphenol oxidase activity in mushrooms. *J. Am. Soc. Horticult. Sci.* **99**:155–158.

Myers, R.A. 1989. Packaging considerations for minimally processed fruits and vegetables. *Food Technol.* **43**(1):129–131.

Nguyen-The, C. and F. Carlin. 1988. Altérations microbiologiques des légumes prêts à l'emploi. Compte-rendu de la Deuxième Conférence Internationale sur les Maladies des Plantes. Bordeaux, 8–10 novembre 1988. **1**:743–750.

Nguyen-The, C. and J.P. Prunier. 1989. Involvement of Pseudomonas in "ready-to-use" salads deterioration. *Int. J. Food Sci. Technol.* **24**:47–58.

Niketic-Aleksic, G.K., M.C. Bourne, and J.R. Stamer. 1973. Preservation of carrots by lactic acid fermentation. *J. Food Sci.* **38**:84–86.

Ponting, J.D., R. Jackson, and G. Watters. 1972. Refrigerated apple slices, perspective effects of ascorbic acid, calcium and sulfite. *J. Food. Sci.* **37**:434–436.

Ranson, L., D.A. Walker, and I.D. Clarke. 1957. The inhibition of succinic oxidase by high CO₂ concentration. *Biochem. J.* **66**:57–p. (Abstr.).

Rolle, R.S. and G.W. Chism. 1987. Physiological consequences of minimally processed fruits and vegetables. *J. Food Qual.* **10**:157–177.

Romo-Parada, L., C. Willemot, F. Castaigne, C. Gosselin, and J. Arul. 1989. Effect controlled atmosphere (low oxygen, high carbon dioxide) on storage of cauliflower (*Brassica oleracea* L., *Botrytis* group). *J. Food Sci.* **54**:122–124.

Rosen, J.C. and A.A. Kader. 1989. Postharvest physiology and quality maintenance of sliced pear and strawberry fruits. *J. Food Sci.* **54**:656–659.

Rouet-Mayer, M.A., J. Philippon, and J. Nicolas. 1993. Enzymatic browning: biochemical aspects. Encyclopedia of Food Science, Food Technology and Nutrition. R. McRae R.K. Robinson and M.J. Sadler (Ed.), New York: Academic Press Vol. 1, 499–506.

Rumpf, G. and H. Hansen. 1973. Gas chromatographische bestimmung löslicher inhaltstoffe. In Controlled atmosphere. Gelagerten Möhren. *Gartenbauwissenschaft* **38**:281–285.

Ryall, A.L. and W.J. Lipton. 1972. Handling transportation and storage of fruits and vegetables. In *Vegetables and Melons*, The AVI Publishing Company, Westport, CT: Vol. 1.

Scandella, D. 1988. 4ème gamme. L'évolution du code des bonnes pratiques professionnelles. Infos-CTIFL. **41**:3–4.

Scandella, D. 1989. Maîtrise de la qualité des produits de 4ème gamme dans la filière de production et de distribution. *Rev. Gén. Froid.* **66**:94–101.

Scandella, D., E. Derens, and R. Benhamias. 1990. 4ème gamme. La chaîne du froid. Infos-CTIFL. **59**:17–22.

Sears, D.F. and R.M. Eisenberg. 1961. A model representing a physiological role of CO₂ at the cell membrane. *J. Gen. Physiol.* **44**:869–887.

Shewfelt, R.L. 1986. Post-harvest treatment for extending shelf-life of fruits and vegetables. *Food Technol.* **40**(5):70–80:89.

Siriphanich, J. and A.A. Kader. 1986. Changes in cytoplasmic and vacuolar pH in harvested lettuce tissue as influenced by CO_2. *J. Am. Soc. Horticult. Sci.* **111**:73–77.

Smith, W.H. 1963. The use of carbon dioxide in the transport and storage of fruits and vegetables. *Adv. Food Res.* **12**:95–146.

Smith, J.P., F.R. Van De Voort, and A. Lambert. 1989. Food and its relation to interactive packaging. *Can. Inst. Food Sci. Technol.* **22**:327–330.

Smock, R.M. 1979. Controlled atmosphere storage of fruits. *Horticult. Rev.* **1**:301–336.

Stewart, J.K. and M. Uota. 1972. Carbon dioxide injury to lettuce as influenced by carbon monoxide and oxygen levels. *HortScience* **7**:189–190.

Tomkins, R.G. 1962. The conditions produced in film packages by fresh fruits and vegetables and the effect of these conditions on storage life. *J. Appl. Microbiol.* **25**:290–307.

Tomkins, R.G. 1967. Assessing suitability of plastic films for packaging fruits and vegetables. *Food Manufacture* **42**:34–38.

Varoquaux, P. 1987. Fruits et légumes de quatrième gamme. *Rev. Prat. Froid Cond. Air.* **654**:161–165.

Varoquaux, P. 1991. Minimally processed potatoes. Unpublished data.

Varoquaux, P. and F. Varoquaux. 1990. Les fruits de 4ème gamme. *Arb. Fruit.* **3**:35–38.

Varoquaux, P., I. Lecendre, F. Varoquaux, and M. Souty. 1990. Change in firmness of kiwi fruit after slicing. *Sci. Alim.* **10**:127–139.

Varoquaux, P., F. Varoquaux, and G. Breuils. 1991. Browning potential of various *Cichorium endivia* cultivars as a function of harvest time. *Lebensm. Wiss. Technol.* **24**:270–273.

Vial, C. 1991. Elaboration de tranches de kiwi de 4ème gamme: stabilité microbiologique—etude des paramètres de qualité au cours de la conservation. Thèse. Décembre.

Watada, A.E., K. Abe, and N. Yamauchi. 1990. Physiological activities of partially processed fruits and vegetables. *Food Technol.* **44**(5):116–122.

Weckel, K.G., B. Seemann, and C.N. We-So. 1964. Effect of postharvest temperature of fresh peas on the quality of canned peas. *Food Technol.* **8**:97–100.

Weichmann, J. 1977a. C.A. storage of celeriac. *Acta Horticult.* **62**:109–118.

Weichmann, J. 1977b. Physiological response of root crops to controlled atmospheres. *Proc. 2nd National Controlled Atmosphere Research Conf. Mich. State Univ. Hort. Rept.* **28**:122–136.

Whitaker, J.R. 1972. *Principles of Enzymology for the Food Sciences.* New York: Marcel Dekker.

Wills, R.B.H., W.B. McGlasson, D. Graham, T.H. Lee, and E.G. Hall. 1989. *Postharvest: An Introduction to the Physiology and Handling of Fruits and Vegetables.* New York: Van Nostrand Reinhold.

Wolfe, S.K. 1980. Use of CO- and CO_2-enriched atmospheres for meats, fish and produce. *Food Technol.* **34**(3):55–58, 63.

Yamauchi, N. and A.E. Watada. 1991. Regulated chlorophyll degradation in spinach leaves during storage. *J. Am. Soc. Horticult. Sci.* **116**:58–62.

Yang, S.F. 1985. Biosynthesis and action of ethylene. *HortScience* **20**:41–45.

Yang, S.F. and M.S. Chinnan. 1988. Modeling the effect of oxygen and carbon dioxide on respiration and quality of stored tomatoes. *Trans. ASAE* **31**:920–925.

Yang, S.F. and N.E. Hoffman. 1984. Ethylene biosynthesis and its regulation in higher plants. *Ann. Rev. Plant Physiol.* **35**:155–189.

Yang, S.F. and H.K. Pratt. 1978. The physiology of ethylene in wounded plant tissues. In *Biochemistry of Wounded Plant Tissues*, Kahl G. (ed.), pp. 595–622. Berlini Walter De Gruyter and Co, Berlin.

Zagory, D. and A.A. Kader. 1988. Modified atmosphere packaging of fresh produce. *Food Technol.* **42**(9):70–77.

7

Microbiological Spoilage and Pathogens in Minimally Processed Refrigerated Fruits and Vegetables

Robert E. Brackett

Introduction

Importance of Minimally Processed Refrigerated Fruits and Vegetables

Minimally processed refrigerated (MPR) fruits and vegetables have always been an important food group in the diet. However, consumers have recently become more aware of the importance of these products in maintaining health. Consequently, consumers are purchasing and eating more fresh produce and demanding a greater variety of these products in the marketplace. This has led food processors to take advantage of modern technology and transportation to satisfy the consumer's demand. Despite improved methods of maintaining quality and shelf-life of MPR produce, a limiting factor to optimum quality is the same as before. That component is the role of microorganisms in the spoilage and safety of MPR produce.

Importance of Microbiology

Microorganisms are an important factor to consider when one is dealing with MPR fruits and vegetables. Bacteria, yeasts, and molds account for up to 15% of postharvest decay (Harvey 1978). In addition, produce that shows obvious microbial growth even without obvious decay is aesthetically unpleasing and is unlikely to be purchased. Consequently, microbial spoilage represents significant economic loss to individuals involved with all aspects of the distribution chain.

Although monetary loss is a strong incentive for considering microbiology, ensuring the safety of consumers should be an even greater motive. An estimated 12.6 million cases of foodborne illness occur each year in the United States (Todd 1989b). Despite consumers' apprehension over so-called artificial chemicals, pathogenic bacteria are the most serious threat to the consumer's health. All members of the food industry share a responsibility to provide consumers with safe, wholesome foods. Profits should always be secondary to safety.

Relatively few types of microorganisms cause the majority of foodborne diseases. Most outbreaks are associated with meats and poultry. Nevertheless, MPR produce items are also occasionally linked to cases of foodborne disease. It is therefore important that this aspect of microbiology be considered in tandem with spoilage problems.

Because microorganisms are so important in affecting the quality and safety of MPR fruits and vegetables, researchers have paid much attention to microbiology research. However, the knowledge gained from such research cannot be fully applied unless the end user has a basic understanding and appreciation for microbiology. The purpose of this chapter is to help provide that understanding.

Microbiology of Minimally Processed Produce

Introductory Microbiology

The term microbiology means different things to different people. The average layperson might equate microbiology with "germs" and disease epidemics. In contrast, a sauerkraut producer might think of lactic acid bacteria when he or she thinks of microbiology. Although they are both correct, microbiology encompasses much more than those narrow definitions.

In its broadest sense, microbiology is simply the study of organisms that are microscopic in size. Thus, any organism that requires a microscope to see could be categorized as a microorganism. However, the food microbiologist is usually concerned only with those microbes that affect the quality or safety of foods. The microorganisms normally of concern are bacteria and fungi, although viruses and parasites are also important.

The viruses and virus-like particles are the simplest and smallest of microorganisms. They are so small, usually <200 nm, that they can be seen only with the help of electron microscopes. Although viruses are categorized as microorganisms, they are not living organisms in the strict sense. That is, they are not capable of independent life. Viruses are simply packets of genetic information that require the biochemical processes of other living organisms (hosts) to reproduce. After infection, viruses utilize the host cells' metabolic processes and nutrients to build new viruses. After the new viruses have been built, the host cell lyses and the new viruses are released to continue the cycle of infection. It is the lysis of host cells that often causes the symptoms of viral disease.

The host organism that a given virus must infect in order to reproduce is often very specific. For example, bacteria, fungi, plants, and animals each have viruses that usually attack only them. Thus, a virus that may be considered a plant pathogen would not be expected to infect a human. Viruses are not capable of growing within a food because they require a live host for reproduction.

Bacteria are probably the best known microorganisms of concern with foods. Unlike viruses, most bacteria are capable of independent life. If conditions are suitable, they are able to metabolize nutrients for required energy, produce cellular components and enzymes, and reproduce. Bacteria are an exceedingly diverse group of organisms. Therefore, making generalizations regarding their characteristics is difficult and exceptions are likely.

Most bacteria reproduce by a process known as binary fission, which simply involves a bacterial cell growing in size and then splitting into two daughter cells. Binary fission allows the population of bacteria to increase exponentially. The time it takes a bacterium to duplicate itself in this manner is called its generation (or doubling) time. The generation time is usually in the range of hours at 20° C but varies with the particular strain of bacterium and incubation temperature. Some bacteria, such as *Clostridium perfringens*, are ca-

Table 7-1
Theoretical Growth of Bacteria with a Generation Time of 20 Min

Time (h)	Number of Cells
0	1
1	8
2	64
3	512
4	4,096
5	3.2×10^4
6	2.6×10^5
7	2.1×10^6
8	1.7×10^7

pable of doubling their populations several times an hour. A true appreciation for the speed: with which bacteria can grow is essential if one is to understand why certain practices diminish the quality of foods. Table 7-1 illustrates the high ultimate theoretical population a bacterium with a generation time of 20 min might achieve in only 8 h.

Fungi are the third important group of microorganisms that affect the quality of fruits and vegetables. These organisms can be divided further into several categories but molds and yeasts are of the greatest concern in foods. Like the bacteria, the fungi are capable of independent life. However, they also differ from bacteria in several important ways. First, the fungi are eucaryotic, meaning they have a highly organized nucleus typical of plants and animals. Second, many fungi are multicellular. This gives molds their fuzzy appearance and mushrooms their distinctive shapes. In general, molds and yeasts are much more tolerant of acidity and reduced moisture than are the bacteria. Molds and yeasts are the fungi of primary concern in fruits and vegetables.

The last group of important microorganisms that will be discussed in this chapter is the parasites. These creatures differ from bacteria and fungi in that they are more closely related to animals than to plants. They are eucaryotic and capable of living an independent life but require a live host to complete their life cycle. However, many parasites have a very complicated life cycle involving several growth phases. Parasites can be a food safety problem but do not otherwise affect the sensory qualities of fruits and vegetables.

Normal Microflora of Vegetables

It is conceivable that almost any microorganism might be found on a given fruit or vegetable in specific circumstances. However, fruits and vegetables often differ substantially in physical and biochemical characteristics. These differences likewise cause differences in microflora normally associated with specific types of produce. In addition, unit operations such as cutting, washing, or peeling can affect the predominant organism on MPR products. Often, a particular bacterium or fungus is simply an innocuous particle on the produce item. Even those microbes that are routinely associated with a particular product may or may not be associated with spoilage of that product. Thus, the predominant microflora associated with fruits and vegetables often has little to do with the quality of that product.

Fresh, raw vegetables characteristically have high water and nutrient contents, and a neutral pH. These characteristics make them capable of supporting the growth of almost any type of microorganism. In general, vegetables are about equally contaminated with bacteria and fungi (Brackett 1987b). Usually, though, it is the gram-negative bacteria that are consistently isolated from fresh vegetables. Table 7-2 lists some of the bacteria that have been isolated from various vegetables. Specific genera of bacteria that are most often isolated from vegetables include *Pseudomonas, Erwinia,* and *Enterobacter.* However, gram-positive bacteria such as *Bacillus* and coryneform bacteria are also frequently found.

The populations of bacteria, also called the microbial load, found on vegetables vary widely. As indicated in Table 7-3, it is not at all unusual to find tens or hundreds of thousands of bacterial cells per gram of raw vegetables. Some vegetables, such as leafy vegetables, may even have millions of bacteria per gram. These products often become heavily contaminated with sand and soil. This soil tends to carry with it many microorganisms. However, carrots and potatoes can contain some of the lowest populations of bacteria, despite being root crops that are in direct contact with soil (Splittstoesser 1970). One should also remember that numbers of bacterial cells that can be found at any given time are affected by extrinsic factors. For instance, environmental conditions immediately before or during harvest (Brackett 1987a; Goepfert 1980); can often affect populations. Thus, the population of microorganisms for a given vegetable could change from day to day. In addition, values such as those listed in Table 7-3 can often be misleading or incomplete. They usually exclude populations of important anaerobic bacteria and provide no

Table 7-2
Bacteria Isolated from Various Vegetables

Vegetable	Organisms Isolated	Reference
Asparagus	*Aeromonas hydrophila*	Berrang, Brackett, and Beuchat (1989a)
Broccoli	*A. hydrophila*	Berrang, Brackett, and Beuchat (1989a)
Cabbage	*Pseudomonas* sp.	Geeson (1979)
Carrots	*Erwinia* sp., *Pseudomonas* sp., *Bacillus* sp.	Buick and Damoglou (1987)
Cauli-flower	*A. hydrophila*	Berrang, Brackett, and Beuchat (1989a)
Collards	*C. freundii, E. cloacae, E. agglomerans, E. coli, Hafnia alvei, Klebsiella oxytoca, S. rubidaea*	Senter, Bailey, and Cox (1987)
Corn	*Enterobacter* sp., *E. agglomerans, E. cloacae, Enterococcus faecalis, E. faecium, Flavobacterium* sp., *Pseudomonas* sp., *Serratia* sp., *Xanthomonas* sp.	Deák et al. (1987)
Cucum-bers	*Citrobacter* sp., *Enterobacter cloacae, Erwinia* sp.	Meneley and Stanghellini (1974)
Lettuce	*C. freundii, C. amalonticus, E. cloacae, E. agglomerans, A. hydrophila, E. aerogenes, Proteus morganai, P. rettgeri, P. vulgaris, P. stuartii*	Riser et al. (1984)
Tomato	*E. agglomerans, E. cloacae, S. marcescens* Corynebacteria, *E. cloacae, Flavobacterium*, Micrococcaeae, *Escherichia* intermedia, Xanthomonas sp.	Senter et al. (1985) Samish et al. (1961)
	Acinetobacter sp., corynebacteria, *E. agglomerans, E. cloacae, Flavobacterium* sp., *Klebsiella* sp., *Lactobacillus* sp., *Micrococcus luteus, Pseudomonas* sp., *Xanthomonas* sp.	Brackett (1988a)
Peas	*E. agglomerans, E. cloacae, S. marcesens*	Senter et al. (1984)
Potato	*Bacillus cereus, B. lichenformis, E. caratovora*	Hayward (1974)

Table 7-3
Populations of Microorganisms Isolated from Various Vegetables

Vegetable	Population Recovered	References
Asparagus	31,600	Berrang, Brackett, and Beuchat (1990)
Beet	3,200	Splittstoesser (1970)
Bell peppers	132,000	Golden, Heaton, and Beuchat (1987)
Broccoli	10,000	Berrang, Brackett, and Beuchat (1990)
	2,500,000	Brackett (1989)
Cabbage	500–100,000	Geeson (1979)
	4–2,000	Splittstoesser (1970)
Carrots	630,000	Buick and Damoglou (1987)
	440	Splittstoesser (1970)
Cauliflower	63,100	Berrang, Brackett, and Beuchat (1990)
Collards	3,200,000–6,300,000	Senter, Bailey, and Cox (1987)
Corn	100	Deák et al. (1987)
	100–100,000	Splittstoesser (1970)
Cucumbers	16,000	Splittstoesser (1970)
Kale	1,200–10,000	Splittstoesser (1970)
Lettuce	100,000–1,000,000	Riser, Grabowski, and Glenn (1984)
Lima beans	1–150	Splittstoesser (1970)
Peas	220–30,000	Splittstoesser (1970)
Potatoes	75–28,000	Splittstoesser (1970)
Tomato	10,000–501,000	Senter et al. (1985)
	64,000	Brackett (1988a)
Snap beans	600–3,000	Splittstoesser (1970)
Southern peas	25,100,000	Senter et al. (1984)
Spinach	2,000–23,000	Splittstoesser (1970)

information about the types of bacteria that make up the population. Populations of bacteria present on vegetables only provide an estimate of microbial load but do not indicate whether that population has beneficial or deleterious effects.

Like bacteria, many different fungi can be isolated from vegetables. Both yeasts and molds are usually isolated from fresh vegetables although little has been published on the former. Various species of the nonfermenting basidiomycetious yeasts, primarily *Cryptococcus* and *Rhodotorula*, commonly appear on fresh vegetables such as cabbage (Geeson 1979), corn (Deák et al. 1987), bell pepper, and tomatoes (Golden, Heaton, and Beuchat 1987). In addition, fermentative yeasts such as *Candida* and *Kloeckera* have been isolated from cabbage (Geeson 1979), corn (Deák et al. 1987), and bell peppers (Golden, Heaton, and Beuchat 1987). Yeast populations can range from $<10^3$ to $>10^6$ cells/g of tissue (Miller 1979). For example, Senter et al. isolated 10^4 yeasts/g from freshly harvested southern peas (Senter et al. 1984) and collard leaves (Senter, Bailey, and Cox 1987). However, obtaining reliable estimates of yeasts in most commodities is difficult because reports usually provide data on total fungal populations only.

The identity of molds isolated from fresh vegetables is more often reported than is the case for yeasts. Webb and Mundt (1978) surveyed 14 different vegetables for molds. They found that the most commonly isolated genera were *Aureobasidium, Fusarium, Alternaria, Epicoccum, Mucor, Chaetomium, Rhizopus*, and *Phoma*. Predominant genera isolated were not affected by cultivar, climatic conditions, location of the growing fields, or the vegetables' height above the ground. Other molds isolated from various fresh vegetables are given in Table 7-4. Molds are generally found in lower concentrations in fresh vegetables than are bacteria. However, it is difficult to find estimates for mold populations alone. Webb and Mundt (1978) reported that populations of molds on fresh vegetables averaged about 42,000–67,000 colony-forming units (CFU) g.

Normal Microflora of Fruits

Fruits primarily differ from vegetables in that they usually have a higher sugar content and a more acidic pH (4.6 or lower). This lower pH and the nature of the organic acids involved usually inhibit the growth of bacteria other than lactic acid bacteria. Consequently, fungi are the predominant microorganisms in fruits (Goepfert 1980).

Many different species of fungi can be isolated from fresh fruits. Although fungi are largely responsible for spoilage of fruits, not all fungi that are isolated are spoilage fungi. Yeasts occurring on fruits are about evenly divided between ascosporogenous and imperfect species (Splittstoesser 1987). *Saccharomyces, Hanseniaspora, Pichia, Kloeckera, Candida*, and *Rhodotorula* are among the most common genera of yeasts found on fruits (Splittstoesser 1987). Predominant

Table 7-4
Molds Isolated from Various Vegetables

Vegetable	Molds Isolated	Reference
Bell peppers	*Aspergillus* sp., *Fusarium* sp.	Golden, Heaton, and Beuchat (1987)
Cabbage	*Alternaria* sp., *Aureobasidium pullulans, Botrytis cinerea, Cladosporium* sp., *Penicillium* sp.	Geeson (1979)
Corn	*A. niger, Cladosporium cladosporioides, Penicillium oxalicum, P. expansum, P. funiculosum*	Deák et al. (1987)
Cucumbers and squash	*Alternaria tenuis, Aureobasidium pullans, Chaetomium fimeti, Epicoccum nigrum, Fusarium* sp., *Mucor* sp., *Phoma* sp., *Rhizopus nigricans*	Webb and Mundt (1978)
Green beans	*A. tenuis, A. pullans, C. fimeti, E. nigrum, Fusarium* sp., *Mucor* sp., *Phoma* sp., *R. nigricans*	Webb and Mundt (1978)
Southern peas	*Alternaria* sp., *Aspergillus* sp., *Cladosporium* sp., *Fusarium* sp., *Phoma* sp.	Senter et al. (1984)
Tomatoes	*Alternaria* sp., *Cladosporium* sp., *Penicillium* sp.	Senter, Bailey, and Cox (1987)
	Geotrichum sp.	Splittstoesser (1987)

molds occurring on fruits include both spoilage and innocuous fungi. Common genera include members of *Aspergillus, Penicillium, Mucor, Alternaria, Cladosporium,* and *Botrytis.*

Populations of fungi on fruits can be quite high. For example, an average of 38,000–680,000 fungi per gram (mostly yeasts) were isolated from Concord grapes (Splittstoesser 1987). In contrast, sound apples contained only about 1,000 yeast cells per gram. Damaged or defective fruits can contain as many as 10 million CFU per gram of fruit.

Importance of Microbial Ecology

Many food scientists only think about microorganisms related to spoilage or safety problems. This perspective of food microbiology is important but it is also too restrictive. Many spoilage and safety problems could be avoided if food scientists took a broader view of food microbiology and also considered *why* bacteria behave the way they do. This view could be called an ecological view and is fundamental to the study of food microbiology. The study of the microbial ecology of foods is not a well recognized branch of food science but has actually been of interest since the 1930s (Mossel 1984). The area has received increased attention in recent years and has resulted in several notable reviews (Hobbs 1986; Skovgaard 1984).

The microbial ecologist views a food as a complex and dynamic ecological niche teeming with life. Within a food there are also many microenvironments. For example, the food–package interface might constitute one microenvironment whereas the interior of the food constitutes another. Because processing and handling of foods affects these microenvironments, the microbes will likewise be affected. The effects of these changes will differ depending on the microorganism in question. Some microbes will be positively affected by the change whereas others might be harmed. The result of these changes in the microflora is often negative, such as spoilage. The changes in the microecology may not be immediately evident but could cause problems indirectly later. The microecology of MPR produce is especially complex because these foods can change the microenvironment of microorganisms via their own respiratory processes. The following discussion will examine the major factors influencing the microbial ecology of fresh fruits and vegetables.

Factors That Affect Microbiology

Source

The product that one is discussing and its source will often determine which organisms are initially present. As mentioned earlier, the microflora of fruits and vegetables often differ appreciably. Vegetables will generally support the growth of any microorganism whereas fruits, because of their high acidity, allow primarily the growth of fungi and aciduric bacteria.

Both the near environment and weather patterns in which fruits and vegetables are produced will affect the type of microorganisms present. For example, one could expect treeborne fruits (e.g., apples) to have a quite different microflora than fruits produced close to the ground (e.g., strawberries). This is because the environment, like food, has a characteristic microflora.

Gram-positive bacteria are the predominant microorganisms in soil. Stolp (1988) estimates that 70% of the 10^6–10^9 bacteria present per cm^3 soil are coryneform bacteria, especially *Arthrobacter*, bacilli, and micrococci. However, fungi are also considered important soil microorganisms, particularly in acid soils (Lynch 1988). Gram-negative bacteria are usually less numerous in soils than gram-positive bacteria but are nevertheless present. Soil and soilborne organisms can gain access to fruits and vegetables by direct contact, by being blown by wind, or even via insects.

In contrast to soil, air serves more as a medium for dispersion than a habitat. Thus, the microflora of air will be composed of those organisms present on dust or water droplets. Microorganisms that have mechanisms to exploit aerial dispersion, such as many fungi, are also likely to be present in air. Air also differs from soil in harboring a relatively small concentration of microorganisms. However, the actual population is affected by humidity and amount of particulates being carried in air. Other important ecological factors that affect the microbial flora are temperature and rainfall. One could expect to isolate more psychrotrophic microorganisms from products grown and harvested in cool climates or seasons. In contrast, one would be more likely to find thermoduric organisms on items grown in tropical regions or harvested during hot seasons.

Rainfall affects microorganisms on fruits and vegetables in several ways. First, heavy rainfall can splash soil from the ground onto low-lying products, thereby increasing the microbial load of those products. In addition, rain also increases the relative humidity and helps to leach nutrients from the plant (Webb and Mundt 1978). The effect of rainfall on recovery of molds was reported by Webb and Mundt (1978). They found that 2.5 cm of rainfall during either of the 3 days preceding harvest increased populations of molds recovered from beans by 72% and cucumbers by 30% as compared to when <2.5 cm rainfall occurred.

Processing

As defined earlier (Chapter 1), processing is basically the forward movement of a food from harvest through marketing. During this movement, products will undergo changes to make them more convenient to use or last longer on store shelves. These changes will also likely change the microflora of the product.

The source and type of raw produce have an important effect on the microflora. However, handling of these products after harvest may be of equal or greater importance. This is because more can be done to control the environment and treatment of fruits and vegetables after harvest.

The form that a MPR fruit and vegetables will eventually take can be quite varied. A minimally processed product could be as simple as packaged fresh tomatoes or as complex as a prepared salad. Despite their final form, most produce items go through similar processing steps such as sorting, grading, and washing. Most minimally processed fruits and vegetables will also be subjected to some sort of temperature-controlled storage. Aside from these common handling steps, some produce products may undergo more specific treatments such as cutting, slicing, or individual packaging. Each of these treatments will affect the quality and microflora of particular products.

Temperature

The temperature at which a food is held is probably the single most important factor affecting microbial growth. Microorganisms, like most other organisms, grow best at an optimum temperature. However, they may be able to grow at temperatures well above or below their optimum temperatures, albeit more slowly. The effect of temperature on growth rate is illustrated in Figure 7-1. Virtually all microbes will behave in this way. However, various groups of microorganism can differ in the range of temperatures over which they can grow.

Microorganisms of concern in foods can be divided into three general groups, although often there is overlap. Those microbes capable of growth at refrigeration temperatures are called psychrotrophs. Psychrotrophs can grow at temperatures as low as freezing but most actually grow best at ambient (about 20–30° C) temperatures. MPR products are often processed under refrigerated conditions and stored refrigerated. Thus, it should not be surprising that psychrotrophic bacteria are especially important in MPR products. Many of the most important spoilage organisms and several human pathogens are psychrotrophic. Thus, individuals concerned with quality and safety of MPR products must be aware of these organisms. Examples of some psychrotrophic microorganisms present in foods are listed in Table 7-5.

Mesophiles grow best at ambient to warm temperatures (about 20–40° C) but poorly or not at all at refrigeration temperatures. In

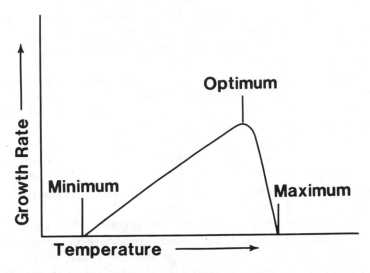

Figure 7-1   Growth of microorganisms in response to temperature (From Brock, Smith, and Madigan 1984.)

Table 7-5
Genera of Bacteria and Fungi that Include Psychrotrophic Strains

Bacteria

Acinetobacter	*Aeromonas*	*Alcaligenes*
Arthrobacter	*Bacillus*	*Chromobacterium*
Citrobacter	*Clostridium*	*Corynebacterium*
Enterobacter	*Erwinia*	*Escherichia*
Flavobacterium	*Klebsiella*	*Lactobacillus*
Leuconostoc	*Microbacterium*	*Micrococcus*
Moraxella	*Proteus*	*Pseudomonas*
Serratia	*Streptomyces*	*Streptococcus*
Vibrio	*Yersinia*	*Listeria*

Fungi

Aspergillus	*Candida*	*Cladosporium*
Cryptococus	*Penicillium*	*Toruplopsis*
Trichothecium	*Rhodotorula*	

addition, many mesophiles have higher maximum growth temperatures than psychrotrophs. Microorganisms, such as *Staphylococcus*
or *Salmonella*, typically associated with warm-blooded animals, are
examples of mesophiles.

Finally, a few types of microorganisms primarily grow at very warm
(greater than about 40° C) temperatures and are called thermophiles. Thermophiles are of little concern with refrigerated foods although they can become a problem in foods that are accidentally
exposed to very warm conditions. Thermophiles should not be con-
fused with thermoduric microorganisms, a group of organisms that
can be important in MPR products. This latter group of microorganisms do not require elevated temperatures for growth but are
capable of surviving high temperatures.

Because most fruits and vegetables are grown or harvested during
warm seasons, mesophiles will often constitute the predominant
microflora. However, storing and processing these foods in a refrigerated environment will gradually select for psychrotrophs. For
example, Brackett (1989) found that only about 0.3% of total aerobic
microorganisms on freshly harvested broccoli were classified as psychrotrophs. However, psychrotrophs comprised about 20% of total
aerobic microorganisms at the end of 6 weeks of storage at 1° C.

Handling

All produce is handled in one way or another during processing.
How the produce is handled can affect the microbiology of the product. One way that handling contributes to the microflora is from
cross-contamination by people or equipment. Fruits and vegetables
are usually placed in containers or vehicles for transportation to
packing or processing facilities. These containers or vehicles can be
a source of microorganisms and contaminate the product (Goepfert
1980). One example of this situation involves the fungus *Geotrichum
candidum*. This organism, commonly known as machinery mold, is
frequently found growing on improperly cleaned harvesting and
processing equipment. Its presence on equipment is considered by
some people (Eisenberg and Cichowicz 1977) to be an indication of
poor sanitation. However, Splittstoesser et al. (1977) found that higher
populations of *Geotrichum* did not always correlate with higher total
microbial populations in processed vegetables.

Handling, particularly if it is done improperly, can damage fresh
produce. Poorly maintained equipment or containers may have burrs
or rough edges that can puncture or abrade the outer skins or peels

Table 7-6
Bacterial Populations Recovered from Vegetables After Cutting[a]

		Bacteria per gram $\times 10^3$	
Operation	Vegetable	Before	After
Cutter	Corn	180	1,300
Slicer	French beans	20	130
Chopper	Spinach	20	120

[a]From Splittstoesser (1973).

of fruits or vegetables (Brackett 1987b). Such damage can allow nutrient-laden juices to leak onto surrounding products and equipment, encouraging microbial growth in these areas. In addition, damaged produce is more susceptible to invasion by spoilage organisms (Goepfert 1980).

Cutting and Slicing

Precut and presliced fresh fruits and vegetables are being increasingly introduced in the marketplace. These products are primarily offered as convenience items for those individuals who do not wish to be bothered with preparation. Slicing or cutting produce will affect the microbiology in several ways. First, cutting allows juices to leak from inner tissues onto equipment and outside of products. These juices often contain nutrients that can be used by microorganisms. This, together with the products' increased surface area that cutting provides, can lead to faster microbial growth. Consequently, higher populations of microorganisms usually develop in cut versus whole produce items. Splittstoesser (1973) found that exposing vegetables to various types of cutting resulted in a six- to seven-fold increase in microbial populations (Table 7-6). Chopping of broccoli (Splittstoesser and Corlett 1980) or cutting of salad vegetables (Priepke, Wei, and Nelson 1976) had similar effects on the microflora.

A second major way that cutting can affect microorganisms is that it circumvents the normal protection provided by outer skins or peelings. Sometimes, microbes that are normally not considered spoilage organisms can serve as such when normal protection mechanisms are eliminated.

Humidity and Water Activity

Microorganisms are like all other living creatures in that they require water. However, it is also vitally important that the water present in a food be available for use by the microbes. The relative amount of water available for use by microorganisms is most often expressed by the term water activity, or a_w. Water activity ranges from 0 (total dryness or complete unavailability to microorganisms) to 1.0 (pure water). The a_w is reduced by increasing the concentration of solutes in the aqueous phase of the food. This is done by either removing water (dehydration) or by adding solutes, such as sugar or salt. For a more thorough discussion of the effect of water activity, the reader is directed to several reviews on the subject (Christian 1980; Gould 1985).

Microbes vary in the minimum water activity necessary for growth and survival. Most bacteria require an a_w of at least 0.90 to grow and many cannot grow below an a_w of 0.95. Most yeasts can grow at a minimum a_w of 0.87 and most molds can grow down to an a_w of only 0.80. Some specialized bacteria and fungi can even grow down to an a_w of 0.65. No microbial growth will occur below an a_w of 0.60 (Christian 1980). Except for a few specialized species, all microbes will grow better at higher water activities than the minimum.

Virtually all fresh fruits and vegetables have an a_w of 0.95 or greater. This is sufficient to allow growth of almost any microorganisms of concern in MPR fruits and vegetables. A related concern that can affect microbial growth is the relative humidity surrounding the product. Low humidity in storage of fruits and vegetables can lead to dehydration and shrinking of the product. Mildly dehydrated produce is more successfully infected by some microbes (Van den Berg and Lentz 1966). In addition, low humidity during storage can also select for development of fungi, which tolerate low a_w environments (Brackett 1987b).

Storage of fruits and vegetables in high humidity can affect the microflora by allowing droplets of condensed moisture to accumulate on the product (Brackett 1987a; Lund 1971). This accumulated liquid can allow any microorganism present to be more easily spread to other produce items and may also serve as a growth broth. Consequently, microbial contamination and growth increase. Brackett (1988a) mentioned that noticeable moisture accumulated on the surface of individually seal-packaged tomatoes. He suggested that this may have been one reason why packaged tomatoes supported higher populations of microorganisms than unpackaged tomatoes.

Acidity and pH

As mentioned earlier, microorganisms differ in their tolerance to acidic pH. Most microorganisms of concern in fruits and vegetables will grow best at near-neutral pH. The growth of some bacteria is limited to neutral conditions but most can grow at pH values of about 4.5 or greater (Corlett and Brown 1980). However, some common bacteria, such as the lactic acid or acetic acid bacteria, can grow at pH 4.0 or less. Fungi are much more tolerant of acidic pH than are bacteria and can grow at pH values as low as 1.5 (Corlett and Brown 1980).

Knowing the relative pH of a fruit or vegetable is helpful in predicting what kinds of microorganisms are likely to grow or become a problem. Fruits, because they usually have pH values of <4.0, are almost exclusively spoiled by fungi. The pH of vegetables, on the other hand, is ordinarily near neutrality and will allow the growth of almost any kind of microorganism. However, bacteria will often have a competitive advantage in vegetables. This is because bacteria grow faster than fungi at neutral pH (Brackett 1987a; Bulgarelli and Brackett 1991). It should also be remembered that some microorganisms produce acid and can therefore affect subsequent growth of other microorganisms.

Antimicrobials

Preservatives used in processed foods are rarely used on fresh, refrigerated fruits and vegetables. However, some produce items are sometimes treated with compounds, such as fungicides, before harvest that are often not thought of as additives. In addition, many produce items are treated with sanitizers during washing or packaging to minimize spoilage. There are growing trends of mixing fresh produce items with other foods and using techniques that greatly extend shelf-life. These trends are increasing the necessity for using preservatives.

The particular effect that an antimicrobial compound will have on the microflora is related to its antimicrobial spectrum. Some compounds are specifically intended for use against fungi and will have little or no effect on bacteria. The result of using such compounds will predictably be a higher proportion of bacteria residing on the product. The bacteriocins are among the newer antimicrobials being proposed for use in foods and have primary activity against gram-positive bacteria (Hurst 1972). Thus, the microflora of foods in which these are used would tend to shift toward gram-negative bacteria. In other cases, such as with most organic acids (Doores 1983), the antimicrobial activity may be more general but is affected by the pH of the food.

Chlorine compounds are quite effective for inactivating microbes in solutions or on equipment. However, their use on fresh fruits and vegetables produces only minor effects on microorganisms. Golden, Heaton, and Beuchat (1987) applied the equivalent of 100 μg available chlorine to bell peppers, tomatoes, peaches, and cantaloupes and determined changes in total microbial populations, and yeasts and molds. They found only small and insignificant differences in either of these groups of microorganisms compared to produce that received no sanitizer treatment. Senter et al. (1985) likewise found that chlorine had little effect on the microflora of tomatoes. In one case, chlorine treatment even increased populations of total aerobic microorganisms. In general, the use of sanitizers on fresh produce items may differ depending on the strength of the compound, method of application, and amount of organic matter present. Dipping soiled produce in solutions containing low concentrations of sanitizers will likely result in cross-contamination of products rather than lowering populations of microorganisms.

Atmosphere

The use of modified or controlled atmospheres for storage of fruits and vegetables has become very popular in recent years. The most common way to modify the atmosphere is to reduce the O_2 while increasing the CO_2 concentration (Brecht 1980). However, there are many changes that can be made to the atmosphere that can rightly be considered modified. In the context of this discussion, modified atmosphere includes any process that causes the gaseous environment of the produce to differ from that of ambient atmospheric conditions.

Microorganisms differ in their sensitivity to gases normally used in modified atmospheres. Nitrogen is often used in modified atmospheres but is primarily used to displace O_2 and has little other direct effects on microorganisms. In contrast, CO_2 has both direct and indirect effects on microorganisms. However, the impact of CO_2 on microbes varies depending on the organism in question, the concentration of gas, and temperature (Clark and Takács 1980). In addition, effects of modified atmospheres can differ in laboratory model systems and on actual commodities (Yackel et al. 1971). The general effects of CO_2 are related to displacement of O_2, reduction of pH, and interference of cellular metabolism (Daniels, Krishnamurthi, and Rizvi 1985). When the O_2 concentration becomes low enough, modified atmospheres can select for facultative or obligate anaerobes.

Gram-negative bacteria, particularly aerobic varieties such as the pseudomonads, are the microorganisms most sensitive to CO_2. In contrast, the anaerobic bacteria and lactic acid bacteria are quite resistant to the gas (Jay 1986c). Among the fungi, molds are sensitive but yeasts comparatively resistant (Daniels, Krishnamurthi, and Rizvi 1985) to CO_2. Usually, concentrations of CO_2 more than about 5% are required for effective inhibition of microorganisms and many applications require much higher concentrations (Daniels, Krishnamurthi, and Rizvi 1980). However, the antimicrobial effect of CO_2 directly increases and decreases with changes in temperature (Jay 1986c).

Produce processors use modified atmospheres with fresh produce to retard ripening (Kader 1986). The desired result of this practice is longer shelf-life and reduced decay. The concentrations of CO_2 used with MPR produce usually range from about 5% to a maximum of about 25% (Brecht 1980). Greater concentrations than this cause damage to most fruits and vegetables (Brecht 1980).

Optimum concentrations of CO_2 for maintaining fruits and vegetables are not always optimum for restricting growth of microorganisms. Deák (1984) studied the effects of modified atmospheres on several microorganisms in culture media and on fruits and vegetables. He discovered that results of experiments with laboratory media did not always predict the best system for use with fruits and vegetables. For example, Deák found that growth of a bacterium (*Flavobacterium*) and three genera of fungi (*Aurobasidium*, *Aspergillus*, and *Penicillium*) on laboratory media was inhibited most by an atmosphere containing 10% CO_2. However, more than 5% CO_2 resulted in increased spoilage of cauliflower. Thus, he suggested that one might need to compromise microbial inhibition slightly and simply use atmospheres best for maintaining overall product quality. Yackel et al. (1971) described similar results and also found that modified atmosphere helped minimize mold spoilage of some fruits but not others. However, they also found that modified atmosphere could not undo the effects of mishandling fruits.

Modified atmospheres used with fresh produce sometimes have no obvious effect on microorganisms. Priepke, Wei, and Nelson (1976) found that populations of total aerobic microorganisms in salad vegetables stored refrigerated in 10.5% CO_2 and 2.25% O_2 differed by only one-tenth of a log cycle. Beuchat and Brackett (1990b) obtained similar results for lettuce stored in an atmosphere of 3% CO_2 and 97% N_2 atmosphere. They also found that atmosphere had no effect on the growth of either total aerobic or psychrotrophic microorganisms. In other cases, microorganisms on fresh produce can be affected. Berrang, Brackett, and Beuchat (1990) found that storing broccoli at $1°$ C in an atmosphere containing 10% CO_2 and 11% O_2 inhibited growth of total aerobic microorganisms by several logs.

Packaging

Packaging is an increasingly important technique that has several features that make it desirable for use with fresh produce. First, it is quite useful from a marketing standpoint because it allows processors to provide labelling information but still allows consumers to see the product. More importantly, it minimizes dehydration of the product, a major cause of deterioration of MPR produce (Ben-Yehoshua 1985). In addition, some packaging schemes are specifically designed to exploit the use of modified atmospheres. Other schemes can unintentionally become modified atmosphere systems as a result of metabolic activity of the product (Brackett 1987a).

The use of packaging can have substantial impact on the microflora of fresh fruits and vegetables. The packaging material itself could conceivably contribute to the microflora if it is sufficiently contaminated. However, packaging's greatest effects are primarily related to its ability to influence the microenvironment of packaged fruits and vegetables. Like modified atmospheres, many of the packaging techniques proposed for fresh fruits and vegetables are designed to increase shelf-life without regard to changes in the microflora. Fruits and vegetables differ from most other foods in that they are living tissues that still maintain active metabolism. In respiring, they expel water, produce some gases, and utilize other gases. Thus, enclosing these foods within a package is especially likely to result in changes to the microenvironment.

Many of the microbial changes that occur within packaged fresh fruits and vegetables result from changes in humidity within the package (Brackett 1987a). Respiration by the plant tissues increases relative humidity and thereby also increases the likelihood for mold growth (Brackett 1987a,b). The increased humidity also increases the likelihood for condensation to occur within the package. This can allow water droplets to form both on the product and on the inner surface of the package, particularly during refrigerated storage.

This accumulation of water droplets can itself affect the microflora. First, droplets can serve as a transport medium and allow microorganisms to more easily be distributed to other parts of the product. In addition, these droplets can dissolve usable carbohydrates leaking from plant tissues and serve as a growth medium. Deák et al. (1987) noted that the atmosphere of shrink-wrapped corn became saturated with moisture. They also surmised that this led to increased growth of microorganisms. The use of water-absorbing materials may help to minimize the amount of water droplets collecting on products and thereby also minimize microbial growth.

Atmospheric gas concentrations can also change when fruits and vegetables are packaged. Consequently, this can also affect the microflora. Sugiyama and Yang (1975) published one of the first reports demonstrating the importance of product respiration on the microflora. In that case, they demonstrated that the metabolic activity of packaged mushrooms changed the atmosphere so much that the obligately anaerobic *Clostridium botulinum* could germinate and grow. Other researchers have also observed an effect of packaging on the atmosphere and microflora but with less dramatic results. Deák et al. (1987) noticed that O_2 and CO_2 concentrations quickly changed after corn was shrink-wrapped. These gases eventually reached 12% and 10%, respectively. The main changes they observed in the microflora were slightly higher populations of aerobic mesophilic microorganisms and yeasts in packaged compared to unpackaged corn. Brackett, in similar experiments with shrink-wrapped tomatoes (1988a), broccoli (1989), and bell peppers (1990) reported only slight changes in the atmospheres.

The enhanced growth of microorganisms in packaged corn and improved shelf-life described by Deák et al. (1987) does not appear to be caused by the drastic changes in atmosphere. Both Golden et al. (1987) and Brackett (1988a, 1989, 1990) confirmed observations of Deák et al. (1987) despite the absence of major atmospheric changes. Brackett further observed that the microflora of tomatoes and broccoli changed from predominantly gram-negative to gram-positive. In contrast, the microflora of unpackaged products were similar to the original products in being predominantly gram-negative.

The atmosphere and microflora of vacuum-packaged produce is also likely to change. Buick and Damoglou (1987) found that the atmosphere of vacuum-packaged fresh carrots changed from ambient to a maximum of about 35% CO_2 and a minimum of about 2% O_2 during storage. The degree of change was greatest at the highest (15° C) and least at the lowest (4° C) storage temperature. They also

Table 7-7
Approximate Lethal Doses of Ionizing Radiation for Various Classes of Microorganisms[a]

Microorganism	Dose (kGy)
Gram-negative bacteria	0.05–7.5
Gram-positive vegetative bacteria	0.05–20
Bacterial endospores	10–50
Molds	1.5–5
Yeasts	3–20
Viruses	>30

[a] Adapted from Brackett (1987a).

found that the microflora expectedly changed from predominantly microaerophilic gram-negative (especially *Erwinia*) to fermentative gram-positive (especially *Leuconostic*) microorganisms. As with other packaging schemes, shelf-life was extended, particularly at the lowest storage temperature.

Irradiation

Low-dose (1 kGy or less) irradiation has been suggested as a minimal processing technique for extending the shelf-life of some fruits and vegetables (Kader 1986). The primary uses of this technique, sometimes known as radurization, are to eliminate insects or inhibit sprouting (Jay 1986b). However, gamma radiation will also affect microorganisms to varying degrees (Table 7-7). Gram-negative spoilage bacteria are among the microorganisms most sensitive to gamma radiation. Thus, forms of vegetable spoilage related to these bacteria might also be expected to be reduced. However, molds and yeasts are among the most resistant organisms. Therefore, irradiation would have less effect in products, such as fruits (Jay 1986b), where these organisms predominate. In addition, irradiation treatments will tend to select for these types of organisms. Deák et al. (1987) observed an effect on the survival of different types of microflora on irradiated sweet corn. They found that a 1 kGy dose of gamma irradiation resulted in an over 3 log decrease in the aerobic mesophilic microorganisms. In contrast, populations of yeasts decreased by only about 1.7 logs and populations of survivors recovered faster than did aerobic microorganisms.

Expected Shelf-Life

The expected shelf-life of refrigerated and minimally processed fruits and vegetables will have a direct effect on the microflora. The time between when a product is harvested and when it is expected to be sold or consumed will often dictate the primary microbiological concern. The potential for foodborne infection could be a main concern with some products intended to be eaten soon after harvest. Thus, one might want to concentrate analysis efforts on detecting organisms such as enteric pathogens. In contrast, long-term storage increases the chance that spoilage will occur. In this case, one might be concerned primarily with spoilage organisms.

Extending shelf-life may allow more time for population shifts to occur or for slow-growing microorganisms, such as psychrotrophs, to grow. Thus, microbiological problems that seem inconsequential during short-term storage may emerge as major problems after long-term storage. For example, Berrang, Brackett, and Beuchat (1989b) found that extending the shelf-life of fresh asparagus allowed *Listeria monocytogenes* to grow to significantly higher populations. Produce processors and distributors should always try to anticipate and have some idea of the basic microflora of their product before it is offered to consumers.

Spoilage

Common Spoilage Problems

Spoilage is another term that is subject to personal interpretation. The broadest definition for spoilage would be any process or condition that makes a food undesirable to consume. These processes could be as diverse as physical damage (e.g., bruising or insect damage), enzymatic activity, senescence, safety problems, or microbial degradation. Of these, physical damage causes the greatest loss. However, this discussion will be limited only to the latter aspect.

Types of Spoilage

Spoilage of fruits and vegetables is often classified according to where or when the spoilage becomes evident. Preharvest or field spoilage refers to those spoilage problems that become obvious before the product is harvested. Traditionally, this has been the domain of the plant pathologists and horticulturists. Such spoilage is primarily of economic concern to producers but otherwise affects processors very little. Therefore, preharvest spoilage problems are not discussed in this chapter.

Spoilage that becomes evident after harvest is often termed postharvest spoilage, or market disease. This is the type of spoilage of most concern for MPR produce. The main problem with categorizing spoilage in this manner is that some microorganisms can cause spoilage to occur both pre- and postharvest. Moreover, some microbiological problems often begin before harvest but do not become apparent until after harvest. Thus, describing spoilage in these ways can often be quite misleading.

Another common way that spoilage problems of fresh fruits and vegetables are categorized is by symptoms such as "wet rot," "watery soft rot," or "black rot." These names are usually quite descriptive of a problem but do not always indicate the microorganism involved. Sometimes several different microorganisms are capable of causing similar spoilage problems. A more accurate way to describe a spoilage problem would include both the spoilage organism and the symptoms, such as *Erwinia caratovora* soft rot.

As stated earlier, fruits and vegetables each have a characteristic indigenous microflora. The same principles apply to spoilage microorganisms. Both fungi and bacteria are important causes of spoilage in MPR vegetables. The high water activity and neutral pH of vegetables make them equally suitable hosts for either type of microorganism. However, the faster growth rate of bacteria usually allows them to more successfully compete with the fungi in these foods. Consequently, bacteria are more often responsible for postharvest spoilage of refrigerated vegetables.

Many different genera of bacteria can spoil fresh and minimally processed vegetables. Some of the more common spoilage genera are listed in Table 7-8. Several excellent reviews of the role of these bacteria in the spoilage of vegetables have been published previously (Lund 1971, 1981, 1982, 1983).

The majority of the bacteria responsible for spoilage of vegetables are gram-negative. Of these, *Erwinia* is among the most aggressive. About five species or subspecies of *Erwinia* are responsible for spoilage of plant products (Lund 1983). However, *E. carotovora* is the species most commonly associated with decay of vegetables. This bacterium causes soft rots in most vegetables but is particularly known for attacking potatoes. The *Erwinia* soft rots initially start as soft,

Table 7-8
General of Spoilage Bacteria Sometimes Associated with Vegetables[a]

Organism	Vegetables Affected
Erwinia	Many vegetables
Pseudomonas	Celery
Cytophaga	Bell pepper, watermelon[b]
Xanthomonas	Beans, cabbage, cauliflower
Corynebacterium	Beans, tomatoes, potatoes
Bacillus	Potato, pepper, tomato
Clostridium	Potato

[a]Lund (1983).
[b]Liao and Wells (1986).

water-soaked areas on the vegetable tissue. As the infection proceeds, the area of rotting expands until complete collapse of the tissue occurs. (Lund 1983).

The fluorescent *Pseudomonas* species, an example of which is *P. marginalis*, are another group of common and important spoilage organisms of refrigerated vegetables. These bacteria are responsible for soft rot decay of many types of vegetables including celery, potato, chicory, lettuce, Chinese chard, and cabbage (Brocklehurst and Lund 1981). Characteristics of *P. marginalis* soft rot spoilage are similar to those of *E. caratovora*. However, the pseudomonads faster growth at refrigeration temperatures makes them more likely to spoil refrigerated produce than would *E. carotovora* (Lund 1982).

Several gram-positive bacteria, most notably clostridia and bacilli (Lund 1982, 1983; Lund, Brocklehurst, and Wyatt 1981), can also cause spoilage of vegetables in the right circumstances. However, these bacteria grow only slowly if at all at refrigeration temperatures. For example, Lund, Brocklehurst and Wyatt (1981) found that the minimum temperature at which spoilage strains of *Clostridium puniceum* grew was about 7° C; most were unable to grow at 10° C or less. Thus, one might find different types of spoilage when vegetables are exposed to abusive temperatures.

Although many different types of fungi can be associated with the spoilage of vegetables (Table 7-9), only a relatively few cause most spoilage problems. Fewer still are able to spoil vegetables at refrigeration temperatures. Pitt and Hocking (1985b) relate that species of *Fusarium, Cladosporium, Penicillium*, and *Thamnidium* will grow and spoil foods at refrigeration temperatures. However, they likewise

Table 7-9
Fungi Sometimes Associated with Spoilage of Vegetables[a]

Organism	Vegetables Affected
Alternaria	Cabbage, carrots, cauliflower, peppers, tomatoes
Aspergillus	Onions, tomatoes
Botrytis	Green beans, cabbage, carrots celery, lettuce, onions, peppers, tomatoes
Candida	Tomatoes
Colletotrichum	Green beans, onions, tomatoes
Fusarium	Asparagus, carrots
Mucor	Celery
Pythium	Green beans, potatoes
Rhizopus	Carrots, tomatoes
Sclerotinia	Carrots, celery

[a]Bulgarelli and Brackett (1990).

specify that psychrotrophic bacteria are more likely to cause spoilage in products (such as vegetables) with a neutral pH. Thus, one is most likely to find fungal spoilage of vegetables when adequate refrigeration is not maintained. Some vegetables are easily damaged by low temperature storage (Shewfelt 1987). Therefore, one could expect the chance for fungal spoilage to become greater in these products, particularly in humid conditions. Indeed, Brackett (1990) observed that mold growth was among the first defects noticed in packaged bell peppers stored at 13° C. In contrast, unpackaged peppers, which were exposed to lower humidity, underwent soft rots but no mold growth. For more details on the fungal spoilage of vegetables, the reader is referred to one of several reviews on the topic (Brackett 1987b; Bulgarelli and Brackett 1991; Pitt and Hocking 1985a).

The normal spoilage flora of refrigerated fruits differs markedly from that of vegetables. Most fruits are sufficiently acidic to limit spoilage primarily to fungi (Splittstoesser 1987). The problem of mold spoilage is also compounded because many fruits must be stored at elevated temperatures to avoid chill injury. More than 20 genera of molds including *Alternaria, Botrytis, Penicillium,* and *Phytophthora* are known to cause spoilage in fruits (Brackett and Splittstoesser 1992). The specific type of fungus that can cause spoilage is often dependent on the fruit in question (Pitt and Hocking 1985a). Some spoilage fungi are highly specialized and will cause decay only in closely related fruits. Others are more generalized in their ability to cause decay in fruits (Pitt and Hocking 1985a). In general, fruits become more susceptible to fungal infection as they become dehydrated (Ben-Yehoshua 1985) or if they become overripe (Pitt and Hocking 1985a). More detailed discussions of fungal spoilage of fruits have been written by Pitt and Hocking (1985b) and Splittstoesser (1987).

Mechanisms of Resistance and Spoilage

Although fruits and vegetables are categorized as perishable, they do possess potent defense mechanisms that keep them from decaying even faster (Pitt and Hocking 1985b). Fruits' and vegetables' first line of defense are peels and skins which serve as physical barriers against invasion by microorganisms. Any breach of these barriers allows microbes access to inner tissues that would normally be inaccessible. Often, damage to outer barriers allow normally saprophytic microorganisms to enter and serve as spoilage microorganisms. An example of this would be sour or wet rots of vegetables caused by *Geotrichum* or *Rhizopus*, respectively. These molds sometimes enter inner vegetable tissues when the common fruit fly, *Drosophila melanogaster*, deposits mold spores along with eggs into cracks or wounds in the vegetable. Similarly, stings and damage from feeding can likewise help insects inoculate produce with microorganisms.

Once damaged, some vegetables can still protect themselves by employing wound-healing mechanisms. These mechanisms allow wounds to be closed or covered with new tissue. This process, sometimes known as lignification (Bulgarelli and Brackett 1991), is especially notable in the case of potato tubers (Friend, Reynolds, and Aveyard 1973).

Some fruits and vegetables also have the ability to resist microbial invasion by producing antimicrobial compounds. In some cases, microbial infections stimulate the plant to produce antimicrobial compounds. The so-called stress metabolites or phytoalexins are one well-known example of such compounds. Celery, for instance, produces phytoalexins known as psoralens in response to *Sclerotinia sclerotiorum* infections (Brackett 1987b).

Although fruits and vegetables have defense mechanisms, many microbes likewise have developed ways to overcome those defense mechanisms. Most notable in this regard is the ability to produce degradative enzymes. Probably the most important of the degradative enzymes are the pectinolytic enzymes such as pectin methyl esterase and polygalacturonase (Brackett 1987a). These enzymes cause degradation of pectins in the middle lamella of the cell. The result is liquification of the plant tissue leading to symptoms such as soft rots. Some of the more common microorganisms that produce pectinolytic enzymes include *E. caratovora* and *P. marginalis* (Lund 1983), *Botrytis, Alternaria, Colletotrichum*, and *Fusarium* (Bulgarelli and Brackett 1991). Other enzymes such as hemicellulase, cellulase, and proteinase are also involved in the spoilage process but are usually secondary to pectinases (Codner 1971). For a further discussion of enzymes involved in fruit and vegetable spoilage, the reader is directed to reviews by Codner (1971) and Chesson (1980).

Minimizing Spoilage

The first step in minimizing spoilage should be to select and keep only the highest quality products. Diseased or damaged products will only serve to contaminate sound products and should therefore be culled as soon as possible. Moreover, culled vegetables should be discarded in such a way that they will not recontaminate equipment or sound products.

Secondly, producers, processors, and distributors need to be conscientious about the cleanliness of equipment and facilities. Accumulated surface grime can serve as nutrients for microorganisms and allow them to form biofilms. For example, *G. candidum* is called "machinery mold" because of its ability to colonize soiled equipment (Eisenberg and Cichowicz 1977; Splittstoesser et al. 1977). In addition, equipment should be maintained in top condition to avoid damaging fruits and vegetables.

Postharvest treatments and storage techniques vary in their effectiveness in reducing spoilage. In general, techniques that maintain fruits and vegetables in top physiological condition will also be effective at reducing spoilage. For example, avoiding desiccation by maintaining adequate relative humidity during storage can reduce the potential for infection of fruits and vegetables by fungi (Brackett 1988a; Van den Berg and Lentz 1966). However, high relative humidities are also more likely to allow condensation to form on produce items, leading to an increased risk of soft rots (Lund 1982).

Safety

Importance of Safety

Most food professionals know that food safety is an important issue. However, fewer individuals fully appreciate their role in ensuring food safety. Food is notable among commerce items in that it is something all people must have to survive. Moreover, most consumers purchase their foods with full trust that the food will be safe to eat. This gives the food industry an ethical responsibility to ensure that this trust is never compromised.

Another important reason for paying close attention to food safety is that foodborne disease can cause catastrophic economic problems for the companies and individuals involved. Todd (1989b) has estimated that over 12 million cases of foodborne disease costing $8.4 billion occur each year in the United States. This comes to an average $670 for each estimated case. Although impressively large, these figures do not even include the cost to food companies resulting from litigation, recall procedures, and lost sales due to adverse publicity. The exact cost to food companies implicated in foodborne disease outbreaks is unknown but can easily run into millions of dollars per company.

Finally, food companies should be concerned with food safety because they have a legal obligation to do so. Virtually every state and nation has laws designed to protect the consuming public to some degree. Penalties for violating these laws can be as minor as having a lot of product impounded or discarded. However, penalties can also be as severe as prison sentences.

Foodborne Illness from Fruits and Vegetables

Not all foods carry equivalent risk as vehicles for foodborne pathogens. Fruits and vegetables, particularly if unprocessed, are among the safest of foods. Todd (1989a) estimated that vegetables and fruits were implicated in only from about 2–5% of foodborne illness cases in Canada in 1983 and 1984. Moreover, raw produce was responsible for fewer than 1% of the reported cases. Bryan (1988b) likewise reported that few cases of illness were linked to vegetables (Table 7-10) and assessed these foods to be low hazard.

There are several reasons why MPR produce is relatively safe when compared to other foods. First, conditions used with fresh produce are usually unfavorable for growth of most pathogens. Only relatively few of the many types of pathogens are capable of growing at the refrigeration temperatures used to store these products. Some items, such as fruits, are acidic enough to prevent growth of pathogens. Second, the normal spoilage organisms in refrigerated produce are usually psychrotrophic and therefore have a competitive

Table 7-10
Foods Associated with Outbreaks of Foodborne Disease,ᵃ 1977–1984

Food Group	Cases	Percentage
Seafoods	393	24.8
Meat	368	23.2
Poultry	155	9.8
Vegetables	78	4.9
Milk and milk products	66	4.2
Baked goods	53	3.3
Beverages	36	2.3
Eggs	35	2.2
Fruits	20	1.3
Other	382	24.0
Total	1,586	100

ᵃAdapted from Bryan (1988b).

advantage over most pathogens. Sometimes this competition can prevent the growth of the pathogens. In other cases, the food simply spoils before it is eaten. Nevertheless, foodborne disease can and does occur with fruits and vegetables. Moreover, Palumbo (1987) warns that refrigeration alone is not sufficient to prevent pathogenic bacteria from growing in foods.

Pathogenic Organisms and Their Characteristics

Fruits and vegetables can serve as vehicles for almost any foodborne pathogenic microorganism and result in disease under the right circumstances. However, only a relatively few pathogenic microorganisms would normally be considered a serious threat with refrigerated fruits or vegetables. Fewer still have ever actually been implicated in cases of illness traced to these foods (Table 7-11). This situation may change, however, as changes in technology and packaging techniques are adopted by the food industry.

Certain gram-negative bacteria are sometimes implicated in enteric diseases associated with fruits and vegetables. These organisms are typically associated with the intestinal tract of man or other animals. Consequently, enteric pathogens are common contaminants of produce that is grown in countries where polluted water is used for irrigation or where sewage or animal manure is used as fertilizer (Brackett and Splittstoesser 1992).

Table 7-11
Bacterial Foodborne Illness Attributed to Fruits and Vegetables[a]

Organism	Disease	Foods Involved
Salmonella typhi	Typhoid	Celery, radishes, lettuce
Salmonella sp.	Salmonellosis	Misc. vegetables, water
Shigella	Shigellosis	Cabbage, lettuce[b]
Vibrio chloerae	Cholera	Vegetables, dates
Listeria monocytogenes	Listeriosis	Cabbage, mushrooms[c]
Bacillus cereus	Enteritis	Green bean salad

[a]Adapted from Brackett (1987a).
[b]Davis et al. (1988).
[c]Junttila and Brander (1989).

Shigella

Shigella is among the most common enteric bacterial pathogens found on fruits and vegetables. For example, one large outbreak of shigellosis was traced to commercially distributed shredded lettuce (Davis et al. 1988). This bacterium causes a serious disease known as shigellosis or bacterial dysentery. Shigellosis is characterized by diarrhea (sometimes bloody), abdominal pain, and fever (Morris 1984). As few as 10 *Shigella* cells may be all that is necessary to cause disease (Morris 1984). Although this bacterium does not grow at refrigeration temperatures, it can survive for extended times at these conditions (Morris 1984).

Salmonella

Salmonella is another important enteric pathogen that can sometimes contaminate fruits and vegetables. Symptoms of *Salmonella* infections can vary from mild diarrhea to potentially life-threatening typhoid fever (Jay 1986a). Salmonellae are similar to the shigellae in that they can survive but do not usually grow at refrigeration temperatures. The usual sources of contamination of fruit and vegetable products are contaminated irrigation or wash water, cross-contamination from other foods (especially meats, poultry, and seafoods), or infected handlers.

Escherichia coli

A third enteric bacterium that is becoming increasingly important are pathogenic, and especially psychrotrophic, strains of *E. coli*. The form of disease normally caused by *E. coli* is typical of "travelers' disease" and can be similar to salmonellosis or shigellosis (Doyle and Padhye 1989). However, a new and more serious form of disease, known as hemorrhagic colitis, has emerged in recent years. Symptoms of this form normally consist of profuse, bloody diarrhea although the disease can progress to include serious kidney damage and death. Hemorrhagic colitis is caused by the relatively newly identified strain (O157:H7) of *E. coli*. Although this strain has so far been associated only with animal products, it is conceivable that the organism could contaminate fruits and vegetables via feces or water. Therefore, fruit and vegetable processors should also be aware of its existence and characteristics.

Aeromonas hydrophila

Another gram-negative bacterium that is a threat in refrigerated produce is *A. hydrophila*. This bacterium most often produces a mild diarrheal illness. However, a more severe form characterized by bloody and mucus-containing diarrhea has also been reported (Stelma 1989). Unlike the preceding gram-negative pathogens, *A. hydrophila* is naturally widespread in nature rather than being a chance fecal contaminant.

A. hydrophila possesses growth characteristics that make it of particular concern in MPR produce. One reason for concern is that *A. hydrophila* is more often found on fresh produce than not. Callister and Agger (1987) surveyed grocery store produce items and found *A. hydrophila* present in virtually every type of vegetable analyzed. Populations of the bacterium at the time of purchase ranged as high as 10^4 cells/g. Berrang, Brackett, and Beuchat (1989a) likewise found naturally occurring *A. hydrophila* on fresh asparagus, broccoli, and cauliflower which they were studying.

A second reason that *A. hydrophila* should be of special concern is that it is a true psychrotroph which can grow at temperatures as low as 1° C (Palumbo 1987). For instance, the bacterium can grow well in vegetables stored at 5° C or less (Callister and Agger 1987, Berrang, Brackett, and Beuchat 1989a).

Finally, *A. hydrophila* is unaffected by modified atmosphere packaging. Berrang, Brackett, and Beuchat (1989a) found that both naturally occurring and artificially inoculated *A. hydrophila* grew equally well on vegetables stored under modified atmospheres or air. The most impressive increase in populations of *A. hydrophila* occurred in asparagus stored at 4° C. Populations were below the level of detection (10^2 cell/g) at initiation of storage. However, they increased to over 10^6 cells/g after 21 days of storage.

Clostridium botulinum

Not all microorganisms of concern are gram-negative. *C. botulinum*, a gram-positive bacterium, is among the most well-known of foodborne pathogens in vegetables. This bacterium produces a potent toxin that causes severe paralysis and death in those who consume it. This disease syndrome, known as botulism, is primarily associated with improperly canned, low-acid foods. The reasons why these foods are a particular problem are related to the growth requirements of the bacterium. It is anaerobic and will usually only grow if the pH is >4.6.

Although conditions favoring the growth of *C. botulinum* are typically found in canned vegetables they may also exist or develop in MPR vegetables. This is especially true when modified atmosphere or barrier packaging is used with respiring products, such as fresh produce. A problem reported by Sugiyama and Yang (1975) involving packaged fresh mushrooms is a classic example of this situation. They suspected that the combination of barrier packaging and the high respiratory activity of the mushrooms could create favorable growth conditions for *C. botulinum*. In testing this hypothesis, they discovered that the bacterium not only grew but produced toxin in the mushrooms. This example clearly demonstrated that *C. botulinum* was more than just a problem in canned foods. Moreover, some strains of *C. botulinum* can grow in temperatures as low as 3.5° C (Hauschild 1989). Thus, it should not be surprising that concern exists that the use of modified atmosphere packaging schemes could increase the risk of botulism (Hintlian and Hotchkiss 1986).

Many food scientists do not realize that acidic foods can constitute a botulism threat. This possibility is primarily of concern in mildly acidic foods such as tomatoes. Mundt and Norman (1982) reported a situation in which molds infecting fresh tomatoes were able to raise the pH of the tomato tissue to as much as 8.1. Draughon, Chen, and Mundt (1988) were later able to demonstrate the growth of *C. botulinum* in fresh tomatoes. Thus, safety should not always be assumed just because a fruit or vegetable is considered acidic.

Listeria monocytogenes

Probably no other pathogen has had as big an impact on the food industry in recent years as has this gram-positive bacterium. Its recognition as a foodborne pathogen and regulations to control it have affected virtually every food commodity, including fruits and vegetables. The reason for concern stems from the nature of the disease, listeriosis. Listeriosis rarely occurs in healthy individuals and is mild in those in whom it is diagnosed. Symptoms normally reported are usually described as transitory flu-like symptoms. However, the disease can be quite severe in individuals whose immune system is for some reason impaired. Pregnant women and their fetuses, the elderly, individuals afflicted with various chronic diseases, and those taking various kinds of medication are at particular risk (Ciesielski et al. 1988). In these individuals, listeriosis often manifests itself as meningitis or encephalitis (Lovett 1989) and is fatal about 30% of the time (Ciesielski et al. 1988).

Although listeriosis is rarely associated with fresh produce, outbreaks and contaminated products have been reported. The first reported major outbreak of listeriosis, involving 41 cases, was traced to cole slaw prepared from cabbage (Schlech et al. 1983). Investigators eventually found that the cabbage had been fertilized with sheep manure from sheep that had a history of listeriosis. The role of fresh produce in listeriosis was later again demonstrated when celery, tomatoes, and lettuce were epidemiologically linked to a listeriosis outbreak in Boston (Ho et al. 1986). More recently, a case of listeriosis was associated with salted mushrooms (Junttila and Brander 1989). Such incidences encouraged the U.S. Food and Drug Administration (Heisick et al. 1989) to extensively survey fresh produce for the presence of *L. monocytogenes*. They found the bacterium in 21% of potatoes, 14% of radishes, and 2% or less in cucumbers and cabbage. In addition, the investigators also found other *Listeria* species in lettuce and mushrooms.

The problem of *L. monocytogenes* in foods, including fruits and vegetables, has been especially troublesome. *L. monocytogenes*, like *A. hydrophila*, possesses characteristics that not only allow it to gain access to foods but to grow well. The bacterium is widespread in the environment, including agricultural habitats (Brackett 1988b). Its primary habitat is thought to be soil and particularly decaying vegetation. In addition, both domestic animals and humans exist as carriers of the organism (Lovett 1989). Thus, there is ample chance for fresh produce to become contaminated with *L. monocytogenes*.

Another characteristic that makes *L. monocytogenes* deserving of concern is that it grows well on vegetables. Conner, Brackett, and Beuchat (1986) demonstrated that it could compete with the indigenous microflora and grow well in cabbage juice, ultimately reaching populations as high as 10^9 cells/ml. Berrang, Brackett, and Beuchat (1989b) found that *L. monocytogenes* grew to populations of more than 10^6 on asparagus, broccoli, and cauliflower stored at an abuse temperature of 15° C. Asparagus was the only one of these vegetables that supported appreciable growth at 5° C. Similar observations have been noted for salad vegetables. *L. monocytogenes* can grow on chopped and packaged (Steinbruegge, Maxey, and Liewen 1988) or shredded and packaged lettuce (Beuchat and Brackett 1990b). However, generalizations about the growth of *L. monocytogenes* cannot be made for all salad vegetables. For example, not only did chopped raw carrots not support growth but were actually bactericidal to *L. monocytogenes* (Beuchat and Brackett 1990a). In contrast, the low pH (4.0) of chopped and whole tomatoes would be assumed detrimental to *Listeria*. Yet, *L. monocytogenes* was able to maintain original populations for up to 2 weeks of storage at 10 or 21° C (Beuchat and Brackett 1991).

Modified atmosphere storage or packaging does not appear to affect the growth of *L. monocytogenes*. Berrang, Brackett and Beuchat (1989b) found that *L. monocytogenes* grew the same on vegetables whether or not they were stored under a modified atmosphere. However, the modified atmosphere did extend the shelf-life of the vegetables and allowed more time for the *L. monocytogenes* to grow. For instance, significantly higher populations of *L. monocytogenes* were present on asparagus stored in a modified atmosphere than asparagus stored in air (Figure 7-2). Thus, vegetable processors should be aware that the apparent sensory quality of a product may not reflect the presence or population of this organism.

Parasites

Foodborne parasites are a well-known hazard in developing countries but have received relatively little attention in developed countries. Nevertheless, parasitic disease can occur in industrialized nations (Jackson 1983). Of the many different types of parasites that exist, only a few are of concern.

Entamoeba histolytica is among the most well known human parasites that can be transmitted by fruits and vegetables. This organism is responsible for the disease known as amebic dysentery or amebiasis. The symptoms of the acute stage of the disease include abdominal cramps, flatulence, diarrhea, bloody feces, and general fatigue. The mortality rate is low (2–3%) and most patients recover fully (Ayres, Mundt, and Sandine 1980). However, the infection can

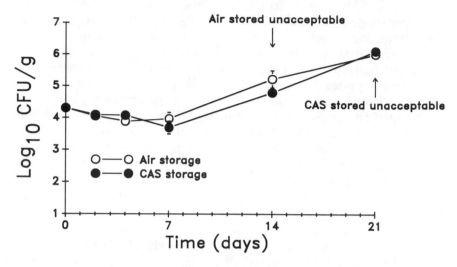

Figure 7-2   Growth of *Listeria monocytogenes* on asparagus stored at 4° C. (Adapted from Berrang, Brackett, and Beuchat 1989b.)

continue for many years in some patients and allow people to become asymptomatic carriers (Barnard and Jackson 1984). In fact, human carriers are thought to be a major source of the organism (Ayres, Mundt, and Sandine 1980). The amoeba gains access to fruits and vegetables via contamination by human or animal carrier, use of polluted water, or from insects. Although *E. histolytica* cysts are readily destroyed by drying, sunlight, and chlorination (Ayres, Mundt, and Sandine 1980), a high degree of sanitation is the best way to prevent the disease.

Giardia lamblia is a flagellated protozoan that can also contaminate fruits and vegetables and cause disease. Giardiasis is similar to amebiasis both in its symptoms and its cause. An estimated 1.5–20% of the American population are carriers of the parasite (Ayres, Mundt, and Sandine 1980) and young people are particularly susceptible (Barnard and Jackson 1984). Barnard and Jackson (1984) mention that raw fruits and vegetables, including lettuce and strawberries, have either been implicated in giardiasis outbreaks or yielded *G. lamblia* cysts. Unlike *Entamoeba*, chlorination is not very effective at destroying *Giardia* cysts.

Ascaris lumbricoides, although less common than the previous parasites, is also a potential problem in fruits and vegetables. However, the use of municipal wastewater and sludges to irrigate or fertilize fresh produce could increase the risk of infections by this organism (Jackson 1977). Unlike *Giardia* and *Entamoeba*, this organism is a roundworm and does not cause diarrheal disease. Infections usually involve development of the worm in the intestinal tract followed by migration to other organs or nerve tissue. Consequently, symptoms may be inapparent or include fever, labored breathing, and cough. Raw vegetables are one of the foods most likely to transmit the parasite (Ayres, Mundt, and Sandine 1980). The eggs of *A. lumbricoides* are very resistant to harsh conditions. They are resistant to drying and many chemical disinfectants, and have been known to survive refrigerated storage for at least 20 years. Thus, techniques normally used in minimal processing of produce will likely be ineffective at destroying the organism.

Viruses

Less is understood about viruses than other foodborne pathogens. However, it is a lack of good methodology rather than importance that has kept them from being studied more fully. Viruses cause a variety of diseases ranging from simple gastroenteritis to poliomyelitis. The majority of viruses associated with fresh produce are thought to be enteroviruses (Larkin 1981), which usually produce the former disease symptoms. However, viruses recovered from raw fruits and vegetables have also included polioviruses, coxsackieviruses, and echoviruses (Larkin 1981). Viruses share a similar cycle of infection to many other foodborne pathogens in that fecal contamination of water or food is the primary route. Once present, viruses may survive long enough to cause disease in consumers. For example, Badawy, Gerba, and Kelley (1985) found rotavirus to survive on vegetables, especially lettuce, for up to a month during refrigerated storage. Although some viruses are destroyed by chlorination (Jay 1986d), fruit and vegetable producers and processors should minimize the chance for contamination by practicing proper sanitation techniques. Additional information on *Yersinia, Campylobacter,* and *Staphylococcus* outbreaks are covered in Chapter 9.

Preventing Foodborne Disease

Because MPR fruits and vegetables are consumed essentially raw, no treatment now allowed will guarantee 100% safety. Still, the chance of microbial foodborne disease can be greatly minimized by applying common-sense practices to maintain a high degree of sanitation. For example, avoid using animal or human waste as fertilizer because these are a major source of pathogens. Similarly, water is a major source of pathogens (Jones and Watkins 1985). Therefore, only the highest quality water available should be used for irrigation and washing of produce.

Another important step in preventing foodborne disease is to be sure that employees and facilities do not contribute to the problem. Employees and handlers should be educated in basic hygienic principles and encouraged to always practice proper personal hygiene. Both facilities and equipment should be kept clean, sanitary, and well-maintained. Finally, a Hazard Analysis Critical Control Point (HACCP) program (Bryan 1988a) should be implemented to ensure that attention is being paid to the most important aspects of the operation. A HACCP program will be most effective if the product has been produced using a systems approach. This means that all aspects from production (or even before) through distribution are considered and controlled.

Summary and Conclusion

Microbiology is one of the most important effects on MPR fruits and vegetables. Microorganisms can adversely affect both sensory qualities and the safety of these products. Many techniques that are presently being used or proposed for use will dramatically change how fruits and vegetables are handled and stored. An appreciation and thorough understanding of microbial ecology can help minimize the chance that new or unexpected microbiological problems will arise. In addition, an increased emphasis on sanitation and the implementation of HACCP programs will reduce microbiological spoilage and safety problems even more.

References

Ayres, J.C., J.O. Mundt, and W.E. Sandine. 1980. Nonmicrobial foodborne illness. In *Microbiology of Foods*, pp. 531–573. San Francisco: W.H. Freeman and Company.

Badawy, A.S., C.P. Gerba, and L.M. Kelley. 1985. Survival of rotavirus SA-11 on vegetables. *Food Microbiol.* **2**:199–205.

Barnard, R.J. and G.J. Jackson. 1984. The transfer of human infections by foods. In *Giardia and Giardiasis*, S.L. Erlandsen and E.A. Mayer (eds.), pp. 365–378. New York: Plenum Press.

Ben-Yehoshua, S. 1985. Individual seal-packaging of fruit and vegetables in plastic film—a new postharvest technique. *HortScience* **20**(1):32–37.

Berrang, M.E., R.E. Brackett, and L.R. Beuchat. 1989a. Growth of *Aeromonas hydrophila* on fresh vegetables stored under a controlled atmosphere. *Appl. Environ. Microbiol.* **55**:2176–2171.

Berrang, M.E., R.E. Brackett, and L.R. Beuchat. 1989b. Growth of *Listeria monocytogenes* on fresh vegetables stored under a controlled atmosphere. *J. Food Prot.* **52**:702–705.

Berrang, M.E., R.E. Brackett, and L.R. Beuchat. 1990. Microbial, color and textural qualities of fresh asparagus, broccoli and cauliflower stored under controlled atmosphere. *J. Food Prot.* **53**:391–395.

Beuchat, L.R. and R.E. Brackett. 1990a. Growth of *Listeria monocytogenes* on carrots as influenced by shredding, chlorine treatment, modified atmosphere packaging, temperature and time. *Appl. Environ. Microbiol.* **56**:1734–1742.

Beuchat, L.R. and R.E. Brackett. 1990b. Growth of *Listeria monocytogenes* on lettuce as influenced by shredding, chlorine treatment, modified atmosphere packaging, temperature and time. *J. Food Sci.* **55**:755–758, 870.

Beuchat, L.R. and R.E. Brackett. 1991. Growth of *Listeria monocytogenes* on tomatoes as influenced by shredding, chlorine treatment, modified atmosphere packaging, temperature and time. *Appl. Environ. Microbiol.* **57**:1367–1371.

Brackett, R.E. 1987a. Microbiological consequences of minimally processed fruits and vegetables. *J. Food Quality* **10**:195–206.

Brackett, R.E. 1987b. Vegetables and related products. In *Food and Beverage Mycology*, L.R. Beuchat (ed.), pp. 129–154. New York: AVI/van Nostrand Reinhold.

Brackett, R.E. 1988a. Changes in the microflora of packaged fresh tomatoes. *J. Food Quality* **11**:89–105.

Brackett, R.E. 1988b. Presence and persistence of *Listeria monocytogenes* in food and water. *Food Technol.* **42**(4):162–164, 178.

Brackett, R.E. 1989. Changes in the microflora of packaged fresh broccoli. *J. Food Quality* **12**:169–181.

Brackett, R.E. 1990. Changes in the microflora of packaged fresh bell peppers. *J. Food Prot.* **53**:255–257, 261.

Brackett, R.E. and D.F. Splittstoesser. 1992. Fruits and vegetables. In *Compendium of Methods for the Microbiological Examination of Foods*, 3rd edit., C. Vanderzant and D.F. Splittstoesser (eds.), pp. 919–927, Washington, D.C.: American Public Health Association.

Brecht, P. 1980. Use of controlled atmospheres to retard deterioration of produce. *Food Technol.* **34**(3):45–50.

Brock, T.D., D.W. Smith, and M.T. Madigan. 1984. The microbe and its environment. In *Biology of Microorganisms*, pp. 239–270. Englewood Cliffs, NJ: Prentice-Hall.

Brocklehurst, T.F. and B.M. Lund. 1981. Properties of pseudomonads causing spoilage of vegetables stored at low temperatures. *J. Appl. Bacteriol.* **50**:259–266.

Bryan, F.L. 1988a. Hazard analysis critical control point: what the system is and what it is not. *J. Environ. Health* **50**:400–401.

Bryan, F.L. 1988b. Risks associated with vehicles of foodborne pathogens and toxins. *J. Food Prot.* **51**:498–508.

Buick, R.K. and A.P. Damoglou. 1987. The effect of vacuum packaging on the microbial spoilage and shelf-life of 'ready-to-use' sliced carrots. *J. Sci. Food Agric.* **38**:167–175.

Bulgarelli, M.A. and R.E. Brackett. 1991. The importance of fungi in vegetables. In *Handbook of Applied Mycology*, Vol. 3: *Foods and Feeds*, D.K. Arora, K.G. Mukerji, and E.H. Marth (eds.), pp. 179–199. New York: Marcel Dekker.

Callister, S.M. and W.A. Agger. 1987. Enumeration and characterization of *Aeromonas hydrophila* and *Aeromonas caviae* isolated from grocery store produce. *Appl. Environ. Microbiol.* **53**:249–253.

Chesson, A. 1980. Maceration in relation to the post-harvest handling and processing of plant material. A review. *J. Appl. Bacteriol.* **48**:1–45.

Christian, J.H.B. 1980. Reduced water activity. In *Microbial Ecology of Foods*, Vol. I, J.H. Silliker, R.P. Elliott, A.C. Baird-Parker, F.L. Bryan, J.H.B. Christian, D.S. Clark, J.C. Olson, Jr., and T.A. Roberts (eds.), pp. 70–91. New York: Academic Press.

Ciesielski, C.A., A.W. Hightower, S.K. Parsons, and C.V. Broome. 1988. Listeriosis in the United States: 1980–1982. *Arch. Intern. Med.* **148**:1416–1419.

Clark, D.S. and J. Takacs. 1980. Gases as preservatives. In *Microbial Ecology of Foods*, Vol. I, J.H. Silliker, R.P. Elliott, A.C. Baird-Parker, F.L. Bryan, J.H.B. Christian, D.S. Clark, J.C. Olson, Jr., and T.A. Roberts (eds.), pp. 170–192. New York: Academic Press.

Codner, R.C. 1971. Pectinolytic and cellulolytic enzymes in the microbial modification of plant tissues. *J. Appl. Bacteriol.* **34**:147–160.

Conner, D.E., R.E. Brackett, and L.R. Beuchat. 1986. Effect of temperature, sodium chloride, and pH on growth of *Listeria monocytogenes* in cabbage juice. *Appl. Environ. Microbiol.* **5**:59–63.

Corlett, D.A., Jr. and M.H. Brown. 1980. pH and acidity. In *Microbial Ecology of Foods*, Vol. I, J.H. Silliker, R.P. Elliott, A.C. Baird-Parker, F.L. Bryan, J.H.B. Christian, D.S. Clark, J.C. Olson, Jr., and T.A. Roberts (eds.), pp. 92–111. New York: Academic Press.

Daniels, J.A., R. Krishnamurthi, and S.S.H. Rizvi. 1985. A review of effects of carbon dioxide on microbial growth and food quality. *J. Food Prot.* **48**:532–537.

Davis, H., J.P. Taylor, J.N. Perdue, G.N. Stelma, Jr., J.M. Humphreys, Jr., R. Rowntree III, and K.D. Greene. 1988. A shigellosis outbreak traced to commercially distributed shredded lettuce. *Am. J. Epidemiol.* **128**:1312–1321.

Deák, T. 1984. Microbial-ecological principles in controlled atmosphere storage of fruits and vegetables. In *Microbial Associations and Interactions in Food*, I. Kiss, T. Deák, and K. Incze (eds.), pp. 9–22. Budapest: Hungarian Academy of Sciences.

Deák, T., E.K. Heaton, Y.C. Hung, and L.R. Beuchat. 1987. Extending the shelf-life of fresh and irradiated sweet corn by shrink-wrapping and refrigeration. *J. Food Sci.* **52**:1625–1631.

Doores, S. 1983. Organic acids. In *Antimicrobials in Foods*, A.L. Branen and P.M. Davidson (eds.), pp. 75–108. New York: Marcel Dekker.

Doyle, M.P. and V.V. Padhye. 1989. *Escherichia coli*. In *Foodborne Bacterial Pathogens*, M.P. Doyle (ed.), pp. 235–281. New York: Marcel Dekker.

Draughon, F.A., S. Chen, and J.O. Mundt. 1988. Metabiotic association of *Fusarium*, *Alternaria*, and *Rhizoctonia* with *Clostridium botulinum* in fresh tomatoes. *J. Food Sci.* **53**:120–123.

Eisenberg, W.V. and S.M. Cichowicz. 1977. Machinery mold-indicator organism in food. *Food Technol.* **31**(2):52–56.

Friend, J., S.B. Reynolds, and M.A. Aveyard. 1973. Phenylalanine ammonia lyases, chlorogenic acid and lignin in potato tuber tissue inoculated with *Phytophtora infestans*. *Physiol. Plant Pathol.* **3**:495–507.

Geeson, J.D. 1979. The fungal and bacterial flora of stored white cabbage. *J. Appl. Bacteriol.* **46**:189–193.

Goepfert, J.M. 1980. Vegetables, fruits, nuts and their products. In *Microbial Ecology of Foods*, Vol. II, J.H. Silliker, R.P. Elliott, A.C. Baird-Parker, F.L. Bryan, J.H.B. Christian, D.S. Clark, J.C. Olson, Jr., and T.A. Roberts (eds.), pp. 606–642. New York: Academic Press.

Golden, D.A., E.K. Heaton, and L.R. Beuchat. 1987. Effect of chemical treatments on microbiological, sensory and physical qualities of individually shrink-wrapped produce. *J. Food Prot.* **50**:673–680.

Gould, G.W. 1985. Present state of knowledge of A_w effects on microorganisms. In *Properties of Water in Foods in Relation to Quality and Stability*, D. Simatos and J.L. Multon (eds.), pp. 229–245. Boston: Martinus Nijhoff Publishers.

Harvey, J.M. 1978. Reduction of losses in fresh market fruits and vegetables. *Annu. Rev. Phytopathol.* **16**:321–341.

Hauschild, A.H.W. 1989. *Clostridium botulinum*. In *Foodborne Bacterial Pathogens*, M.P. Doyle (ed.), pp. 111–189. New York: Marcel Dekker.

Hayward, A.C. 1974. Latent infections by bacteria. *Annu. Rev. Phytopathol.* **12**:87–97.

Heisick, J.E., D.E. Wagner, M.L. Nierman, and J.T. Peeler. 1989. *Listeria* spp. found on fresh market product. *Appl. Environ. Microbiol.* **55**:1925–1927.

Hintlian, C.B. and J.H. Hotchkiss. 1986. The safety of modified atmosphere packaging: a review. *Food Technol.* **40**(12):70–76.

Hobbs, G. 1986. Ecology of food microorganisms. *Microb. Ecol.* **12**:15–30.

Ho, J.L., K.N. Shands, G. Friedland, P. Eckind, and D.W. Fraser. 1986. An outbreak of type 4b *Listeria monocytogenes* infection involving patients from eight Boston hospitals. *Arch. Intern. Med.* **146**:520–524.

Hurst, A. 1972. Interactions of food starter cultures and food-borne pathogens: the antagonism between *Streptococcus lactis* and sporeforming microbes. *J. Milk Food Technol.* **35**:418–423.

Jackson, G.J. 1977. Recycling of refuse into the food chain: the parasite problem. In *Proceedings of the Conference on Risk Assessment and Health Effects of Land Application of Municipal Wastewater and Sludges*, B.P. Sagik and C.A. Sorber (eds.), pp. 116–131. San Antonio, TX: Center for Applied Research and Technology.

Jackson, G.J. 1983. Examining food and drink for parasitic, saprophytic and free-living protozoa and helminths. In *CRC Handbook of Foodborne Diseases of Biological Origin*, R. Miloslav (ed.), pp. 247–255. Boca Raton: CRC.

Jay, J.M. 1986a. Foodborne gastroenteritis caused by *Salmonella* and *Escherichia*. In *Modern Food Microbiology*, pp. 489–514. New York: Van Nostrand Reinhold.

Jay, J.M. 1986b. Food preservation using irradiation. In *Modern Food Microbiology*, pp. 297–316. New York: Van Nostrand Reinhold.

Jay, J.M. 1986c. Intrinsic and extrinsic parameters of foods that affect microbial growth. In *Modern Food Microbiology*, pp. 33–60. New York: Van Nostrand Reinhold.

Jay, J.M. 1986d. Other proven and suspected food-borne pathogens. In *Modern Food Microbiology*, pp. 541–575. New York: Van Nostrand Reinhold.

Jones, F. and J. Watkins. 1985. The water cycle as a source of pathogens. *J. Appl. Bacteriol. Symp. Suppl.* **59**:27S–36S.

Junttila, J. and M. Brander. 1989. *Listeria monocytogenes* septicemia associated with consumption of salted mushrooms. *Scand. J. Infect. Dis.* **21**:339–342.

Kader, A.A. 1986. Potential applications of ionizing radiation of postharvest handling of fresh fruits and vegetables. *Food Technol.* **40**(6):117–121.

Larkin, E.P. 1981. Food contaminants-viruses. *J. Food Prot.* **44**:320–325.

Liao, C.-H. and J.M. Wells. 1986. Properties of *Cytophaga johnsonae* strains causing spoilage of fresh produce at food markets. *Appl. Environ. Microbiol.* **22**:1261–1265.

Lund, B.M. 1971. Bacterial spoilage of vegetables and certain fruits. *J. Appl. Bacteriol.* **34**:9–20.

Lund, B.M. 1981. The effect of bacteria on post-harvest quality of vegetables. In *Quality in Stored and Processed Vegetables and Fruit*, P.W. Goodenough and R.K. Arkin (eds.), pp. 287–300. New York: Academic Press.

Lund, B.M. 1982. The effect of bacteria on post-harvest quality of vegetables and fruits, with particular reference to spoilage. In *Bacteria and Plants*, Soc. Appl. Bacteriol. Symp. Ser. No. 10, M.E. Rhodes-Roberts and F.A. Skinner (eds.), pp. 133–153. New York: Academic Press.

Lund, B.M. 1983. Bacterial spoilage. In *Post-Harvest Pathology of Fruits and Vegetables*, C. Dennis (ed.), pp. 219–257. New York: Academic Press.

Lund, B.M., T.F. Brocklehurst, and G.M. Wyatt. 1981. Characterization of strains of *Clostridium puniceum* sp. nov., a pink-pigmented, pectolytic bacterium. *J. Gen. Microbiol.* **122**:17–26.

Lovett, J. 1989. *Listeria monocytogenes*. In *Foodborne Bacterial Pathogens*, M.P. Doyle (ed.), pp. 283–310. New York: Marcel Dekker.

Lynch, J.M. 1988. The terrestrial environment. In *Microorganisms in Action: Concepts and Applications in Microbial Ecology*, J.M. Lynch and J.E. Hobbie (eds.), pp. 103–131. Boston: Blackwell Scientific Publications.

Meneley, J.C. and M.E. Stanghellini. 1974. Detection of enteric bacteria within locular tissue of healthy cucumbers. *J. Food Sci.* **39**:1276–1268.

Miller, M.W. 1979. Yeasts in food spoilage: an update. *Food Technol.* **33**(1):76–80.

Morris, G.K. 1984. *Shigella*. In *Compendium of Methods for the Microbiological Examination of Foods*, 2nd edit. M.L. Speck (ed.), pp. 343–350. Washington: American Public Health Association.

Mossel, D.A.A. 1984. Half a century of microbial ecology of foods. In *Microbial Associations and Interactions in Food*, I. Kiss, T. Deák, and K. Incze (eds.), pp. 3–7. Budapest: Hungarian Academy of Sciences.

Mundt, J.O. and J.M. Norman. 1982. Metabiosis and pH of moldy fresh tomatoes. *J. Food Prot.* **45**:829–832.

Pitt, J.I. and A.D. Hocking. 1985a. Spoilage of fresh and perishable foods. In *Fungi and Food Spoilage*, pp. 365–381. New York: Academic Press.

Pitt, J.I. and A.D. Hocking. 1985b. The ecology of fungal food spoilage. In *Fungi and Food Spoilage*, pp. 5–18. New York: Academic Press.

Palumbo, S.A. 1987. Can refrigeration keep our foods safe? *Dairy Food Sanit.* **7**:56–60.

Priepke, P.E., L.S. Wei, and A.I. Nelson. 1976. Refrigerated storage of prepackaged salad vegetables. *J. Food Sci.* **41**:379–382.

Riser, E.C., J. Grabowski, and E.P. Glenn. 1984. Microbiology of hydroponically-grown lettuce. *J. Food Prot.* **47**:765–769.

Samish, Z., R. Etinger-Tulczynska, and M. Bick. 1961. Microflora within healthy tomatoes. *Appl. Microbiol.* **9**:20–25.

Schlech, W.F., P.M. Lavigne, R.A. Bortolussi, A.C. Allen, E.V. Haldane, A.J. Wort, A.W. Hightower, S.E. Johnson, S.H. King, E.S. Nicholls, and C.V. Broome. 1983. Epidemic listeriosis-evidence for transmission by food. *N. Engl. J. Med.* **308**:203–206.

Senter, S.D., J.S. Bailey, and N.A. Cox. 1987. Aerobic microflora of commercially harvested, transported and cryogenically processed collards *(Brassica olearacea)*. *J. Food Sci.* **52**:1020–1021.

Senter, S.D., N.A. Cox, J.S. Bailey, and W.R. Forbus, Jr. 1985. Microbiological changes in fresh market tomatoes during packing operations. *J. Food Sci.* **50**:254–255.

Senter, S.D., N.A. Cox, J.S. Bailey, and F.I. Meredith. 1984. Effects of harvesting, transportation, and cryogenic processing on the microflora of southern peas. *J. Food Sci.* **49**:1410–1411, 1437.

Shewfelt, R.L. 1987. Quality of minimally processed fruits and vegetables. *J. Food Quality* **10**:143–156.

Skovgaard, N. 1984. Vegetables as an ecological environment for microbes. In *Microbial Associations and Interactions in Food*, I. Kiss, T. Deák, and K. Incze (eds.), pp. 27–33. Budapest: Hungarian Academy of Sciences.

Splittstoesser, D.F. 1970. Predominant microorganisms on raw plant foods. *J. Milk Food Technol.* **33**:500–505.

Splittstoesser, D.F. 1987. Fruits and fruit products. In *Food and Beverage Mycology*, L.R. Beuchat (ed.), pp. 101–128, New York: AVI/van Nostrand Reinhold.

Splittstoesser, D.F. 1973. The microbiology of frozen vegetables. *Food Technol.* **27**(1):54–60.

Splittstoesser, D.F. and D.A. Corlett, Jr. 1980. Aerobic plate counts of frozen blanched vegetables processed in the United States. *J. Food Prot.* **43**:717–719.

Splittstoesser, D.F., M. Groll, D.L. Downing, and J. Kaminski. 1977. Viable counts versus the incidence of machinery mold *(Geotrichum)* on processed fruits and vegetables. *J. Food Prot.* **40**:402–405.

Steinbruegge, E.G., R.B. Maxey, and M.B. Liewen. 1988. Fate of *Listeria monocytogenes* on ready to serve lettuce. *J. Food Prot.* **51**:596–599.

Stelma, G.N., Jr. 1989. *Aeromonas hydrophila*. In *Foodborne Bacterial Pathogens*, M. P. Doyle (ed.), pp. 1–19. New York: Marcel Dekker.

Stolp, H. 1988. The natural environments of microorganisms. *Microbial Ecology*, pp. 114–151. New York: Cambridge University Press.

Sugiyama, H. and K.H. Yang. 1975. Growth potential of *Clostridium botulinum* in fresh mushrooms packaged in semi-permeable plastic film. *Appl. Microbiol.* **30**:964–969.

Todd, E.C.D. 1989a. Foodborne and waterborne disease in Canada—1984. Annual Summary. *J. Food Prot.* **52**:503–511.

Todd, E.C.D. 1989b. Preliminary estimates of costs of foodborne disease in the United States. *J. Food Prot.* **52**:595–601.

Van den Berg, L. and C.P. Lentz. 1966. Effect of temperature, relative humidity, and atmospheric composition on changes in quality of carrots during storage. *Food Technol.* **20**:104–107.

Webb, T.A. and J.O. Mundt. 1978. Molds on vegetables at the time of harvest. *Appl. Environ. Microbiol.* **35**:655–658.

Yackel, W.C., A.I. Nelson, L.S. Wei, and M.P. Steinberg. 1971. Effect of controlled atmosphere on growth of mold on synthetic media and fruit. *Appl. Microbiol.* **22**:513–516.

8

Nutritional Quality of Fruits and Vegetables Subject to Minimal Processes

Marie A. McCarthy and Ruth H. Matthews

Introduction

Minimally processed refrigerated (MPR) fruits and vegetables are slightly modified fruits and vegetables that retain characteristics of freshness during expanded shelf-life. Fresh fruits and vegetables, which are used to prepare MPR fruits and vegetables, supply over one-fourth of the ascorbic acid and about one-fourth of the vitamin A in the American diet (USDA 1990).

Initially, MPR fruits and vegetables are prepared by one or more unit operations—peeling, slicing, etc.—followed by a partial preservation treatment such as minimal heat, chemical, or irradiation treatment. Next, MPR fruits and vegetables may undergo some kind of controlled atmosphere (CA), modified atmosphere (MA), or vacuum packaging (VP) and are then maintained at a temperature above the freezing point during storage and transit. For safety and to retain the highest sensory and nutritional quality, MPR fruits and vegetables must be maintained at cool or refrigerator temperatures throughout their preparation, preservation, distribution, and marketing (Wiley 1989, personal communication).

Chapter 2 summarizes the use of the many available forms of MPR fruits and vegetables. A large variety of MPR fruits are used whole or peeled, prepared, pitted, halved, sliced, diced, and shredded either as a snack or as an ingredient in fruit cocktails, fruit pies, fruit salads, fruit soups, fruit cakes, fruit gelatins, fruit puddings, and fruit sauce/puree/juice. MPR whole, podded, peeled, cut, sliced, diced, and shredded vegetables can also be used as snacks and ready-to-cook vegetables or ingredients in stew, salad, soup, sandwiches, sauce and gravy, puree and juice, and pizza toppings. Those that are used as a whole product will usually have been given a minimal preservation treatment (Chapter 3).

Most reviews of fresh and MPR fruits and vegetables have been concerned with market quality as determined objectively and subjectively by color, flavor, and texture measurements. In this chapter, however, only nutritive value of fresh and MPR fruits and vegetables is addressed and these relate primarily to losses in ascorbic acid and Vitamin A. Shewfelt (1987) has emphasized that little was known concerning the nutritional consequences of minimal processing and the situation generally is very similar today. Studies on maturity and cultivar effects, transportation and marketing conditions, and preparation practices related to nutritional quality of fresh fruits and vegetables are reviewed in the following sections with an attempt to suggest similar trends for MPR fruits and vegetables. The effects of CA or MA and refrigerated storage, irradiation, and edible films on nutritional quality of fresh and MPR fruits and vegetables are also examined.

Maturity and Cultivar Effects

When fresh fruits and vegetables are selected to prepare MPR products, it is especially important to examine the raw intact produce used from the standpoint of maturity and cultivar. Maturity is an important factor to be considered when shipping produce, since immature fruits and vegetables are more firm and less susceptible to injury. As fruits and vegetables mature and are stored, ascorbic acid levels generally decrease (Augustin et al. 1978; Matthews, Crill, and Locasio-1974; Nagy 1980). However, Kader, Heintz, and Chordas (1982) and Salunkhe, Deshpande, and Do (1968) found that fully ripe peaches had higher ascorbic acid levels than immature peaches. Mature bell peppers also contained higher ascorbic acid levels than those harvested green (immature) (Matthews, Locasio, and Ozaki 1975). Vitamin A generally increases with maturity (Kader, Heintz, and Chordas 1982; Matthews, Crill, and Locasio-1974; Salunkhe, Deshpande, and Do 1968). On the other hand, investigators disagree about the levels of ascorbic acid and vitamin A in tomatoes ripened on and off the vine (Betancourt, Stevens, and Kader 1977; Matthews, Crill, and Locasio-1974; Pantos and Markakis 1973).

The effect of cultivar on MPR fruits and vegetables should also be considered. Ascorbic acid and vitamin A contents of raw fruits and vegetables (Brecht et al. 1976; Watada, Aulenbach, and Worthington 1976) differ according to cultivar and other factors. Brecht et al. (1976) reported on ascorbic acid contents of eight cultivars of ripened tomatoes (12.5 mg–22.5 mg per 100 g), whereas Watada, Aulenbach, and Worthington (1976) reported that 11 cultivars of ripe tomatoes ranged from 13.7 to 31.8 mg/100 g ascorbic acid. Vitamin A values of 10 cultivars of ripe tomatoes ranged from 667 to 955 IU/100 g, but the vitamin A value found for another cultivar, Caro Red, was very high (6,983 IU/100 g) (Watada, Aulenbach, and Worthington 1976). These values in a brief way indicate the great importance maturity and cultivar will have on nutritional levels of products subsequently treated by minimal processes with extended shelf-life.

Transportation and Marketing Conditions

Shipping is a major factor in the preservation of nutrients in raw and intact fruits and vegetables after harvest. At the present time, studies on the effects of transportation and marketing on nutritive value have not been conducted with MPR fruits and vegetables. A review of transportation and marketing studies conducted on intact fresh fruits and vegetables, however, should serve as a guide to nutrient retention in MPR fruits and vegetables.

Freshly harvested fruits and vegetables may be sold where they are grown at roadside stands or transported short or long distances before being marketed. Fruits and vegetables purchased from roadside stands are assumed to have higher nutrient values than those obtained from supermarkets. Ascorbic acid and beta-carotene contents of tomatoes from roadside stands were found in studies by Bushway et al. (1989) and Bushway, Yang, and Yamani (1986) to be significantly higher than levels of the same nutrients in supermarket

Table 8-1
Ascorbic Acid and Beta-Carotene Content of Tomatoes from Roadside Stand and Supermarket 100 gm, edible portion[a]

Nutrients and Units	Tomatoes		
	Roadside Stand	Supermarket	Contrast[b]
Ascorbic acid	mg	13.7	11.5	S
Beta-carotene	μg	623.2	241.0	S

[a] Adapted from Bushway, Yang, and Yamani 1986; Bushway et al. 1989.
[b] S, Significant at the .05% level.

tomatoes (Table 8-1). As the authors state, however, tomato samples in the ascorbic acid study (Bushway et al. 1989) were harvested the night before or the same day as purchased, and in the carotenoid study the same day as harvested (Bushway, Yang, and Yamani 1986). Supermarket tomato samples in both studies were harvested at least 7–10 whole days prior to purchase.

For optimum quality, fruits and vegetables are canned in the same local area as they are harvested. Snap beans for canning may be shipped overnight in open trucks with mesh sides to circulate air (Massey 1983). Massey analyzed samples of the 1982 crop of Bush Blue Lake snap beans for ascorbic acid and vitamin A content. Snap beans from New York were harvested a short time before analyses, and the other samples, 9–12 h earlier. The ascorbic acid value of snap beans from the nearby area (10 mg/100 g) was slightly higher than values for beans shipped from out of state (8–9 mg/100 g). Vitamin A values for snap beans from New York (516 IU/100 g) and New Jersey (527 IU/100 g) were similar and higher than for snap beans grown in Virginia (394 IU/100 g).

In another study, Klein and Perry (1982) found no effect of shipping on the ascorbic acid values of five vegetables (cabbage, carrots, celery, corn, and tomatoes). Although the vegetables were obtained wholesale in six different cities, they often originated in the same growing area. Ascorbic acid variability, however, could not be attributed to differences in either transportation time or growing season.

It is often assumed that the vitamin content of fruits and vegetables remains constant during marketing. Some studies that have examined the effect of postharvest handling on the ascorbic acid content of fruits and vegetables include those of Hudson, Butter-

Table 8-2
Ascorbic Acid Content of Green Peppers at Three Marketing Levels 100 gm, Edible Portion[a]

Marketing Levels	Ascorbic Acid	
	Mean Value (mg/100 g)	Range (mg/100 g)
Wholesale	119	70–165
Retail	118	60–197
Stored	114	35–162

[a]Adapted from Hudson, Butterfield, and Lachance 1985.

field, and Lachance (1985a), Hudson, Mazur, and Lachance (1985b), Hudson, Cappellini, and Lachance (1986), and Hudson and Lachance (1986).

Hudson, Butterfield, and Lachance (1985a) analyzed ascorbic acid in sweet peppers from wholesale and retail markets and simulated consumer storage and found little variation in the average ascorbic content during the three marketing stages (see Table 8-2). Individual retail samples had the largest range of ascorbic acid values.

Hudson, Mazur, and Lachance (1985b) found in a study of strawberries grown in California and Florida that ascorbic acid values were about 65 mg/100 g for wholesale, retail, and simulated consumer storage. Freshly harvested New Jersey grown strawberries stored at 5.5°C, however, decreased from 62 mg to 53 mg/100 g after 4 days and to 33 mg/100 g after 7 days.

As seen in the above review, transportation and marketing conditions can affect the ascorbic acid and vitamin A content of intact fresh fruits and vegetables. The same trends shown in intact fresh fruits and vegetables should also be evident in MPR fruits and vegetables. It is expected, however, that ascorbic acid and vitamin A values of MPR fruits and vegetables would be somewhat lower than the values of intact fresh fruits and vegetables.

Initial Preparation

According to Watada, Abe, and Yamauchi (1990), top quality fresh fruits and vegetables should be selected without bruises, skin breaks, injuries, and other mechanical damages. Any break in plant tissue can cause changes in physiological activities or infection by pathogens, followed by deterioration. In the preparation of MPR fruits and vegetables, trimming, peeling, cutting, slicing, and other physical actions can also cause injury and damage to the tissues (see Chapter 2). Furthermore, MPR fruits and vegetables subjected to various preservation hurdles can undergo injury and damage (see Chapter 3).

Tissue is bruised less when cut with a sharp knife than with a dull knife. Less bruising preserves more quality and nutritive value. Ohta and Sugawara (1987) found that the quality of lettuce stored at 5°C was more stable if shredding was done by slicing with a sharp knife. For 2 h, raw cabbage shredded by either a Hobart machine or a slaw cutter retains about 85% of its ascorbic acid (Wood et al. 1946).

Quantitative nutrient data are needed when a mild heat preservation treatment is applied to MPR fruits and vegetables. Information on the ascorbic acid and vitamin A retention of fresh fruits and vegetables cooked in a minimum amount of water, however, is available (USDA 1984) and should serve as a good indicator of nutrient retention in MPR fruits and vegetables. Heat-treated tomatoes, which are acid in pH, retain almost all of their ascorbic acid, whereas dark green leafy vegetables retain only 60% of their ascorbic acid. Potatoes and sweetpotatoes, root/bulb/high starch content vegetables, other vegetables, and fruits have an average ascorbic acid retention of about 75%. On the other hand, heat-treated fruits and vegetables retain almost all of their vitamin A.

CA, MA, and Refrigerated Storage

Data that determine the effects of CA, MA, and refrigerated storage on the nutritive value of MPR fruits and vegetables are not, as yet, available. Nutrient data obtained from CA, MA, and refrigerated storage studies on intact fruits and vegetables, however, can be used to estimate the nutrient retention of MPR fruits and vegetables.

Controlled and Modified Atmosphere Storage

For over 50 years, CA or MA storage has been used to extend the shelf-life of many intact fruits including apples, bananas, kiwifruit, and strawberries (Lewis and Shibamoto 1986). CA and MA storage require lowering the O_2 level, adjusting CO_2 level, and controlling the ethylene level. The CA and MA storage can occur in a completely sealed warehouse, in a large shipping container, or in individual packages (Labuza and Breene 1989). The smaller packaging units are usually designated as modified atmosphere packaging (MAP). Controlled atmosphere packaging (CAP) would be rarely used in MPR foods; however, a freshly pressed orange juice deaerated and then N_2 flushed in a hermatically sealed glass bottle might qualify as CAP.

With CA storage, the gas atmosphere must be adjusted constantly to control changes in respiration of the food or growth of microorganisms. In the more prevalent MA storage, a predetermined atmosphere is used in the package, but this atmosphere changes with respiration of the food, gas permeability of packaging material, and growth of microorganisms. When VP is used, most of the air is removed, and CO_2 from respiration of the food or growth of microorganisms increases (Stiles 1989), which may cause anaerobiosis in the package.

As shown by Perdue (1989), fruits and vegetables lend themselves well to MAP. Individual shrinkwrapping slows respiration, extends the shelf-life, and retains moisture. Several different kinds of MA systems, such as atmosphere-controlled warehouses, sea vans, railroad cars, and trailer trucks, are used for intact apples and pears. Nitrogen-flushed packaging is used for the shipment of boxed lettuce, cleaned and ready for use, to hotels, restaurants, and institution markets, whereas bulk shredded and chopped lettuce, generally VP packed, is shipped to fast-food restaurants for salads.

CA is preferred over MA when specified levels of O_2 and CO_2 must be precisely controlled (Zagory and Kader 1989). The effects of CA storage on the ascorbic acid and vitamin A contents of fruits and vegetables have been studied by Burgheimer et al. (1967), Delaporte (1971), Kurki (1979), Wang (1983), and Weichmann (1983). Ascorbic acid levels of fruits and vegetables stored under CA vary with atmosphere, commodity, and storage temperature (Watada 1987). Vitamin A values in fruits and vegetables can be retained when CA conditions maintain low O_2 with high relative humidity (Zagory and Kader 1989).

An atmosphere of 5–6% CO_2 and 2–3% O_2 is generally used in the United States for CA apple storage (Watada 1991, personal communication). In a study conducted in France by Delaporte (1971), however, one cultivar of apples, Reinett du Mans, was stored in a CA of 3% O_2 and 97% N_2 at 15°C up to 85 days. As expected, as-

Table 8-3
Ascorbic Acid and Vitamin A Content of Stored Leeks 100 g, Edible Portion[a]

Storage Conditions	Ascorbic Acid Content (mg/100 g)	Vitamin A Content (IU/100 g)
Relative humidity over 95%		
Temperature = 0° C		
Controlled atmosphere[b]:		
0 month	37.2	2525
4 months	20.2	1350
Cold storage[c]:		
0 months	37.2	2525
4 months	24.1	62

[a]Adapted from Kurki 1979.
[b]$O_2 = 1\%$, $CO_2 = 10\%$.
[c]Normal air.

corbic acid content decreased with time. The values for this cultivar (14.9–24.1 mg/100 g) compare favorably with ascorbic acid values for apples (3–20 mg/100 g) reported in a French food composition table (Randoin et al. 1961).

Wang (1983) studied the effect of high-CO_2 (low O_2) atmospheres on ascorbic acid content of Chinese cabbage and found that ascorbic acid levels were not affected under 10 or 20% CO_2 for 5–10 days. Ascorbic acid losses were accelerated under higher levels of 30%–40% CO_2.

In another study on vitamin content in vegetables, Kurki (1979) studied the effects of CA storage and cold air storage on ascorbic acid and vitamin A content of the Tropita cultivar of leeks grown in Finland (Table 8-3). After 4 months, ascorbic acid content of leeks (20.2–24.1 mg/100 g) stored under CA and in cold storage showed little difference. The vitamin A values for leeks stored under CA (1350 IU/100 g) were higher than when held in cold storage (62 IU/100 g) as reported by Kurki (1979).

In CA-stored fruits and vegetables, minerals are concentrated (Zagory and Kader 1989) because moisture is lost. Perring and Pearson (1987) reported a redistribution of calcium in CA-stored apples and found also that both CA-stored and air-stored apples were similar. Changes in the mineral content of cauliflower have been reviewed by Weichmann (1986); real losses in mineral content were minimal.

Refrigerated Storage

As discussed by Klein (1987), most fresh fruits and vegetables are stored just above the freezing point to retard respiration and transpiration. Both temperature and humidity must be carefully controlled to prevent wilting and maintain crispness. Today, supermarkets often use misters and sprinklers in produce cases to prevent wilting. After 72 h of storage in a refrigerated produce display cabinet, misted broccoli retains 75% of its ascorbic acid compared with 55% ascorbic acid retention for unmisted broccoli (Barth et al. 1990).

Fresh intact fruits and vegetables generally retain ascorbic acid when refrigerated for a short time. For example, in the few studies reported by Nagy (1980), ascorbic acid is retained well in refrigerated fresh processed single-strength and reconstituted citrus juices for about 4 weeks; only a minimal amount of ascorbic acid is lost when juices are stored in open containers (glass, plastic, or cans). Leafy vegetables, such as kale, retained 60% of their ascorbic acid when stored at 0°C for up to 3 weeks (Ezell and Wilcox 1959). Fresh lima beans refrigerated for 48 h retained 100% ascorbic acid when stored in the pod and only 85% ascorbic acid when shelled (Eheart et al. 1946).

Irradiation

Regulations on the use of ionizing radiation for the treatment of food were published in the Federal Register of May 2, 1990 (FDA 1990). In the context of this book irradiation is considered a preservation method for MPR fruits and vegetables. Fresh fruits and vegetables may be irradiated to inhibit or delay maturation or senescence and to control pest infestation at dosages up to 1 kiloGray (kGy) = 100 kilorad (krad) (FDA 1990).

Papayas may be irradiated at 1.0 kGy; nectarines, peaches, and plums (stone fruits) at 0.3 kGy; and oranges and lemons at 0.50–0.75 kGy (Moy and Nagai 1985). Sprouting potatoes and other root vegetables, such as onions and garlic, can be prevented for at least 6 months by dosages of 0.02–0.15 kGy (Moy 1989). Ripening of papayas, mangoes, and bananas may be delayed with doses of 0.12–0.75 kGy (Moy 1989).

Although many irradiation studies with fruits and vegetables have been concerned with the extension of shelf-life, some studies have been conducted on the effects of irradiation on nutritive value of fruits and vegetables. Maxie, Sommer, and Brown (1964), Beyers, Thomas, and VanTonder (1979), Lu et al. (1986), and Tajima, Branco, and Todoriki (1988) studied levels higher than 1 kGy. Others used lower levels (Ghods et al. 1976; Salem 1974; Schwimmer, Weston, and Makower 1958). Recently, fruit and vegetable studies, such as Lodge, Hogg, and Fletcher (1985), Curzio, Croci, and Ceci (1986), Lu et al. (1986), and Tajima, Hossain, and Todoriki (1988), have been primarily concerned with the effect of irradiation doses of 1.0 kGy or less on ascorbic acid and vitamin A values.

Beyers, Thomas, and VanTonder (1979) irradiated four cultivars of mangoes and two cultivars of papayas at 0.75 kGy and found little difference between the ascorbic acid and vitamin A values of control and irradiated fruits. Lu et al. (1986) irradiated two cultivars of sweetpotatoes, Jewel and Georgia Jet, with several irradiation doses ranging from 0.1 kGy to 2.0 kGy and found that vitamin A was retained throughout the radiation treatment. Ascorbic acid was retained at 0.1 and 0.5 kGy levels, and only minimal losses (5–10%) were seen at 0.8–2.0 kGy. Sensory evaluation tests, however, showed that baked sweetpotatoes were unacceptable at irradiation levels of 0.5 kGy and above.

Edible Films

Although information on the nutrient retention of MPR fruits and vegetables preserved by edible coatings is not yet available, this area is very promising. Edible coatings can act as barriers to prevent loss of flavor, texture, and nutrients (Krochta et al. 1988).

A casein-based film—with a small amount of ascorbic acid added for increased protection against browning—kept small pieces of sliced and peeled apples fresh for 6 days while undipped apple pieces shriveled and turned brown in a few hours (Pavlath 1990, personal communication; USDA 1989). Avocados protected by edible films remained fresh for 6 days without blackening (Pavlath 1990, personal communication). With the trend toward buying foods that are ready to use and easily stored, edible coatings should prove a boon to consumers, restaurants, and others in the food industry who wish to purchase presliced and packaged products (USDA 1989).

Another edible film made of vegetable oil, cellulose, and an emulsifier can act as an antioxidant atmospheric barrier. In a laboratory experiment with mature green tomatoes, only 40% of the tomatoes treated with the film ripened after 14 days of storage compared with

100% ripening for untreated tomatoes. Results with oranges and carambolas were also excellent. This emulsified edible film should prove to be an invaluable aid to the fresh and minimally processed fruit and vegetable industry in preventing spoilage (Sanchez 1990).

Summary

Almost all of the studies published on MPR fruits and vegetables have been market quality studies. Except for irradiation studies, data on the nutrient content and nutrient retention of MPR fruits and vegetables are generally sparse. Studies that are concerned with the effect of maturity and cultivar, transportation and marketing conditions, preparation operations, preservation methods, CA and MA storage and packaging, refrigerated storage, and edible films on the nutritive value and the nutrient retention of MPR fruits and vegetables are now needed.

Acknowledgments

The authors wish to thank Avril Gonsalves and Sherri Johnson for their technical assistance.

References

Augustin, J., S.R. Johnson, C. Teitzel, R.B. Toma, R.L. Shaw, R.H. True, J.J. Hogan, and R.M. Deutsch 1979. Vitamin composition of freshly harvested and stored potatoes. *J. Food Sci.* **43**:1566–1570.

Barth, M.M., A.K. Perry, S.J. Schmidt, and B.P. Klein 1990. Misting effects on ascorbic acid retention in broccoli during cabinet display. *J. Food Sci.* **55**:1187–1188, 1191.

Betancourt, L.A., M.A. Stevens, and A.A. Kader 1977. Accumulation and loss of sugars and reduced ascorbic acid in attached and detached tomato fruits. *J. Am. Soc. Horticult. Sci.* **102**:721–723.

Beyers, M., A.C. Thomas, and A.J. VanTonder 1979. Gamma irradiation of subtropical fruits. 1. Compositional tables of mango, papaya, strawberry, and litchi fruits at the edible-ripe stage. *J. Agric. Food Chem.* **27**:37–42.

Brecht, P.E., L. Keng, C.A. Bisogni, and Munger, H.M. 1976. Effect of fruit portion, stage of ripeness and growth habit on chemical composition of fresh tomatoes. *J. Food Sci.* **41**:945–948.

Burgheimer, F., J.N. McGill, A.I. Nelson, and M.P. Steinberg. 1967. Chemical changes in spinach stored in air and controlled atmosphere. *Food Technol.* **21**:109–111.

Bushway, R.J., A. Yang, and A.M. Yamani. 1986. Comparison of alpha- and beta-carotene content of supermarket versus roadside stand produce. *J. Food Quality* **9**:437–443.

Bushway, R.J., P.R. Helper, J. King, B. Perkins, and M. Krishnan. 1989. Comparison of ascorbic acid content of supermarket versus roadside stand produce. *J. Food Quality* **12**:99–105.

Curzio, O.A., C.A. Croci, and L.N. Ceci 1986. The effects of radiation and extended storage on the chemical quality of garlic bulbs. *Food Chem.* **21**:153–159.

Delaporte, N. 1971. [Effect of oxygen content on the ascorbic acid amount of apples during storage-controlled atmosphere]. 1971. *Lebens.-Wiss. Technol.* **4**:106–112.

Eheart, J.F., R.C. Moore, M. Speirs, F.F. Cowart, H.L. Cochran, O.A. Sheets, L. McWhirter, M. Gieger, J.L. Bowers, P.H. Heinze, F.R. Hayden, J.H. Mitchell, and R.L. Carolus 1946. Vitamin studies on lima beans. *Southern Coop. Series Bull.* **5**, 24 pp.

Ezell, B.D. and M.S. Wilcox 1959. Loss of vitamin C in fresh vegetables as related to wilting and temperature. *J. Agric. Food Chem.* **7**:507–509.

FDA. 1990. 21 CFR Part 179. Irradiation in the production, processing, and handling of foods: Final Rule. *Fed. Reg.* **55**:18538–18544.

Ghods, F., F. Didevar, E. Hamidi, and B. Malekghassemi 1976. The influence of gamma-irradiation on potatoes and onions. *Lebensmittel Ernahrung* **29**:81–84.

Hudson, D.E. and P.A. Lachance 1986. Ascorbic acid and riboflavin content of asparagus during marketing. *J. Food Quality* **9**:217–224.

Hudson, D.E., J.E. Butterfield, and P.A. Lachance 1985a. Ascorbic acid, riboflavin, and thiamine content of sweet peppers during marketing. *HortScience* **20**:129–130.

Hudson, D.E., M.M. Mazur, and P.A. Lachance 1985b. Ascorbic acid, riboflavin, and thiamine content of strawberries during postharvest handling. *HortScience* **20**:71–73.

Hudson, D.E., M. Cappellini, and P.A. Lachance 1986. Ascorbic acid content of broccoli during marketing. *J. Food Quality* **9**:31–37.

Kader, A.A., C.M. Heintz, and A. Chordas 1982. Postharvest quality of fresh and canned clingstone peaches as influenced by genotypes and maturity at harvest. *J. Am. Soc. Horticult. Sci.* **107**:947–951.

Klein, B.P. 1987. Nutritional consequences of minimal processing of fruits and vegetables. *J. Food Quality* **10**:179–183.

Klein, B.P. and A.K. Perry. 1982. Ascorbic acid and vitamin A activity in selected vegetables from different geographical areas of the United States. *J. Food Sci.* **47**:941–945, 948.

Krochta, J.M., J.S. Hudson, W.M. Camirand, and A.E. Pavlath. 1988. Edible films for lightly-processed fruits and vegetables. Paper No. 88-6523 read at 1988 International Winter Meeting of the American Society of Agricultural Engineers, 13–16 December, at Hyatt Regency, Chicago, IL.

Kurki, L. 1979. Leek quality changes in CA-storage. *Acta Horticult.* **93**:85–89.

Labuza, T.P. and W.M. Breene. 1989. Applications of "active packaging" for improvement of shelf-life and nutritional quality of fresh and extended shelf-life foods. *J. Food Process. Preserv.* **13**:1–69.

Lewis, D.C. and T. Shibamoto. 1986. Shelf life of fruits. In *Handbook of Food and Beverage Stability*, G. Charalmbous (ed.), pp. 353–389. Orlando: Academic Press.

Lodge, N., M.G. Hogg, and G.C. Fletcher. 1985. Gamma-irradiation of frozen kiwifruit pulp. *J. Food Sci.* **50**:1224–1226.

Lu, J.Y., S. White, P. Yakubu, and P.A. Loretan. 1986. Effects of gamma radiation on nutritive and sensory qualities of sweet potato storage roots. *J. Food Quality* **9**:425–435.

Massey, L.M., Jr. 1983. Nutritive quality of long-distance shipped green beans for processing. *J. Food Sci.* **48**:1564–1565.

Matthews, R.F., P. Crill, and S.J. Locasio. 1974. Beta-carotene and ascorbic acid contents of tomatoes as affected by maturity. *Proc. Florida State Horticult. Soc.* **87**:214–216.

Matthews, R.F., S.J. Locasio, and H.T. Ozaki. 1975. Ascorbic acid and carotene contents of peppers. *Proc. Florida State Horticult. Soc.* **88**:263–265.

Maxie, E.C., N.F. Sommer, and D.S. Brown. 1964. Radiation Technology in Conjunction with Postharvest Procedures as a Means of Extending the Shelf Life of Fruits and Vegetables. Report of Feb. 1, 1963-Jan. 30, 1964. Prepared for the Division of Isotope Development, U.S. Atomic Energy Comm. by Dept. of Pomology, U. California, Davis, with the cooperation of Dept. of Vegetable Crops, Davis, and Plant Biochemistry, Riverside, 166 pp.

Moy, J.H. 1989. Irradiation processing of fruits and vegetables. Status and prospects. In *Quality Factors of Fruits and Vegetables*, J.J. Jen (ed.), pp. 329–336. Chemistry and Technology, ACS Symposium Series 405, Washington, DC: American Chemical Society.

Moy, J.H. and N.Y. Nagai. 1985. Quality of fresh fruits irradiated at disinfestation doses. In *Radiation Disinfestation of Food and Agricultural Products*. Honolulu, HI: Hawaii Inst. Trop. Agric. Human Resources, U. Hawaii, 428 pp.

Nagy, S. 1980. Vitamin C content of citrus fruit and their products: a review. *J. Agric. Food Chem.* **28**:8–18.

Ohta, H. and W. Sugawara. 1987. Influence of processing and storage conditions on quality stability of shredded lettuce. *Nippon Shokuhin Kogyo Gakkaishi* **34**:432–438.

Pantos, C.E. and P. Markakis. 1973. Ascorbic acid content of artificially ripened tomatoes. *J. Food Sci.* **38**:550.

Perdue, R.R. 1989. MAP: shoppers wooed with fresh ideas. *Can. Packag.* **42**:26–28,31.

Perring, M.A. and K. Pearson. 1987. Redistribution of minerals in apple fruit during storage: the effect of storage atmosphere on calcium concentration. *J. Sci. Food Agric.* **40**:37–42.

Randoin, L., P. LeGallic, Y. Dupuis, and A. Bernardin, in collaboration with Duchene, G., and P. Brun. 1961. *Tables de Composition des Aliments*. Third Edition. Institut Scientifique d'Higiene Alimentaire, Centre National de la Recherche Scientifique. J. Lanore Editeurs, Paris, France.

Salem, S.A. 1974. Effect of gamma irradiation on the storage of onions used in the dehydration industry. *J. Sci. Food Agric.* **25**:257–262.

Salunkhe, D.K., P.B. Deshpande, and J.Y. Do. 1968. Effects of maturity and storage on physical and biochemical changes in peach and apricot fruits. *J. Horticult. Sci.* **43**:235–242.

Sanchez, D. 1990. Keep it under an edible coat. *Agric. Res.* **38**:4–5.

Schwimmer, S., W.J. Weston, and R.U. Makower. 1958. Biochemical effects of gamma radiation on potato tubers. *Arch. Biochem. Biohpys.* **75**:425–434.

Shewfelt, R.L. 1987. Quality of minimally processed fruits and vegetables. *J. Food Quality* **10**:143–156.

Stiles, M.E. 1989. Controlled atmosphere storage: microbiology. In *Proceedings of the International Conference on Microwavable Foods.* Atlanta, GA: Micro-Ready Foods.

Tajima, M., L.R. Branco, and S. Todoriki. 1988. Comparative effect of gamma irradiation and heat treatment on vitamin C content of grapefruit. *Food Irradiat.* **23**:62–65.

Tajima, M., M.M. Hossain, and S. Todoriki. 1988. Effect of low dose irradiation on the free amino acid, glucose, and ascorbic acid contents of potato. *Food Irradiat.* **23**:1–3.

USDA. 1984. Provisional Table on Percent Retention of Nutrients in Food Preparation. SI. Rev., 2 pp.

USDA. 1989. New Edible Coatings May Protect Fresh Food. USDA News Release. July 17, 1989.

USDA. 1990. Primary Data Set, Weighted Grams Consumed in Nationwide Food Consumption Survey (1987–1988). U.S. Dept. of Agriculture, Human Nutrition Information Service, Hyattsville, MD (Unpublished data).

Wang, C.Y. 1983. Postharvest responses of Chinese cabbage to high CO_2 treatment or low O_2 storage. *J. Am. Soc. Horticult. Sci.* **108**:125–129.

Watada, A.E. 1987. (Chapter 22. Vitamins. In Postharvest Physiology of Vegetables, Weichmann, J. ed. pp. 435–468. New York, Marcel Dekker.

Watada, A.E., K. Abe, and N. Yamauchi. 1990. Physiological activities of partially processed fruits and vegetables. *Food Technol.* **44**(5):116, 118, 120–122.

Watada, A.E., B.B. Aulenbach, and J.T. Worthington. 1976. Vitamins A and C in ripe tomatoes as affected by stage of ripeness at harvest and by supplementary ethylene. *J. Food Sci.* **41**:856–858.

Weichmann, J. 1983. CO_2 partial pressure in the storage atmosphere and vitamin C content of brussels sprouts. *Gartenbauwissenschaft* **48**:13–16.

Weichmann, J. 1986. The effect of controlled-atmosphere storage on the sensory and nutritional quality of fruits and vegetables. In *Horticult. Rev.* **8**:101–127.

Wood, M.A., A.R. Collings, V. Stodola, A.M. Burgoin, and F. Fenton. 1946. Effect of large-scale food preparation on vitamin retention: cabbage. *J. Am. Dietetic Assoc.* **22**:677–682.

Zagory, D. and A.A. Kader. 1989. Chapter 4. Quality maintenance in fresh fruits and vegetables by controlled atmospheres. In *Quality Factors of Fruits and Vegetables*, Chemistry and J.J. Jen (ed.), pp. 174–187. Technology, ACS Symposium Series 405, Washington, DC: American Chemical Society.

9

Regulatory Issues Associated with Minimally Processed Refrigerated Foods

D.M. Dignan

Introduction

MPR foods are foods with added value and convenience. They may have been peeled, sliced, diced, or chopped; they may be blanched, pasteurized, or partially cooked. They are stored and marketed under refrigeration in combination with other treatments such as modified atmosphere or vacuum packaging for shelf-life extension. In addition to many traditional foods, such as milk and orange juice which are minimally processed and refrigerated, other examples of MPR foods include cooked pasta and vegetable salads; uncooked pasta; packaged sandwiches; chopped or shredded lettuce or cabbage; various forms of prepeeled fresh potatoes; baked goods; fresh fish, meat, or poultry; and partially prepared or cooked entrees or complete meals.

Brody (1987) has noted that controlled atmosphere (CA) technology to extend shelf-life has been diminishing as other processes and technologies such as modified atmosphere (MA), vacuum, gas scavengers, and synergistic thermal pasteurization are enlisted to preserve quality and freshness over ever-extending periods of shelf-life. The careful and systematic research conducted by universities, agricultural experiment stations, and supply and user trade associations in the 1950s, 1960s, and early 1970s ensured new but successful systems of fresh food distribution. As a result, the shelf-lives of billions of pounds of apples, pears, tomatoes, lettuce, and beef, pork, and chicken were extended annually. Developments in vacuum shrink skin packaging for various foods, for containers, and for pallet packs have also done their part to ensure a more diversified and better quality food supply. Primarily, these developments have been for industrial and institutional usage. Although little is known about the microbiological safety of this technology, experience has demonstrated that CA/MA/vacuum packaging can reliably deliver safe products that have a like-fresh quality or at least are close facsimiles. These early experiences and successes implied that the principles of reduced oxygen/high carbon dioxide packaging might also be applicable to consumer foods and food packaging systems.

Circumstances in the 1980s led to the fulfillment of that expectation. Retort pouches and aseptic packaging technologies fell short of premarket projections and forecasts. Furthermore, external business forces influenced many packaging supply concerns to diversify, expand product range, and generate rapid profit and growth. Thus, the initial push for MRP foods came not from a consumer demand for "fresh," but from a group of technology suppliers and manufacturers who saw a market potential. This impetus was accelerated further when it became obvious that discretionary income was rising, fewer meals were being prepared in the home, and that "fresh" was being perceived as better than canned or frozen, or as "less processed." According to Brody (1987) a possible drawback of this market identification is that some suppliers and manufacturers or processors may be less than fully informed. He states that the safety issues and regulatory concerns have not been clearly identified or fully clarified to satisfy concerns of industry and public health officials about consumer protection.

Generally, food law addresses itself to issues of public health and economic protection. The public health concerns stemming from minimally processed refrigerated (MPR) foods are essentially microbiological and chemical in nature. The safeguard against economic deception in food has always been truthful labeling. This chapter briefly examines the microbiological hazards associated with the production and distribution of MPR foods and touches on the question of food additives, particularly those indirect additives that might migrate from recent advances in packaging technology that help make MPR foods attractive choices.

With these thoughts in mind, it is fairly clear that regulatory issues associated with MPR foods can cover a wide spectrum of interests and range in consideration from what constitutes good manufacturing practice for MPR foods to shelf-life and the accuracy of time–temperature indicators. It is also clear that the regulatory issues of MPR foods must be examined in a broader context. Thus information in this chapter necessarily includes a population of refrigerated foods more extensive than just fruits and vegetables; however, many of the concepts and concerns put forth apply to MPR fruit and vegetable products although sometimes other food products are used as examples.

Minimally Processed Refrigerated Fruits and Vegetables

Huxsoll and Bolin (1989) have stated that "minimally processed fruits and vegetables are products that have attributes of convenience and fresh-like quality." They indicate that forms vary widely, depending on the nature of the unprocessed commodity and how it is normally consumed. MRP fruits and vegetables are defined in Chapter 1. Rolle and Chism (1987) and Shewfelt (1987) have pointed out that minimal processing often increases product perishability rather than making it more stable. As an example, consider that trimmed heads of iceberg lettuce have a shelf-life of 40 days stored at 1.7° C (Singh, Yang, and Salunkhe 1972), whereas chopped or shredded lettuce bagged for use in green salads in restaurants or institutional feeding situations has a shelf-life of only 26 days at the same temperature (Bolin et al. 1977).

Convenience without the necessary shelf-life, when centralized processing is coupled to widespread distribution, is of little or no use. Therefore, to combat the perishability, a preservation procedure is applied. This consists primarily of two parts: preservation and packaging.

Preservation (See Chapter 4)

The preservation processing step may consist of one or more of the following available technologies or procedures. They are low-temperature refrigerated storage, which is beneficial in many ways and is, in most cases, the most effective preservative treatment applied to minimally processed foods. Chemical preservatives may alleviate undesirable changes in like-fresh appearance or quality and stave off the onset of spoilage due to molds or yeasts. Mild heat pasteurization treatments or partial cooking may be useful in reducing enzymatic deterioration and microbial load. Modification of pH and reduction of water activity are often used in combination with pasteurization to extend shelf-life; however, these treatments, in order to be effective alone, can also change the commodity to such an extent that the like-fresh characteristics and quality are no longer discernible.

Irradiation is preservation technology that demonstrates potential for extending shelf-life and lessening perishability; however, the irradiation dosages required to bring about reduction in microbial load can result in softened tissue which is more easily invaded by destructive microbial agents.

CA, MA, vacuum packaging, and hypobaric storage are other technologies that have been used to extend the shelf-life and quality of foods. In CA and MA storage and packaging, the levels of O_2 and CO_2 are adjusted to either inhibit or retard the reaction rates for such basic biochemical activities as respiration, senescence, and tissue softening. For CA or MA to be effective, each commodity and packaging or storage system must be studied separately to determine optimum gas levels.

Interestingly, an "old" process is being considered as suitable for use with new foods. This is biocontrol, based on the "Wisconsin process" developed in the late 1970s to prevent botulinal toxin formation in temperature-abused meat products (Tanaka et al. 1985). As applied to MPR foods, products would be inoculated with lactic acid-producing organisms which would grow and change product pH in case of refrigeration failure or other temperature abuse. While not fully developed for certain foods and technologies, contained biocontrol may become a powerful product development and product safety tool.

Ultimately, the recommended preservation procedure may be a combination of two or more of the above treatments. The multiple treatment approach has been variously referred to as the "hurdle" approach or "multiple barrier" approach. The preferred end result is to use treatments that are either additive or synergistic in delaying the onset of spoilage that results from either enzymatic degradation or microbiological activity.

A significant point about MPR foods is that they are not "commercially sterile." Because refrigeration is part of the preservation process, the foods are sensitive to temperature and consumer abuse and are limited in shelf-life. The potential for consumers to mishandle the products is considerable, especially if the products are perceived by consumers as shelf-stable. Optimal storage temperatures for minimally processed food range between 0° and 4° C with an upper maximum limit near 7° C.

Refrigeration, which is relied on to ensure that MPR foods safely achieve their intended shelf-life, unfortunately is the component, barrier, or part of the preservation scheme that is most difficult to control. Manufacturers of such foods must understand that, at some point during manufacture, storage, distribution, display, or consumer handling, proper refrigeration probably will not be maintained. The reasons for such occurrences include shipping or receiving delays, mechanical problems with refrigeration equipment, and improper loading or stocking in display cases (Davidson 1987).

Normally, foods that rely exclusively on refrigeration to extend their shelf-life soon spoil under temperature abuse; spoilage is usually sufficient to deter consumption. However, when other treatments such as vacuum packaging or modified atmosphere are used for overall preservation and shelf-life extension, this environment, during conditions of temperature abuse, may allow the selective development of pathogens or their toxins without the accompanying traditional organoleptic signs of spoilage.

Packaging (See Chapter 4)

Food packaging for MPR foods, particularly retail sized packages, is dominated by innovation in plastics packaging and has undergone remarkable changes in recent years. New packaging materials and techniques have produced seemingly endless possibilities for manufacturing, packaging, and marketing, and have created, as a result, a wider variety of foods than ever before. Inroads by plastics into arenas traditionally held by steel, aluminum, glass, and paperboard are visible in all segments of the food industry. Cabes (1985) projected that by 1991, plastics would account for 26.5% of all containers in the marketplace. Glass and metal combined were predicted to constitute 27.9% of food containers in 1991, down from 52.4% in 1981.

Consumers, as part of the force driving this switch to plastics, are demanding higher quality, fresher tasting, more convenient foods. In response to this demand, packaging technologists have developed a whole range of plastic containers that can go from the retail display case to the oven to the table. Not only do MPR food packages frequently function as cooking containers, but occasionally packages, such as those using microwave susceptor technology, may even have a function in cooking the food.

The expanding role of today's food packages draws attention to new areas of concern. Multilayer plastic packaging materials and microwave susceptors used at higher and higher temperatures lead to questions about migration of food packaging components to food. The Food and Drug Administration's (FDA's) concerns relative to these matters are discussed later in this chapter.

Microbiological Hazards of MPR Foods as Related to Outbreaks of Various Pathogens

The unique characteristics of certain MPR fruits and vegetables may affect or enhance the growth of pathogenic microorganisms. Partial cooking or pasteurizing extends the marketable shelf-life of many foods. Although these heat processes kill normal spoilage organisms and the vegetative forms of pathogens, they may also actually promote growth of remaining spore-forming pathogens by eliminating competition. During further processing, assembly, and packaging, pathogens may recontaminate already heated or pasteurized foods. Because many common spoilage organisms are obligate aerobes, the combination of controlled or modified low oxygen atmosphere can delay spoilage; but packaging designed to exclude oxygen could enhance growth of spore-forming anaerobic or microaerophilic bacteria. The extended shelf life of these products may allow time for psychrotrophic pathogens, such as type E *C. botulinum*, to multiply to numbers large enough to cause illness. However, adequate sanitation and use of heat or refrigeration to inhibit microbial growth prevents most bacterial food poisoning. The following discussion is limited to members of the genera *Clostridium*, *Listeria*, *Yersinia*, *Campylobacter*, and *Staphylococcus*. Other bacteria capable of causing food poisoning could become a problem if the food is contaminated and preservative barriers are abused. (See Chapter 7 for additional details.)

Clostridium

Probably the most significant threat to public health is *Clostridium botulinum*. Ingestion of minute amounts of botulinal toxin results in illness and may cause death. *Clostridium botulinum* organisms are gram-positive motile rods, 0.6–1.4 μm wide by 3–20 μm long (Cato, George, and Finegold 1986). *C. botulinum* organisms are inhibited by 6.5% NaCl and grow between pH 4.6 and 8.5. These organisms form an oval or spherical endospore that is extremely heat resistant. *C. botulinum* organisms are ubiquitous in nature, occurring as part of the normal soil microflora, and in animal, bird, and fish intestines.

There are seven toxin types—A, B, C, D, E, F, and G—all heat-labile. Types A and B are found most frequently in food poisoning cases, although type F was isolated in a case of infant botulism (Cato, George, and Finegold 1986). Illness results from ingestion of the toxin, a potent neurotoxin, causing blurred vision, nausea, and muscle weakness and may result in death (MacDonald et al. 1985).

Proteolytic strains of *C. botulinum* (all type A, some B and F) require temperatures above 10° C for growth and toxin production (Sperber 1982), although optimum growth occurs between 30 and 40° C (Cato, George, and Finegold 1986). Unless refrigerated foods are temperature abused, only minimal risk of botulism exists from these strains. However, nonproteolytic strains (all type E, some B and F) can grow and produce toxin even at refrigeration temperatures of 3–4° C (Abrahamsson, Gullmar, and Molin 1966; Eklund, Wieler, and Poysky 1967; Solomon, Kautter and Lynt 1982). For this reason, nonproteolytic strains may pose a botulism risk in MPR vegetables.

Most of the cases of botulism in the United States result from un-derprocessing of home-canned foods. An anaerobe, *C. botulinum*, grows well in hermetically sealed containers, in food interiors, or in oil-immersed food. Usually, the putrid smell associated with growth of *C. botulinum* results in the food being rejected as undesirable; however, in many cases of illness, enough growth occurred to permit toxin production, but the food did not show overt signs of spoilage. Boiling food may be sufficient to inactivate existing toxin because botulinal toxins are very heat-labile.

Several recent outbreaks of botulism were traced to minimally processed nonrefrigerated vegetable products. These cases were atypical, because the illness did not result from ingestion of under-processed or postprocessing contaminated canned foods. Con-

sumption of chopped garlic in oil (St. Louis et al. 1988) resulted in
36 cases of type B botulism, from a restaurant in Vancouver, B.C.
Epidemiological studies showed a relationship between illness and
consumption of one of two types of meat sandwiches. The one ingredient common to both sandwiches was garlic-buttered bread.
Garlic used in the garlic butter had been chopped, covered with
soybean oil, and stored for months at *room temperature*. Because garlic
has a strong odor, the smell associated with growth of a nonproteolytic *C. botulinum* strain was difficult to detect. Slow progression
of type B botulism in this outbreak made diagnosis difficult, but,
luckily, no patients died.

Garlic was inoculated with the same type B strain of *C. botulinum*
isolated from the outbreak in Vancouver and held at *room temperature* (Solomon and Kautter 1988). Toxin was detected after 30 days,
although the garlic appeared and smelled acceptable.

Ingestion of sauteed onions caused a botulism outbreak resulting
in hospitalization of 28 people in Peoria, Illinois in 1983 (MacDonald
et al. 1985). Fresh raw onions were sauteed and served on a patty
melt sandwich in a restaurant. After they were sauteed, the onions
were poured into a pan, covered by a layer of melted margarine,
and allowed to stand in a *warm place* (41° C) throughout the day.
The onions were not reheated before the sandwiches were prepared. The wrapper of a sandwich taken home by one of the patients contained *C. botulinum* type A toxin. Cultures of raw onions
obtained from the restaurant produced *C. botulinum* type A organisms. Anaerobic conditions created by the margarine layer and incubation at *warm temperatures* created an ideal environment for *C.
botulinum* growth.

Additional cases of botulism have occurred from food other than
canned foods. Following an outbreak of botulism, potato salad was
suspected as the food poisoning vehicle. In studies with inoculated
foil-wrapped baked potatoes (Sugiyama et al. 1981), spores of *C.
botulinum* survived baking at 260° C for 45 min. When incubated at
room temperature, potatoes became toxic in 3–7 days. If leftover
baked potatoes are used in potato salad, they should be refrigerated
like any other perishable, cooked food.

Inoculated pack studies were conducted with *C. botulinum* in vacuum-packed cooked potatoes (Notermans, Dufrenne, and Keijbets
1981). Pouches of peeled, cut potatoes were evacuated, sealed, and
then heated in a water bath at 95° C for 40 min. *C. botulinum* strains
grew and the potatoes became toxic before overt signs of spoilage,
when stored at 15 or 20° C. Strains of types A, B, and E grew and

produced toxin at 10° C, although in this study growth of all types was inhibited at 4° C. Although the product causes no health risk when stored at 4° C, it could be a problem if temperature abused. Vacuum-packed cooked potatoes could be a significant health risk because they might be used without recooking in a potato salad. In another study, potatoes were treated with ascorbic acid and citric acid before vacuum packaging (Notermans, Dufrenne, and Keijbets 1985). When potatoes were dipped in solutions of ascorbic or citric acid and stored for 70 days at 15° C, growth and toxin production did not occur. Treating vacuum packaged foods with additives such as citric, ascorbic, or sorbic acid could help ensure their safety.

C. botulinum and Modified Atmosphere Packaging

Dignan (1984) studied growth and toxin production of *C. botulinum* in raw diced potatoes treated with sulfur dioxide and packaged under modified atmosphere. Potatoes were first placed in an atmosphere of 0, 10, or 100% gaseous SO_2 for 3 min. After SO_2 treatment, containers were evacuated, and the atmosphere replaced with 100% CO, 100% CO_2, or a mixture of 5% CO, 25% CO_2, and 70% air. Treatment with 100% SO_2 reduced the pH of potatoes to below 4.6, and consequently inhibited growth of *C. botulinum*. After exposure to 10% SO_2, potatoes stored at 25° C in 100% CO or CO_2 became toxic in 7 days, whereas appearance and odor remained "like-fresh." Without SO_2, potatoes in all atmospheres became toxic and spoiled in 7–14 days, although 100% CO or CO_2 delayed the onset of spoilage and toxin production.

Vacuum packaging has been considered as a technique to increase the storage life of many fresh vegetables. However, whenever vacuum packaging is used to extend shelf-life, hazards from pathogenic anaerobes should be considered. Johnson (1979) inoculated pouches of cut celery with types A, B, and E spores of *C. botulinum*. Pouches were evacuated, flushed with nitrogen, sealed, and stored at 7 or 21° C for up to 8 weeks. Although none of these celery samples became toxic, when nutrient broth was added to celery in pouches, toxin was found after 8 weeks at 21° C, demonstrating that for *C. botulinum* to grow and produce toxin, adequate nutrients must be available.

Listeria

Listeria organisms are distributed widely in nature and can be isolated from soil, water, humans, and a variety of animals. Typically, infection with *Listeria* results in flu-like septicemia, and/or menin-gitis (Ho et al. 1986). Listeriosis victims are typically immunosup-pressed individuals such as chemotherapy patients, pregnant women, or the very young or very old. The disease can be extremely serious, as evidenced by the death of 29% of the patients in one epidemic (Fleming et al. 1985).

Several characteristics of *Listeria monocytogenes* make this organism of concern to producers of MPR foods. *Listeria* are aerobic to fac-ultatively anaerobic and may flourish in packaging designed to ex-clude oxygen. Bacteria of the genus *Listeria* are short, gram-positive rods, 0.4–0.5 μm in diameter by 0.5–2 μm long (Seeliger and Jones 1986). They are non-spore-formers and motile with a few peritri-chous flagella when grown at 20–25° C. *Listeria* organisms grow at a pH between 5.6 and 9.6 (Gray and Killinger 1966), can metabolize glucose, and tolerate up to 10% NaCl.

Following an outbreak of listeriosis in several Boston hospitals, epidemiological studies implicated raw celery, tomatoes, and lettuce as possible vehicles for the illness (Ho et al. 1986). This conclusion was based upon common consumption patterns among victims, al-though *Listeria* was not isolated from the suspected foods. Stein-bruegge, Maxcy, and Liewen (1988) showed *L. monocytogenes* can grow when inoculated on lettuce. Although variable, growth occurs at 5 and 12° C, and may be affected by other, naturally occurring, competing organisms.

An outbreak of listeriosis with 41 cases in the Maritime Provinces of Canada was linked to consumption of coleslaw made from cab-bage that had been fertilized with contaminated sheep manure (Schlech et al. 1982). In one case, the same serotype, 4B, was iden-tified in a patient and isolated from coleslaw in the patient's refrig-erator. Subsequently, several researchers studied the growth of *Lis-teria* in cabbage and cabbage juice. Beuchat et al. (1986) found that *L. monocytogenes* strains Scott A and LCDC 81-861 increased from 1.6×10^4 to 2.6×10^3 colony-forming units (CFU)/g raw cabbage when held at 5° C for 25 days. However, the number of viable *Lis-teria* organisms declined during storage, when heat-sterilized cab-bage was inoculated and held for 42 days at 5° C. Conner, Brackett and Beuchat (1986) demonstrated that cabbage and cabbage juice could support the growth of *L. monocytogenes*. They found *L. mon-ocytogenes* grew well at pH 5.0, although others describe pH 5.6 as the lower limit of growth (Gray and Killinger 1966). *L. monocytogenes* organisms reduced the pH of cabbage juice to 4.14 before growth ceased.

Listeria monocytogenes is psychrotrophic, with a wide growth temperature range of 1–45° C, although optimum growth occurs between 30 and 37° C (Seeliger and Jones 1986). Thermotolerance data on *L. monocytogenes* have generally indicated a relative heat resistance compared to other non-spore-formers (Bunning et al. 1988; Doyle et al. 1987, Mackey and Bratchell 1989), this characteristic, together with an ability to grow at refrigeration temperatures, albeit slowly, has caused concern about this pathogen's presence in minimally processed food (Mackey and Bratchell 1989).

Yersinia

As psychrotrophic pathogens, *Yersinia* organisms are of concern in MPR refrigerated foods. All species of *Yersinia* may grow between 4 and 42° C, although the optimum growth temperature is 28–29° C. Members of this genus are facultative anaerobes and may proliferate in modified atmosphere packaging.

Members of the genus *Yersinia* (Bercovier and Mollaret 1984) range from non-spore-forming gram-negative rods to coccobacilli, 0.5–0.8 μm in diameter by 1–3 μm long. *Yersinia* organisms associated with foodborne illness are nonmotile when grown at 37° C, but are motile with peritrichous flagella when grown at temperatures below 30° C. They ferment glucose and many other sugars. *Y. enterocolitica* can tolerate up to 5% NaCl and survive between pH 4 and 10, with optimum pH of 7.2–7.4.

Illness caused by *Y. enterocolitica* includes pseudoappendicitis, gastroenteritis, terminal ileitis, mesenteric lymphadenitis, arthritis, and septicemia. The organisms are found on food of animal origin and can be isolated from healthy humans and animals. One member of the genus, *Y. kristensii* (Schiemann 1988), when grown under aeration at 6° C produces a heat-stable enterotoxin.

In a study of the microbial flora of packaged salad vegetables, bacteria of the genus *Yersinia* were isolated from all specimens tested (Brocklehurst, Zaman-Wong, and Lund 1987). Most of the *Yersinia* organisms isolated were identified as *Y. enterocolitica* and all but one strain were considered nonpathogenic.

Tofu consumption resulted in an outbreak of yersiniosis in Seattle, WA (Aulisio et al. 1983). The tofu was contaminated by unchlorinated well water used during manufacture.

Campylobacter

Members of the genus *Campylobacter* present a potential hazard in foods packaged to exclude oxygen because they are microaerophilic, requiring an environment with 3–15% oxygen and 3–5% carbon dioxide (Smibert 1984). *Campylobacter jejuni* is characterized by gram-negative non-spore-forming rods, 0.2–0.5 µm wide by 0.5–5 µm long. Rods are motile with a single polar flagellum at one or both ends. As chemoorganotrophs, these organisms are unable to ferment or oxidize carbohydrates. These bacteria are commonly found in food, water, unpasteurized milk, and the blood and feces of humans infected with *C. jejuni*. Infection with *C. jejuni* may cause fever and enteritis in humans. Because *C. jejuni* grows at temperatures of 42–45° C, but is unable to multiply at 25° C, it could grow only in temperature-abused MPR foods.

C. *jejuni* and *C. coli* are practically indistinguishable biochemically. The species differ mainly in that *C. jejuni* can hydrolyze hippurate and *C. coli* cannot. Most investigations of foodborne illness caused by *Campylobacter* discuss both species.

Foodborne illness caused by members of the genus *Campylobacter* is usually associated with animal products (Harris, Weiss, and Nolan 1986a), although reports of several food poisoning cases implicate foods of other origin. Harris et al. (1986c) reported a possible association of mushroom consumption with enteritis caused by *C. jejuni* and *C. coli*. Doyle and Schoeni (1985) isolated *C. jejuni* in wrapped, fresh mushrooms. Of 200 packages of mushrooms obtained from retailers in a survey, 3% contained *C. jejuni*.

Following an outbreak of *Campylobacter* enteritis at a boys' summer camp in Connecticut, birthday cake was implicated as the vehicle of transmission. The findings were based on epidemiological studies, although cultures of cake and icing mixes were negative. None of the cake suspected of causing food poisoning remained available for testing. The salads served at camp also may have been the source of *Campylobacter* because an infected food-handler responsible for salad making had been ill with *C. jejuni* enteritis (Blaser et al. 1982).

C. *jejuni* and *C. coli* are common contaminants of animal products, most prevalent in raw, uncooked poultry products. A survey of markets in King County, Washington, showed 23.1% of chicken and 17.2% of game hens were positive for *C. jejuni/coli* (Harris et al. 1986b). *C. jejuni/coli* was the most common organism identified in the survey. Fewer than 5% of specimens contained *Yersinia* or *Sal-*

monella. Epidemiological studies of 225 cases of *C. jejuni/coli* enteritis found an increased risk associated with consumption of under-cooked chicken (Harris, Weiss, and Nolan 1986a). The risk of *Campylobacter* enteritis may be increased if fruits and vegetables are prepared on the same work surface as poultry products, or if they are served as part of a multiple-component entree, such as chicken breasts with broccoli.

Staphylococcus

Several unique properties of *Staphylococcus aureus* make it a concern in discussions of MPR foods. These organisms are *not heat-tolerant* and are *unable to grow at refrigeration* temperatures. However, if foods are contaminated with *S. aureus* following cooking but before packaging, growth is possible with temperature abuse. Because *S. aureus* lives in the nasal membranes, perineum, skin, gastrointestinal tract, and genital tract of warm-blooded animals (Kloos and Schleifer 1986), carriers or infected food handlers may easily transmit these organisms to food. If food is contaminated and temperature abused before cooking, heating will destroy the bacteria, but the heat-stable enterotoxin may remain and cause illness.

S. aureus are gram-positive, nonmotile, non-spore-forming cocci, 0.5–1 μm in diameter (Kloos and Schleifer 1986). They are facultative anaerobes but grow more rapidly in the presence of oxygen. This species grows well in up-to-10% NaCl and can tolerate up-to-15% NaCl. Growth occurs between 10 and 45° C, although the optimum growth temperature is 30–37° C. *S. aureus* ferments most sugars. The pH range for growth of *S. aureus* is between 4.5 and 9.3 with an optimum range of 7.0–7.5.

S. aureus produces five types of heat-stable enterotoxin—A, B, C, D, and E. Typical symptoms of food poisoning from *S. aureus* enterotoxin begin 1–4 after ingestion, and include nausea, vomiting, diarrhea, headaches, fatigue, and abdominal cramps (Lindroth et al. 1983).

For *S. aureus* to produce toxin and cause illness, the food must support the growth of these organisms. Following a case of staphylococcal food poisoning, investigators studied the growth of *S. aureus* in wild mushrooms (Lindroth et al. 1983). Mushrooms were contaminated with *S. aureus* and then stored for 3 days at 15 and 21° C. Within 3 days, *S. aureus* grew to numbers large enough to detect enterotoxin. The food poisoning outbreak occurred when the mushrooms were contaminated, held at room temperature, and then cooked. The dish suspected of causing food poisoning contained staphylococcal enterotoxin but no live organisms.

A study of the microflora of potato-topped meat pies showed that both cooked and uncooked pies contained *S. aureus* (Thomas and Masters 1988). When the pies were stored at either 4 or 37° C, outward signs of spoilage were not evident. If this type of pie were temperature abused, the potential would exist for staphylococcal food poisoning.

Morita and Woodburn (1983) studied growth and toxin production by *S. aureus* in a variety of salads. Macaroni, potato, soymeat, and chicken salads were inoculated with *S. aureus*, incubated at 37° C, and tested for toxin after 8 or 24 h. Three types of salad dressings were tested on all varieties of salad. Most salads contained enterotoxin after 8 h, although growth and toxin production were highest in macaroni and potato salad. Higher enterotoxin concentration resulted in salads with either no dressing or a water dressing. A lower initial pH in salads with a commercial dressing or vinegar dressing contributed to lower levels of enterotoxin.

A survey of pumpkin pie revealed *S. aureus* in one of four pies purchased from retail outlets (Wyatt and Guy 1981). Because the interior of the pies reaches 108° C during cooking, any viable staphylococcal organisms would be a result of recontaminating the surface of cooked product. The primary tools for prevention of growth and enterotoxin production by *S. aureus* include use of proper sanitary procedures and refrigeration of products.

Regulatory Issues Associated with Minimally Processed Foods

Sanitation

Besides the basic provisions of the Food, Drug, and Cosmetic Act, the U.S. Food and Drug Administration has promulgated Good Manufacturing Practice Regulations (GMPs) designed to minimize risk to public health from improper handling, storage, distribution, or processing of fruits and vegetables and other foods. In addition, certain provisions of the Meat Inspection regulations (9 CFR 318) and the Poultry Products Inspection regulations (9 CFR 381) also relate to sanitary food production.

All MPR foods will include refrigeration as one of the hurdles or barriers to maintain product safety and quality. Consequently, such foods are considered refrigerated foods. Because there is no specific good manufacturing practice regulation for refrigerated foods at this time, manufacturers need to concern themselves only with the requirements found in Title 21 Code of Federal Regulates (CFR) part 110, Current Good Manufacturing Practice in Manufacturing, Packing, or Holding Human Food. This GMP is sometimes called the "Umbrella GMP" because it addresses everything from plant and equipment construction to personnel hygiene.

Likewise there are at present no GMP regulations for the manufacture of smoked foods or foods with extended shelf-life as a result of controlled or modified atmosphere packaging. Until such time as the need or demand for GMPs for food products preserved by these means becomes apparent, manufacturing should be conducted so as to comply with the requirements of 21 CFR 110.

In addition to FDA's "Umbrella GMP," the United States Department of Agriculture's Food Safety and Inspection Service (FSIS) recently issued Policy Memo (PM) 110 for products containing more than 2% meat or poultry requiring processors of refrigerated food to submit detailed processing procedures along with the application for label approval. These food products may have fruit or vegetable content. PM 110 also requires manufacturers to have a USDA approved Partial Quality Control Program (PQCP) prior to final label approval. The PQCP must contain a detailed description of ingredient storage controls; product formulations and preparation procedures; container filling and sealing practices; any heat treatment (time/temperature), including a description of the equipment used; any other treatments applied; cooling (time/temperature); lot identification procedures; finished product storage conditions; in-plant quality control procedures; and a record of maintenance procedures.

When taken in context, these regulations and policies indirectly ensure that risk to public health does not increase due to insanitary processing or handling procedures. Although the absence of specific regulations can facilitate rapid introduction of MPR foods into the marketplace, companies must recognize and assume the responsibility of minimizing the risks to consumer and industry reputation imposed by the presence or growth of potentially harmful microorganisms.

What is more likely is that FDA and USDA will address specific issues for MPR fruits and vegetables as they arise. In some instances that has already occurred. The FDA and USDA have already issued positions or policies on certain minimally processed foods. As a result of the illnesses caused by the presence of *C. botulinum* toxin in chopped garlic in oil, the FDA issued a letter to processors of chopped garlic in oil urging that the product be acidified, if marketing and storage is intended to occur at *room temperature*. In the letter, FDA stated that it was prepared to charge that any product relying entirely on refrigeration for safety during storage, distribution, and retailing was adulterated under Section 402(a)(4) of the Act, in that it had been prepared, packed, or held under insanitary conditions whereby it may have been rendered injurious to health. FDA also stated that it would no longer consider the product as safe, even if labeled "Keep Refrigerated," if the product did not contain an additional barrier to microbial growth. FDA stated the product represents a special hazard because it is unlikely to appear spoiled, even if it is temperature abused.

Another instance of addressing specific problems or practices is the FDA Division of Retail Food Protection's position on "sous vide." Sous vide is a process where entrees, typically meats, fish, and *vegetables* are cooked in plastic bags that have been vacuumed and sealed. After cooking, the product is quickly cooled and stored under refrigeration. This cooking and preparation system has been marketed widely with claims of a 6-week shelf-life to restaurant and delicatessen operators. The FDA's Division of Retail Food Protection issued a letter to State and local health officials advising that such procedures should be practiced only in establishments recognized as food processing facilities (Schwarz 1988). FDA expressed its belief that in a retail food service establishment without controls associated with a food processing plant, vacuum packaging followed by cooking and refrigeration would constitute an unnecessary and significant public health hazard.

A National Advisory Committee on Microbiological Criteria for Foods working group examining meat and poultry has issued recommendations for refrigerated foods containing cooked, uncured meat or poultry products that are packaged for extended refrigerated shelf-life and that are ready-to-eat or prepared with minimal additional heat treatment. The group believes these types of products are of concern because of the ability of *L. monocytogenes* to grow at refrigerated temperatures, toxin production by *C. botulinum*, and other microbiological hazards associated with temperature abuse. The working group recommends that producers of these types of products operate with a scientifically sound HACCP program. Procedures would be required to demonstrate a thermal process sufficient to reduce the initial population of *L. monocytogenes* by decimal log cycles, as well as procedures sufficient to demonstrate control of toxin production by nonproteolytic and proteolytic *C. botulinum*, including psychrotrophic species. The recommendations also address packaging systems, distribution, labeling, education, and research. It is reasonable to expect that, over time, other microbiological criteria will also be developed by similar committees for other minimally processed foods.

Packaging Safety Considerations (See Also Chapter 4)

The Federal Food, Drug, and Cosmetic Act places the responsibility for assessing the safety of food packaging materials on the FDA. Substances that are unintentional components of food as a result of their use or presence in food packaging are considered to be indirect food additives and legally require premarket safety approval via the food additive petition process, that is, food additives require safety evaluation prior to their actual use. During this petition process to amend the food additive regulations, FDA evaluates information to support the safety of the proposed food additive. FDA requires industry to perform extraction tests to determine the nature and amount of packaging materials and components of packaging materials likely to migrate to food and to supply appropriate toxicological data for the migrants. To reach appropriate conclusions about the safety of food packaging materials, the extraction test procedures must be able to reliably predict migration levels in likely food packaging applications. Approval for the use of a food additive takes the form of a regulation that specifies the conditions (such as temperature, type of food, etc.) of safe use.

Although the conditions of use for food packaging materials are limited in a food additive regulation, they still represent the maximums that safety data can support when migration potential is considered. In general, increased migration of components of food packaging materials results from its use at increased temperatures or with foods of increased fat content. In premarket approval, the amount of toxicological data necessary to demonstrate the safety of any food additive depends on the consumer's probable total dietary intake. For a food packaging material the data requirements increase as the amount of likely migration increases, and the regulation must permit only those conditions of use that have been demonstrated to be safe.

FDA's regulations for food packaging materials are specific with regard to permitted use conditions, but they are generic regarding the particular material used to package food. That is, food additive regulations are *not* licenses; they sanction a particular material with certain specifications and not a particular company's product. As long as a company's material is used in accordance with the terms and specifications in the regulation, further approval from FDA is not required.

The system of generic regulation for food packaging materials can give rise to concerns that result from new technology. Examples occur in the areas of microwaveable food packages and packages containing microwave heat susceptors. Most of the indirect food additive regulations concerned with food packaging materials were established prior to the development of the technology to make packages suitable for microwave heating. FDA was not able to predict the great extent to which microwaving of packaged food was occurring and will continue to occur. The susceptor package provides the type of heating that is necessary for browning or crisping food in the microwave oven. A variety of susceptors have been developed, but the essential component is a metallized film (usually limited to polyethylene terephthalate, PET) which absorbs microwave energy, becomes very hot in a very short period of time, and acts like a small frying pan in the microwave oven. Depending on the specific application (pizza tray, popcorn bag, etc.) the metallized film is also laminated to paper and/or paperboard with one or more types of adhesive.

The following is a list of some of the pertinent food packaging regulations for the type of constructions just described:

21 CFR 175.105   Adhesives
21 CFR 176.170   Components of paper and paperboard in contact with aqueous and fatty foods
21 CFR 177.1390   Laminate structures for use at temperatures of 250° F and above
21 CFR 177.1630   Polyethylene phthalate polymers

At the time that these regulations were issued, FDA scientists never anticipated the very high temperatures attained by susceptor packaging. Consequently, the safety data provided for the materials described in these regulations may not cover the levels of migration observed with microwave susceptors. Research performed in FDA's Indirect Additives Laboratory indicated that migration of some of the susceptor packaging components could be substantial (Begley and Hollifield 1989).

Time–Temperature Indicators

Regulatory agencies can also be expected to encourage, and perhaps require, greater reliance on "use by" or "sell by" dating or some other similar mechanism to ensure that extended shelf-life products remain safe and wholesome. Manufacturers will need a complete and thorough understanding of their products' shelf-lives to implement a useful and meaningful system. By necessity, this will require manufacturers to examine their distribution systems and to monitor the effectiveness of their in-store personnel; to educate supermarket personnel; and to select dates based not only on the product's microbiological and quality attributes, but also on tested consumer storage and handling practices. This last point is particularly important, initially because consumers may perceive products as shelf-stable instead of shelf-life extended; or may not be familiar with the technology. To alleviate some of this confusion, time–temperature indicators or integrators may be justified, so long as they are accurate, to alert regulatory and quality control personnel and more importantly distributors and retailers, as well as consumers, to the fact that temperature abuse has occurred.

Several types of devices record or monitor changes in temperature: temperature indicators, time–temperature integrators, and time–temperature integrator/indicators (Byrne 1976). Temperature indicators change if a certain temperature is reached but are unable to indicate the length of exposure to a particular temperature. Time–temperature integrators react gradually to show the cumulative effects of time and temperature. Ideally, a colored end-point corresponds with the end of a product's shelf-life. Time–temperature integrator/indicators work like a thermometer, with a colored line advancing in direct proportion to storage temperature. The line advances more quickly at higher temperatures. Time–temperature integrator/indicators show the extent of temperature abuse, rather than a specific end-point. The use of these terms is not consistent in the literature, however, and many prefer to lump all devices that combine the effects of time and temperature under the category, time–temperature indicators. This terminology is used throughout the remainder of this discussion.

One type of time–temperature indicator consists of an enzyme and pH indicator dye separated by a film from the substrate. The time–temperature indicator is activated by breaking the film and mixing the reaction components. The rate of enzyme hydrolysis depends on time and temperature. As the substrate is used, the pH change results in a color change; the color is revealed when the usable shelf-life has expired.

Refrigeration is one of the foremost tools for inhibiting or slowing the growth of pathogenic microorganisms. Unfortunately, refrigeration temperatures used in practice often exceed recommended values ($<7.2°$ C). In a survey of temperatures of home refrigerators, over 20% exceeded $10°$ C (Van Garde and Woodburn 1987). Temperatures in retail establishments vary and may depend on position within the case or proximity to fluorescent lights.

Many refrigerated foods are marked with "use by" or "sell by" dates. Although these give the consumer guidelines for use of a safe product, they do not give the temperature history. Spoilage and pathogen growth increases when storage temperature increases. Because temperature abuse is one of the most critical factors in the growth of pathogenic microorganisms, ideal food packaging might contain some outward sign demonstrating past temperature history. Time–temperature indicators could be useful in this way, to record or somehow reveal a product's temperature history. Unfortunately not enough research information has been developed for MPR fruits and vegetables.

Consumer Considerations

In recognition that consumers must bear some responsibility for protecting their own health, USDA and FDA are presently participating in a joint effort to study consumer attitudes and knowledge of the hazards posed by improper handling of risk-imposing foods. The study is designed to include a survey of in-home refrigeration temperatures and in-home food preparation, handling, and holding practices. Results of the study will be used to alert industry to potential product dangers created by uninformed consumers; they will serve as a basis to develop education programs for consumers on how to store, handle, and prepare MPR fruits and vegetables that exhibit extended shelf-life but are not truly commercially sterile.

Industry Initiatives

Hazard Analysis/Critical Control Point (HACCP) Systems

HACCP systematically evaluates the potential for microbial hazards in manufacturing and distribution; it estimates or quantifies, to the best possible extent, the associated risk. Having identified hazards and estimated their risk, critical control points are subsequently identified and the necessary monitoring programs put in place. HACCP evaluations should be performed for each specific minimally processed food product. The HACCP approach should be considered and practiced by all MPR food manufacturers. In addition to participating in working groups of the National Advisory Committee on Microbiological Criteria for Foods, the industry is conducting other significant efforts in the areas of HACCP to ensure safe and wholesome minimally processed foods of high quality. The work of the National Food Processors Association (NFPA) in this area has been significant.

NFPA recognized some concerns and issues about MPR foods whose shelf-lives are extended by refrigeration in combination with other preservative procedures or techniques, and suggested certain factors to consider in establishing good manufacturing practices (Refrigerated Foods and Microbiological Criteria Committee, 1988). The committee recommended the use of 4.4° C in place of 7.2° C as the upper limit for refrigerated products. While the committee recognized that 4.4° C at present may be unrealistic for practical application, they endorsed the concept as a desirable goal. During product development the committee suggested using pathogen inoculation studies to verify process effectiveness. Temperature abuse testing with inoculated samples is recommended to test the limits of the preservative barrier. The participation of persons knowledgeable in heating, cooling, and refrigeration procedures is also encouraged. To complete the list, the committee recommended considering the processing equipment, product and ingredient flow, monitoring and recording devices, and overall plant sanitation. The committee also suggested evaluating food ingredients and establishing microbiological specifications wherever necessary to minimize risk. The "Manufacturing Guidelines for the Production, Distribution, and Handling of Refrigerated Foods" (National Food Processors Association Microbiology and Food Safety Committee, 1989) represents another, yet significant, industry effort. These guidelines address product and process development, predistribution, distribution, retailing, and food service, with HACCP principles clearly emphasized. As such, the guidelines represent a responsible approach to food safety.

To further these kinds of approach, Agriculture Canada is examining the feasibility of using expert system technology to automate use of HACCP in the chilled food industry (Finnegan 1989).

Echoing a previously expressed viewpoint that end-point analysis will not necessarily ensure a safe product, this group has noted that a preventive approach such as HACCP must be utilized. Considering the resource demands that HACCP might place on small and medium size concerns, expert system technology is being examined as a means to alleviate strain and decrease the risk of product development and chilled food production. A feasibility study has been started to determine if HACCP principles can be automated, using a selected product, namely lasagna with a beef and cheese sauce. A prototype is in the development stage as a proof-of-concept model. In its final form, the expert system will be an affordable personal computer that is both compatible and accessible to Canadian government inspection personnel.

In addition to HACCP, the industry is also initiating other steps to ensure the safe and economical production, distribution, and storage of MPR foods (Keller 1989). An example is the Campbell Soup Company's select supplier program to control ingredients. Another example is a practice called high-risk/low-risk manufacturing. Here extensive sanitation practices and precautions are taken in what is defined as a high-risk zone, such as an assembly operation between cooking and final package sealing. Further advances in mechanization are also important; these are needed particularly in areas that rely heavily on human handling or assembly. One possibility is the use of computer-aided robotics.

Modeling

The information available on bacterial spoilage of foods is not always useful because few standardized testing or reporting procedures exist. Systematic studies on the specific effects of treatments, and treatment interactions in food matrices, are rare because studies are extensive, time consuming, and expensive. Furthermore, if a formulation change is made, a whole new series of tests may be necessary. When the force behind microbiological preservation studies is merely to be "first to market," is not surprising that the studies are sufficient only to ensure stability and safety without providing a full understanding of how preservation occurs.

Researchers in food microbiology (Genigiorgis 1981; Gibson, Bratchell, and Roberts 1988) have been developing procedures and tools that could prove useful in predicting the safety and shelf-life of MPR foods. Gibson, Bratchell, and Roberts (1988) modeled the combined effects of pH, sodium chloride, and storage temperature on the growth of salmonellae in a laboratory medium. Tanaka et al. (1986) tested the effect of percent moisture, salt, pH, and additives, such as sorbate, on inhibiting the germination and growth of C. *botulinum* spores in pasteurized cheese spreads.

As progress in computer capabilities and user friendly software continues, other microbiologists can be expected to contribute models based on either probability or kinetics. Both types of models allow researchers to predict the effects of varying treatments; the choice ultimately depends on both intended use and the bacteria of concern. For example, probability models appear to be the model of choice for C. *botulinum* because no growth of the organism can be tolerated. In instances where the growth dynamics of an organism in a product is critical, kinetic models may be useful. Kinetic models may grow in popularity because they provide more information about both products and organisms. Such information is needed to ensure that "use by" dates, time–temperature indicators, and product quality are synchronized. Ultimately, and perhaps, most importantly, with model development, food scientists will be able to design safety and stability into MRP foods including MPR fruits and vegetables, as is done at present with low-acid canned food process design, rather than being limited to analysis of finished product.

Conclusion

Consumer demand for convenience and added value means that MPR foods including fruits and vegetables with extended shelf-life will play a significant role in the future of the United States food supply. Thus, an understanding of the interplay between microorganisms and MPR foods during manufacture, storage, and distribution is critical. Because these foods rely on processing and preservation schemes that do not render them commercially sterile, their inherent microbiological safety requires that refrigeration and other appropriate barriers remain in place. To ensure that MPR foods are distributed, sold, and stored in a safe and uncompromising manner, the food industry, regulatory authorities, and consumers need to exercise continued vigilance and caution.

References

Abrahamsson, K.B. Gullmar, and N. Molin. 1966. The effect of temperature on toxin formation and toxin stability of *Clostridium botulinum* type E in different environments. *Can. J. Microbiol.* **12**:385–394.

Anon. 1989. US Department of Health and Human Services Press Release, P89-20, Attachment B.

Aulisio, C.C.G., J.T. Stanfield, S.D. Weagant, and W.E. Hill. 1983. Yersiniosis associated with tofu consumption: serological, biochemical and pathogenicity studies of *Yersinia enterocolitica* isolates. *J. Food Protect.* **46**:226–230.

Begley, T. and H. Hollifield. 1989. FDA laboratory study of susceptor packaging. Presented at the AOAC National Meeting, September 24–27, St. Louis, MO.

Bercovier, H. and H.H. Mollaret. 1984. Genus XIV. *Yersinia*. In *Bergey's Manual of Systematic Bacteriology*, Vol. 1, N.R. Krieg and J.G. Holt (eds.), pp. 498–506. Baltimore: Williams & Wilkins.

Beuchat, L.R., R.E. Brackett, D.Y.Y. Hao, and D.E. Conner. 1986. Growth and thermal inactivation of *Listeria monocytogenes* in cabbage and cabbage juice. *Can. J. Microbiol.* **32**:791–795.

Blaser, M.J., P. Checko, C. Bopp, A. Bruce, and J.M. Hughes. 1982. *Campylobacter* enteritis associated with foodborne transmission. *Am. J. Epidemiol.* **116**:886–894.

Bolin, H.R., A.E. Stafford, A.D. King, and C.C. Huxsoll. 1977. Factors affecting the storage stability of shredded lettuce. *J. Food Sci.* **42**:1319–1321.

Brocklehurst, T.F., C.M. Zaman-Wong, and B.M. Lund. 1987. A note on the microbiology of retail packs of prepared salad vegetables. *J. Appl. Bacteriol.* **63**:409–415.

Brody, A.L. 1987. In the beginning: the whys and hows of market entry in controlled/modified atmosphere packaging. Presented at the Third International Conference on Controlled/Modified Atmosphere/Vacuum Packaging, September 16–18, Itasca, IL.

Bunning, V.K., C.W. Donnelly, J.T. Peeler, E.H. Briggs, J.G. Bradshaw, R.G. Crawford, C.M. Beliveau, and J.T. Tierney. 1988. Thermal inactivation of *Listeria monocytogenes* within bovine milk phagocytes. *Appl. Environm. Microbiol.* **54**:364–370.

Byrne, C.H. 1976. Temperature indicators—the state of the art. *Food Technol.* **30**(6):66–68.

Cabes, L.J. 1985. Plastic packaging used in retort processing: control of key parameters. *Food Technol.* **39**(12):57–60.

Cato, E.P., W.L. George, and S.M. Finegold. 1986. Genus *Clostridium*. In *Bergey's Manual of Systematic Bacteriology*, Vol. 2, P.H.A. Sneath, N.S. Mair, M.E. Sharpe, and J.G. Holt (eds.), pp. 1157–1160. Baltimore: Williams & Wilkins.

Conner, D.E., R.E. Brackett, and L.R. Beuchat. 1986. Effect of temperature, sodium chloride, and pH on growth of *Listeria monocytogenes* in cabbage juice. *Appl. Environm. Microbiol.* **52**:59–63.

Davidson, W.D. 1987. Retail store handling conditions for refrigerated foods. Presented at a Technical Session "New Extended Shelf-Life: Low-acid Refrigerated Foods" at the 80th Annual Convention of the National Food Processors Association, January 26, Chicago, IL.

Dignan, D.M. 1984. Evaluation of the botulism hazard from diced raw potatoes preserved by gas exchange. Ph.D. Dissertation. University of Maryland, College Park.

Doyle, M.P. and J.L. Schoeni. 1985. Isolation of *Campylobacter jejuni* from retail mushrooms. *Appl. Environm. Microbiol.* **51**:449–450.

Doyle, M.P., K.A. Glass, J.T. Beery, G.A. Garcia, D.J. Pollard, and R.D. Schultz. 1987. Survival of Listeria monocytogenes in milk during high-temperature, short-time pasteurization. *Appl. Environm. Microbiol.* **53**:1433–1438.

Eklund, M.W., D.I. Wieler, and F.T. Poysky. 1967. Outgrowth and toxin production of nonproteolytic type B *Clostridium botulinum* at 3.3 to 5.6 C. *J. Bacteriol.* **93**:1461–1462.

Finnegan, N. 1989. Development of a HACCP based expert system for chilled foods. Presented at the Annual Conference of the Canadian Institute of Food Science and Technology, June 4–7, Quebec, ON.

Fleming, D.W., S.L. Cochi, K.L. MacDonald, J. Brondum, P.S. Hayes, B.D. Plikaytis, M.B. Holmes, A. Audurier, C.V. Broome, and A.L. Reingold. 1985. Pasteurized milk as a vehicle of infection in an outbreak of listeriosis. *N. Engl. J. Med.* **312**:404–407.

Genigiorgis, C.A. 1981. Factors affecting the probability of growth of pathogenic microorganisms in food. *J. Am. Vet. Med. Assoc.* **179**:1410–1417.

Gibson, A.M., N. Bratchell, and T.A. Roberts. 1988. Predicting microbial growth: growth responses of salmonellae in a laboratory medium as affected by pH, sodium chloride and storage temperature. *Int. J. Food Microbiol.* **6**:155–178.

Gray, M.L. and A.H. Killinger. 1966. *Listeria monocytogenes* and Listeric infections. *Bacteriol. Rev.* **30**:309–382.

Harris, N.V., N.S. Weiss, and C.M. Nolan. 1986a. The role of poultry and meats in the etiology of *Campylobacter jejuni/coli* enteritis. *Am. J. Public Health* **76**:407–411.

Harris, N.V., D. Thompson, D.C. Martin, and C.M. Nolan. 1986b. A survey of *Campylobacter* and other bacterial contaminants of pre-market chicken and retail poultry and meats, King County, Washington. *Am. J. Public Health* **76**:401–406.

Harris, N.V., T. Kimball, N.S. Weiss, and C. Nolan. 1986c. Dairy products, produce and other non-meat foods as possible sources of *Campylobacter jejuni* and *Campylobacter coli* enteritis. *J. Food Protect.* **49**:347–351.

Ho, J.L., K.N. Shands, G. Friedland, P. Eckind, and D.W. Fraser. 1986. An outbreak of type 4b *Listeria monocytogenes* infection involving patients from eight Boston hospitals. *Arch. Intern. Med.* **146**:520–524.

Huxsoll, C. and H.R. Bolin. 1989. Processing and distribution alternatives for minimally processed fruits and vegetables. *Food Technol.* **43**(2):124–128.

Johnson, C.E. 1979. Behavior of *Clostridium botulinum* in vacuum-packed fresh celery. *J. Food Protect.* **42**:49–50.

Keller, S. 1989. What is R&D's future role in the quality and safety of refrigerated foods. Presented at the Refrigerated Food Symposium, April 5–6, Rosemont, IL.

Kloos, W.E. and K.H. Schleifer. 1986. Genus IV. *Staphylococcus*. In *Bergey's Manual of Systematic Bacteriology*, Vol. 2, P.H.A. Sneath, N.S. Mair, M.E. Sharpe, and J.G. Holt (eds.), pp. 1015–1019. Baltimore: Williams & Wilkins.

Lindroth, S., E. Strandberg, A. Pessa, and M.J. Pellinen. 1983. A study on the growth potential of *Staphylococcus aureus* in *Boletus edulis*, a wild edible mushroom, prompted by a food poisoning outbreak. *J. Food Sci.* **48**:282–283.

MacDonald, K.L., R.F. Spengler, C.L. Hatheway, N.T. Hargrett, and M.L. Cohen. 1985. Type A botulism from sauteed onions. *JAMA* **253**:1275–1278.

Mackey, B.M. and N. Bratchell. 1989. The heat resistance of *Listeria monocytogenes*. *Lett. Appl. Microbiol.* **9**:89–94.

Morita, T.N. and M. Woodburn. 1983. Enterotoxin C_2 production by *S. aureus* in entree salads. *J. Food Sci.* **48**:243–245.

National Food Processors Association Microbiology and Food Safety Committee. 1989. Guidelines for the Development, Production, Distribution, and Handling of Refrigerated Foods. Washington, DC.

Notermans, S., J. Dufrenne, and M.J.H. Keijbets. 1981. Vacuum-packed cooked potatoes: toxin production by *Clostridium botulinum* and shelf life. *J. Food Protect.* **44**:572–575.

Notermans, S., J. Dufrenne, and M.J.H. Keijbets. 1985. Use of preservatives to delay toxin formation by *Clostridium botulinum* (type B, strain Okra) in vacuum-packed, cooked potatoes. *J. Food Protect.* **48**:851–855.

Post, L.S., D.A. Lee, M. Solberg, D. Furgang, J. Specchio, and C. Graham. 1985. Development of botulinal toxin and sensory deterioration during storage of vacuum and modified atmosphere packaged fish fillets. *J. Food Sci.* **50**:990–996.

Refrigerated Foods and Microbiological Criteria Committee of the National Food Processors Association. 1988. Safety considerations for new generation refrigerated foods. *Dairy Food Sanit.* **8**:5–7.

Rolle, R.S. and G.W. Chism, III. 1987. Physiological consequences of minimally processed fruits and vegetables. *J. Food Quality* **10**:157–177.

Schiemann, D.A. 1988. Examination of enterotoxin production at low temperature by *Yersinia* spp. in culture media and foods. *J. Food Protect.* **51**:571–573.

Schlech, W.F., P.M. Lavigne, R.A. Bortolussi, A.C. Allen, E.V. Haldane, A.J. Wort, A.W. Hightower, S.E. Johnson, S.H. King, E.S. Nicholls, and C.V. Broome. 1982. Epidemic listeriosis—evidence for transmission by food. *N. Engl. J. Med.* **308**:203–206.

Schwarz, T.L. 1988. Letter of January 13 to R.E. Harrington, National Restaurant Association. Division of Retail Food Protection, US Food and Drug Administration, Washington, DC.

Seeliger, H.P.R. and D. Jones. 1986. Genus *Listeria*. In *Bergey's Manual of Systematic Bacteriology*, Vol. 2, P.H.A. Sneath, N.S. Mair, M.E. Sharpe, and J.G. Holt (eds.), pp. 1235–1245. Baltimore: Williams & Wilkins.

Shewfelt, R.L. 1987. Quality of minimally processed fruits and vegetables. *J. Food Quality* **10**:143–156.

Singh, B., C.C. Yang, and D.K. Salunkhe. 1972. Controlled atmosphere storage of lettuce. 1. Effects on quality and respiration rate of lettuce heads. *J. Food Sci.* **37**:48–51.

Smibert, R.M. 1984. Genus *Campylobacter*. In *Bergey's Manual of Systematic Bacteriology*, Vol. 1, N.R. Krieg and J.G. Holt (eds.), pp. 111–118. Baltimore: Williams & Wilkins.

Solomon, H.M. and D.A. Kautter. 1988. Outgrowth and toxin production by *Clostridium botulinum* in bottled chopped garlic. *J. Food Protect.* **51**:862–865.

Solomon, H.M., D.A. Kautter, and R.K. Lynt. 1982. Effect of low temperatures on growth on nonproteolytic *Clostridium botulinum* types B and F and proteolytic type G in crabmeat and broth. *J. Food Protect.* **45**:516–518.

Sperber, W.H. 1982. Requirements of *Clostridium botulinum* for growth and toxin production. *Food Technol.* **36**(12):89–94.

St. Louis, M.E., S.H.S. Peck, D. Bowering, G.B. Morgan, J. Blatherwick, S. Banerjee, G.D.M. Kettyls, W.A. Black, M.E. Milling, A.H.W. Haushcild, R.V. Tauxe, and P.A. Blake. 1988. Botulism from chopped garlic: delayed recognition of a major outbreak. *Ann. Intern. Med.* **108**:363–368.

Steinbruegge, E.G., R.B. Maxcy, and M.B. Liewen. 1988. Fate of *Listeria monocytogenes* on ready to serve lettuce. *J. Food Protect.* **51**:596–599.

Sugiyama, H., M. Woodburn, K.H. Yang, and C. Movroydis. 1981. Production of botulinum toxin in inoculated pack studies of foil-wrapped baked potatoes. *J. Food Protect.* **44**:896–898.

Tanaka, N., L.M. Meske, M.P. Doyle, E. Traisman, D. Thayer, and R.W. Johnston. 1985. Plant trials of bacon made with lactic acid bacteria, sucrose and lowered sodium nitrite. *J. Food Protect.* **48**:679–686.

Tanaka, N., E. Traisman, P. Plantinga, L. Finn, W. Flom, L. Meeke, and J. Guggisberg. 1986. Evaluation of factors involved in antibotulinal properties of pasteurized process cheese spreads. *Food Protect.* **49**:526–531.

Thomas, C.J. and F. Masters. 1988. Microbial spoilage of pre-cooked potato-topped pies. *J. Appl. Bacteriol.* **64**:227–234.

Van Garde, S.J. and M.J. Woodburn. 1987. Food discard practices of householders. *J. Am. Diet. Assoc.* **87**:322–329.

Wyatt, J.C. and V.H. Guy. 1981. Growth of *Salmonella typhimurium* and *Staphylococcus aureus* in retail pumpkin pies. *J. Food Protect.* **44**:418–421.

Appendix

Recommended Storage Temperatures for Refrigerated Food Products and Ingredients

Table 1
Ideal Refrigeration Temperature for Product Categories

Commodity	Temperature
Dairy	32–40° F (0–4.4° C)
Milk	
Eggs	
Butter, Margarine	
Sour Cream	
Cottage Cheese	
Meats, fresh	30–34° F (−1.1 to 1.1° C)
Roasts	
Steaks	
Chops	
Hamburger	
Sausage	
Processed Meats	
Poultry	30–34° F (−1.1 to 1.1° C)
Chicken	
Turkey	
Duck	
Goose	
Seafood	30–34° F (−1.1 to 1.1° C)

Table 1   Continued

Shrimp
Lobster
Mollusc
Fish (fresh and smoked)

Salads	32–40° F (0–4.4° C)

Table 2
Ideal Refrigerated Storage Temperature for Vegetables

Commodity	Temperature	Comments
Artichoke	32° F (0° C)	
Asparagus if stored	32° F (0° C)	Chilling injury
	36° F (2.2° C)	if held more than 10 days below 36° F (2.2° C)
Avocado	40–55° F (4.4–12.8° C)	
Fuerte var	45° F (7.2° C)	
Beans, lima	32–40° F (0–4.4° C)	
Beans, snap	45–50° F (7.2–10° C)	
Beets	32° F (0° C)	
Broccoli	32° F (0° C)	
Brussels sprouts	32° F (0° C)	
Cabbage	32° F (0° C)	
Carrots	32° F (0° C)	
Cauliflower	32° F (0° C)	
Celery	31–32° F (−0.6 to 0° C)	
Corn	32° F (0° C)	
Cucumber	45–50° F (7.2–10° C)	
Eggplant	45–50° F (7.2–10° C)	
Greens, leafy	32° F (0° C)	
Horseradish	30–32° F (−1.1 to 0° C)	
Leeks, green	32° F (0° C)	
Lettuce	32–33° F (0–0.6° C)	
Mushrooms	32° F (0° C)	
Onion, dry	32° F (0° C)	
Onion, green	32° F (0° C)	
Okra	45–50° F (7.2–10° C)	
Olives	45–50° F (7.2–10° C)	
Peas, green	32° F (0° C)	
Pepper, sweet	45–50° F (7.2–10° C)	

Table 2　Continued

Potato	40–70° F (4.4–21.1° C)	
Early, immature		
Late, mature	38–40° F (3.3–4.4° C)	
Radish	32° F (0° C)	
Rutabaga	32° F (0° C)	
Spinach	32° F (0° C)	
Squash, winter and 　pumpkin	50–55° F (10–12.8° C)	
Squash, summer	32° F (0° C)	Chilling may
if stored	45–50° F (7.2–10° C)	occur if held more than one week below 45° F (7.2° C)
Sweet potato	55–60° F (12.8–15.6° C)	
Tomato		
Mature green	55–70° F (12.8–21.1° C)	
Firm ripe	45–50° F (7.2–10° C)	Quality reduced when held be- low 35° F (1.7° C)
Turnip	32° F (0° C)	
Turnip greens	32° F (0° C)	

Adapted from "Commercial Cooling of Fruits and Vegetables," Manual 43, California Agricultural Experimental Station Extension Service, University of California.

Table 3
Ideal Refrigerated Storage Temperature for Fruits

Commodity	Temperature
Apple	30–31° F (−1.1 to −0.6° C)
Chilling sensitive varieties	38–40° F (3.3–4.4° C)
Apricot	31–32° F (−0.6 to 0° C)
Banana	56–58° F (13.3–14.4° C)
Berries:	31–32° F (−0.6 to 0° C)
(bush-, blue-, straw-)	
Cherry, sour	32° F (0° C)
Cherry, sweet	30–32° F (−1.1 to 0° C)
Citrus:	
Grapefruit	58–60° F (14.4–15.6° C)
Lemon	58–60° F (14.4–15.6° C)
Limes	45–50° F (7.2–10° C)
Orange	38–44° F (3.3–6.7° C)

Table 3 Continued

Tangerine and other mandarins	32° F (0° C)
Coconuts	32–35° F (0–1.7° C)
Dates	32° F (0° C)
Figs	31–32° F (−0.6 to 0° C)
Grapes	30–31° F (−1.1 to −0.6° C)
Mangoes	55° F (12.8° C)
Melons:	
Honeydew	45–50° F (7.2–10° C)
Cantaloupe	32–40° F (0–4.4° C)
Watermelon	40–50° F (4.4–10° C)
Papayas	31–32° F (−0.6 to 0° C)
Peach and nectarine	32° F (0° C)
Pears	29–31° F (−1.7 to −0.6° C)
Persimmon	40° F (4.4° C)
Pineapple	45–47° F (7.6–8.3° C)
Plums and prunes	31–32° F (−0.6 to 0° C)
Pomegranate	32° F (0° C)
Quinces	32° F (0° C)

Adapted from "The Commercial Storage of Fruits, Vegetables, and Florist and Nursery Stocks," Agriculture Handbook Number 66, United States Department of Agriculture, U.S. Govt. Printing Office, Washington, DC.
Courtesy National Food Processors Association, Washington, DC.

Index*

---

*Page numbers printed in *italics* refer to tables or figures